Medical Radiology

Diagnostic Imaging

For further volumes:
http://www.springer.com/series/4354

Medical Radiology

Diagnostic Imaging

Series Editors

Albert L. Baert
Maximilian F. Reiser
Hedvig Hricak
Michael Knauth

For further volumes:
http://www.springer.com/series/4354

Caroline Keyzer • Pierre Alain Gevenois
Editors

Imaging of Acute Appendicitis in Adults and Children

Springer

Editors
Caroline Keyzer M.D., Ph.D.
Department of Radiology
Hôpital Erasme, Université libre de Bruxelles
Route de Lennik 808
1070 Brussels
Belgium
e-mail: caroline.keyzer@erasme.ulb.ac.be

Pierre Alain Gevenois M.D., Ph.D.
Department of Radiology
Hôpital Erasme, Université libre de Bruxelles
Route de Lennik 808
1070 Brussels
Belgium
e-mail: pierre.alain.gevenois@erasme.ulb.ac.be

ISSN 0942-5373
ISBN 978-3-642-17871-9 e-ISBN 978-3-642-17872-6
DOI 10.1007/978-3-642-17872-6
Springer Heidelberg Dordrecht London New York

Library of Congress Control Number: 2011935930

Cover design: eStudio Calamar, Berlin/Figueres

Printed on acid-free paper

Springer is part of Springer Science+Business Media (www.springer.com)

Preface

The appendix is considered as a vestigial organ, with no known physiological role, that has been accepted as the origin of a potentially life threatening but easily treatable inflammatory disease of the right lower quadrant of the abdomen only at the end of the nineteenth century. Appendectomy for acute appendicitis is since then still the most frequently performed emergency surgical procedure. Despite the fact that this surgical procedure is so frequently and easily performed, its indication was, till recently, the result of equilibrium between the negative appendectomy rate and the appendiceal perforation rate. It has been advocated that imaging could play an important role in ruling out acute appendicitis, preventing negative appendectomy and in confirming acute appendicitis. Nevertheless, even if various diagnostic imaging techniques, especially ultrasonography (US) and computed tomography (CT), are widely available and diagnostic features very well known in each technique, the impact of medical imaging on the clinical work-up of patients suspected of acute appendicitis remains a matter of debate. In addition, among the radiology community, there are still debates addressing the questions of the most appropriate technique (US vs. CT), in men or in women, in children or in adults, with or without intravenous contrast injection, at standard or at low radiation dose. In addition, the possible impact of imaging on cost-effective care has to be taken into account. Selected on the only basis of their scientific contributions in the field and on the impact of these contributions, recognized international experts have accepted to address all these issues in this handbook. This book, entirely dedicated to the appendix and acute appendicitis in adults and children, sets out to be a guide for radiologists, emergency physicians, and surgeons, beginners as well as experienced ones. We want to express our sincere gratitude to all renowned radiologists, emergency physicians, and surgeons who have contributed to this book with great enthusiasm and support.

Brussels, Belgium

Caroline Keyzer
Pierre Alain Gevenois

Contents

Part I

Introduction

Historical Background, Anatomy and Function, Etiology and Epidemiology

Caroline Keyzer

Contents

Abstract

This introduction presents the history of the recognition of the appendix as the organ responsible for a disease with a high mortality rate in the previous century and called acute appendicitis. This history reveals examples of resistance to changing concepts and brilliant early observations that were not easily accepted in the medical community. The anatomy of the appendix is nowadays well known but its function remains unclear. Acute appendicitis is the most common cause of acute abdominal pain that requires surgery but, for a disease that is prevalent and apparently simple, there is currently little that is well established on its etiology.

1 Historical Background

Acute appendicitis is a very common acute abdominal disease but it took several centuries to understand its pathogenesis. Berengario da Capri first described the vermiform appendix in humans in 1521 but it was illustrated in 1492 by Leonardo da Vinci in his anatomic drawings that were not published before the 18th century (Prystowsky et al. 2005; Williams 1983) (Fig. 1). Despite these early description and drawings, the role of the appendix in acute inflammatory diseases of the right iliac fossa—that could even lead to death—was only recognized and accepted by the surgical lobby in the late 19th century. Till then, it was indeed considered that the disease we currently know as acute appendicitis was one of the cecum, named typhlitis, even if most of the pathologic description of typhlitis

C. Keyzer (✉)
Department of Radiology, Hôpital Erasme,
Université Libre de Bruxelles,
Route de Lennik, 808,
1070 Brussels, Belgium
e-mail: caroline.keyzer@erasme.ulb.ac.be

C. Keyzer and P. A. Gevenois (eds.), *Imaging of Acute Appendicitis in Adults and Children*,
Medical Radiology. Diagnostic Imaging, DOI: 10.1007/174_2011_210, © Springer-Verlag Berlin Heidelberg 2011

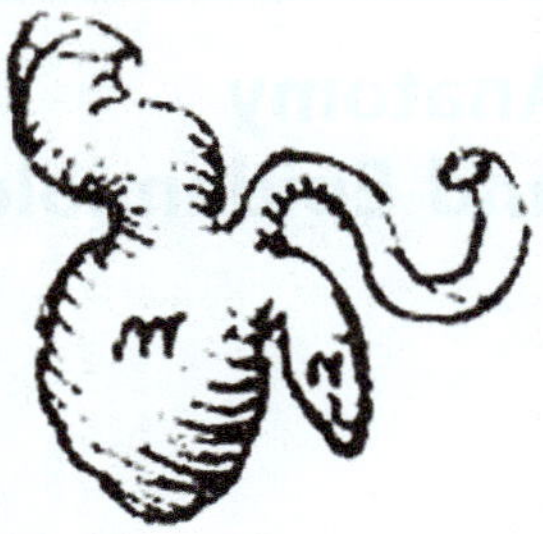

Fig. 1 Annotated drawing of the appendix by Leonardo da Vinci: "The appendix n, of the colon n m, is a part of the cecum and is capable of contracting and dilating so that excessive wind does not rupture the cecum" (from O'Malley and Saunders 1983, Leonardo da Vinci on the human body, p.185)

reported that the appendix was inflamed and/or perforated. It was indeed believed that the communication between the appendix and a neighboring abscess was a secondary phenomenon and that the cecum should be far more likely responsible of the disease than the appendix itself, the appendix being only considered as a vestigial organ (Williams 1983; McBurney 1891; Carmichael 1985). The controversy between the French physician François Melier and the leading, and known as arrogant, French surgeon Guillaume Dupuytren in the early 19th century is a nice example of resistance to changing concepts. Melier indeed suggested to surgically remove the appendix as a treatment for this acute right lower quadrant (RLQ) inflammatory disease but he was openly criticized by Dupuytren who considered that the appendix was not responsible for any relevant disease, persisting to state that it began in or around the cecum (Prystowsky et al. 2005; Williams 1983). Despite several descriptions of successful treatment of acute appendicitis by early appendectomy, the treatment for right lower quadrant inflammatory disease in the late 19th century consisted of plasters, cathartics, and opiates but the nonoperative mortality was not lower than nearly 100% (Carmichael 1985).

In 1886, a paper by Reginald H. Fitz from Harvard Medical School marked a turning point in the recognition and treatment of acute appendicitis (Prystowsky et al. 2005; McBurney 1891; Carmichael 1985). In this paper, R.H. Fitz wrote that "in most fatal cases of typhlitis the cecum is intact while the appendix is ulcerated and perforated" and thus suggested the appendix as the cause of most inflammatory diseases of the RLQ (Prystowsky et al. 2005; Carmichael 1985; Fitz 1886). He described the clinical features of appendicitis—a term that he coined—and most importantly, he advocated prompt surgical laparotomy and appendectomy in case of early recognition of acute appendicitis. If appendectomy could not be done within the first day after the onset of the symptoms, he recommended that "the resulting abscess, as a rule intraperitoneal, should be incised as soon as it becomes evident" (Carmichael 1985; Fitz 1886). After the death of R.H. Fitz, the Dean of Harvard Medical School, in reference to Fitz's accomplishments, claimed, "Many have sought truth, but it is rare to have found and taught it is so clearly that the lives of thousand and thousands were saved thereby" (Carmichael 1985).

A few years after the paper by R.H. Fitz, Charles McBurney of New York described the symptoms and clinical signs of acute appendicitis, including the elective point of tenderness that bears his name, and he also suggested early surgical intervention (McBurney 1891). In 1894, McBurney described the lateral muscle splitting for appendectomy, the so-called McBurney incision (McBurney 1894). Nowadays appendectomy is the most frequent urgent surgical intervention performed in the Western World with about 300,000 procedures/year in the United States (De Frances et al. 2006).

2 Anatomy and Function

The embryological developments of the cecum and appendix are closely related to that of the midgut. The cecum is the result of a bulging of the caudal limb of the primary intestinal loop. This bulging is divided into two parts with different growth rates. The distal part will fail to grow in thickness and will be narrower than the proximal part. This distal long and narrow part, looking like a worm, will become the "*vermiform appendix*" (Balthazar 2000; Prenant 1912). The appendix starts first at the apex of the cecum but with the asymmetrical growth of the cecal bud, the root of the appendix will be deported to the medial aspect of the cecum, below the ileo-cecal valve. There are huge variations in the course of the appendix against the cecum and the terminal ileum: it can run along all the aspects of the cecum and the tip of the appendix can lie in the pelvis or extend across the abdominal cavity in the left lower (and even upper) quadrant (Ahmed et al. 2007; Wagner et al. 1996). There is also a great variation in length of the appendix ranging from 2 to

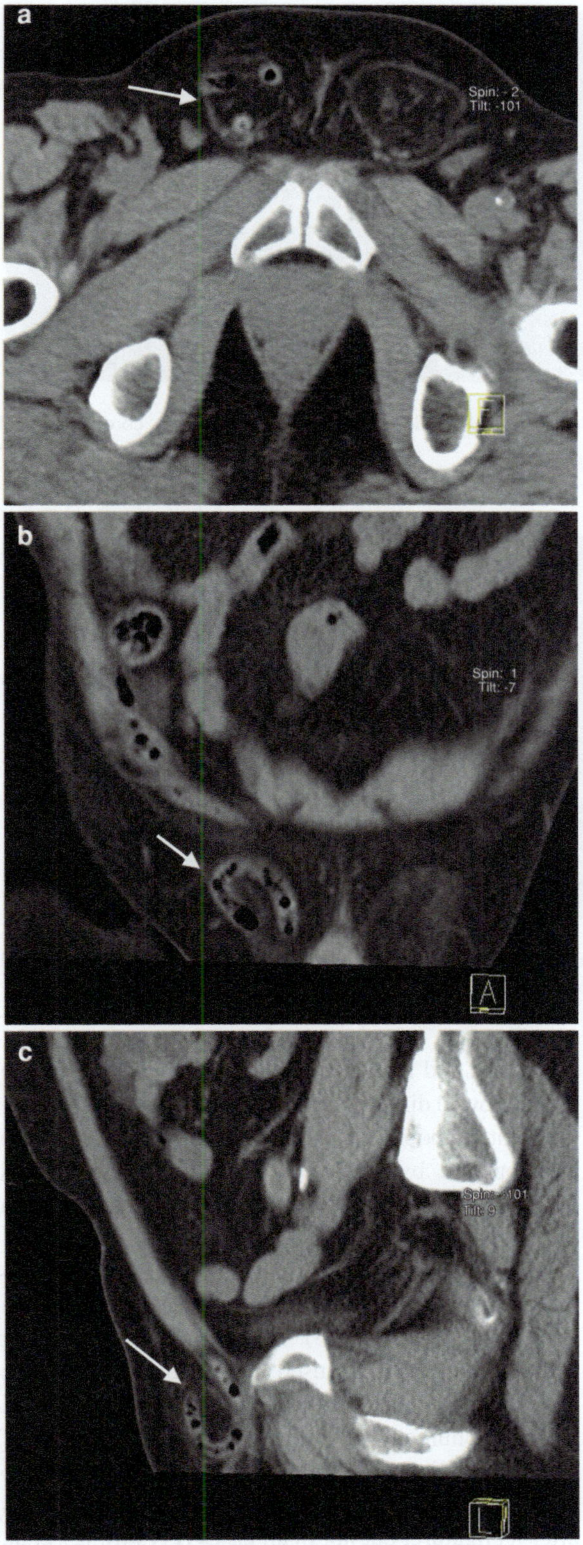

Fig. 2 **a, b, c** Normal appendix located in a right inguinal hernia (*arrow*) seen on axial (**a**), coronal (**b**), and sagittal CT images (**c**)

25 cm with an average of 9 cm (Ahmed et al. 2007; Wakeley and Childs 1950; Williams 1994). These anatomical variations, illustrated in Figs. 2, 3, 4, 5, are responsible for the wide variability of symptoms observed when the appendix is inflamed.

Duplication of the appendix may occur but it is quite rare. Duplication is of three types: 1) Type A consists of partial duplication on a normally localized appendix with a single cecum; 2) Type B consists of a single cecum with two separate appendices; and 3) Type C consists of a duplicated cecum each with its own appendix (Peddu and Sidhu 2004; Wallbridge 1962).

In humans, the role of the appendix is not definitely established (Dasso et al. 2000; Fisher 2000). As the appendix contains abundant lymphoid tissue and is close to the entrance of the colon—thereby exposed to large amounts of antigens—it could play an immune role. In rabbits, the appendix contains 50% of Gut Associated Lymphoid Tissue (GALT) but the proportion of GALT in the human appendix is unknown (Dasso et al. 2000). Moreover, neonatal appendectomy in rabbits reduces the antibody response and the repertoire diversity. However, even if the appendix of adult humans and rabbits are similar in many respects, they differ in amount of lymphoid tissue, follicular structure, and developmental distribution of T-cells (Dasso et al. 2000). It could thus be not appropriate to compare humans and rabbits in terms of the immune role of their appendix. Such an immune role has also been suggested by epidemiological studies that showed that individuals who had an appendectomy for appendicitis are at lower risk for ulcerative colitis than those who had no appendectomy (Andersson et al. 2001). In the same line, a mouse model of ulcerative colitis has suggested that appendectomy could prevent colonic inflammation by reducing the production of antibodies against the cytoskeletal protein tropomyosin expressed on colonocytes (Colombel et al. 2008).

3 Etiology and Epidemiology

With a lifetime risk ranging from 6 to 9%, acute appendicitis is the most frequent acute non traumatic abdominal disease requiring surgery (Addiss et al. 1990). The annual incidence of acute appendicitis ranges from 90 to 140 per 100,000 individuals depending on studies (Körner et al. 1997; Livingston

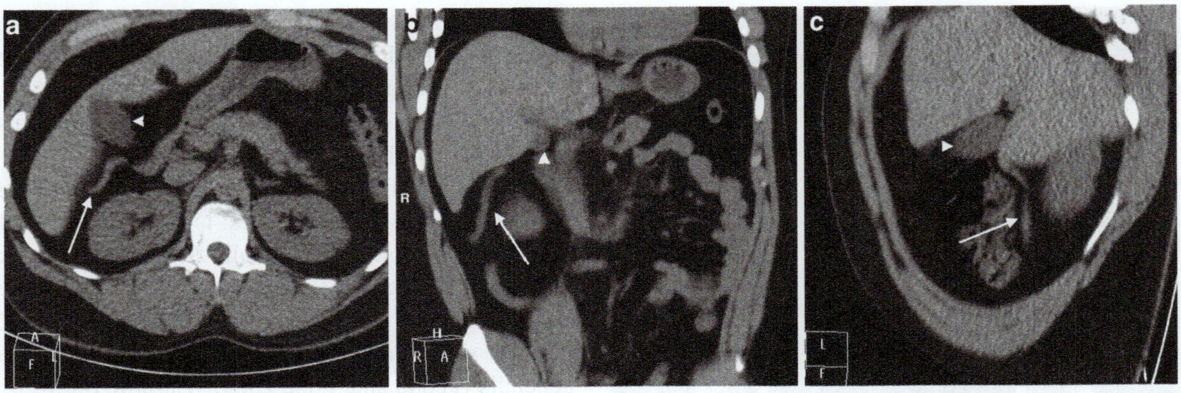

Fig. 3 **a, b, c** Normal appendix located in the subhepatic space, close to the gallbladder (*arrow*) seen on axial (**a**), coronal (**b**), and sagittal oblique CT reformations (**c**)

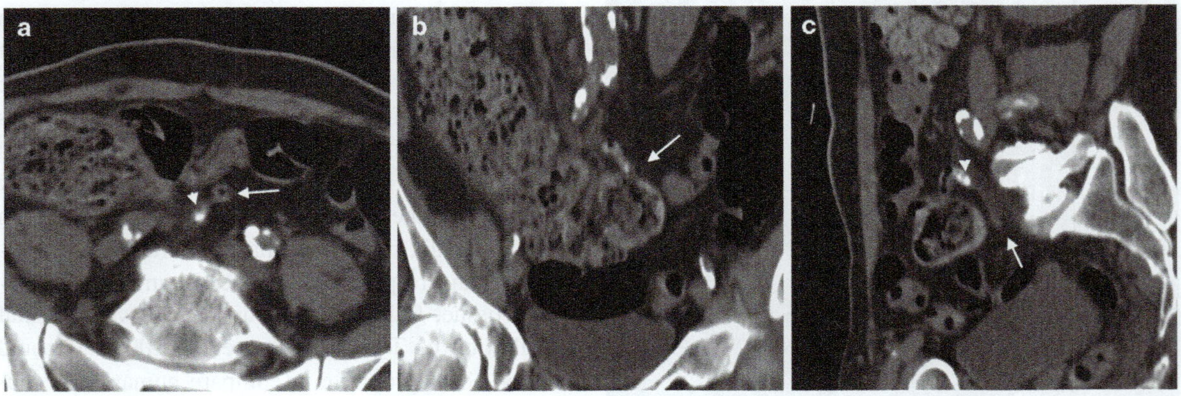

Fig. 4 **a, b, c** Centro-abdominal normal appendix (*arrow*), containing an appendicolith (*arrowhead*), located in the medio-sagittal plane and anterior to the aortic bifurcation, seen on axial (**a**), coronal (**b**), and sagittal CT reformations (**c**)

et al. 2007). The mean age of patients ranges from 20 to 30 years, the maximum incidence is observed between 10 and 20 year-old (Addiss et al. 1990; Flum et al. 2001), men are more risk at than women (ratio: 1.4/1), as white than non-white people (ratio: 1.5/1), acute appendicitis occurs more frequently in summer than in winter (Addiss et al. 1990; Alvarado 1986), and acute appendicitis progresses to perforation more frequently in children and elderly patients (Wagner et al. 1996; Addiss et al. 1990; Körner et al. 1997; Hale et al. 1997).

The non-perforated acute appendicitis rate fell from the early 1970s to a nadir in 1995, after which it began rising for both women and men. On the other hand, in both women and men, the perforation rate increased slightly with time, and the negative appendectomy rate remained low and constant (Livingston et al. 2007). The perforated and non-perforated acute appendicitis have thus followed different epidemiologic trends suggesting different pathophysiologies (Livingston et al. 2007) as supported by studies discussed in "Appendicitis Perforation Rates and Time Interval between Symptom Onset and Surgery" by T.S. Menes and N. Bickell.

While acute appendicitis is a prevalent and apparently simple disease, its etiology is not well known (Prystowsky et al. 2005). It is usually believed that acute appendicitis is caused by the obstruction of the appendiceal lumen. This belief originates from animal and even human studies investigating the effect of appendiceal ligature of the normal appendix leading to an inflammatory response in the appendix a few hours after its ligature, but not in all cases (Prystowsky et al. 2005; Dachman et al. 1987; Wangensteen and Dennis 1939). There are indeed various causes of acute

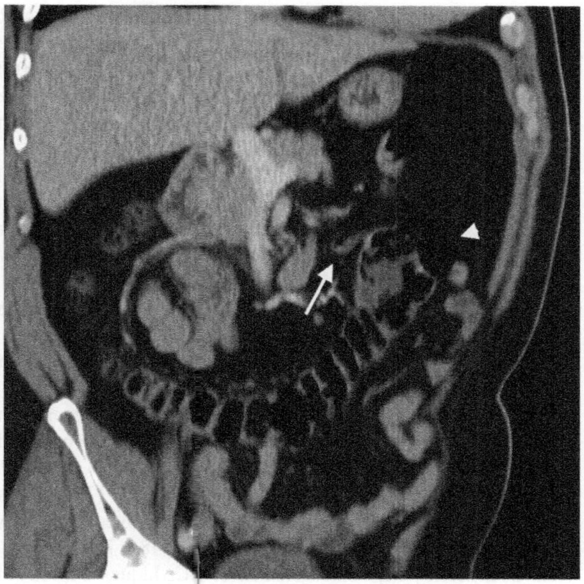

Fig. 5 Normal appendix (*arrow*) and cecum (*arrowhead*) located in the left upper abdominal quadrant on a coronal CT reformation

appendicitis that all lead to bacterial invasion of the appendicular wall secondary to mucosal ulceration (Prystowsky et al. 2005; Carr 2000). Acute appendicitis usually (or always) results from injury of its mucosa and spread from that injury through its wall (Carr 2000; Butler 1981). The mucosal ulceration occurs early in the evolution of the disease and could be induced by viral infection followed by bacterial invasion. This idea could be supported by the observation of endemic clustering of acute appendicitis (Carr 2000).

Demonstrable obstruction, by fecalith or by lymphoid hyperplasia, is frequently absent in acute appendicitis (Butler 1981). Conversely, obstruction does not necessarily produce acute appendicitis (Hale et al. 1997; Wangensteen and Dennis 1939; Butler 1981) and appendicolith—incidentally discovered in 27% of the autopsies (Andreou et al. 1990)—seems to play no role in the initiation of the disease but only in potentiating the increase in pressure within the appendiceal lumen, facilitating necrosis and further perforation, appendicoliths being indeed often found in association with gangrenous appendicitis (Wakeley and Childs 1950; Hale et al. 1997; Jones et al. 1985). The role of obstruction in the pathogenesis of acute appendicitis has also been studied by measuring perioperatively the pressure within the appendiceal lumen (Arnbjornsson and Bengmark 1984). This pressure is not elevated in approximately 70% of patients with phlegmonous appendicitis suggesting that obstruction is not a causative agent of acute appendicitis but might develop as a result of the inflammatory process (Arnbjornsson and Bengmark 1984).

Diet could also play a role in the occurrence of acute appendicitis. Is has been inferred that low fiber diet leads to fecalith formation which in turn predisposes to acute appendicitis (Jones et al. 1985), explaining the higher incidence of acute appendicitis in Western countries than in developing countries. This hypothesis is, however, not supported by epidemiological studies that showed that in urban South Africans who have even a lower fiber intake than Caucasian people, the incidence of acute appendicitis remains lower than that in Caucasians (Carr 2000; Walker and Segal 1995).

Hygienic, genetic, and environmental features could also be components of the susceptibility to acute appendicitis but they are difficult to separate from each other and from dietary influences (Carr 2000; Andersson et al. 1979; Basta et al. 1990; Papadopoulos et al. 2008; Williams et al. 1998). Finally, ischemia by lack of blood supply, and impaction of foreign bodies within the appendix (i.e., lead shot from wild game), although unusual, can cause acute appendicitis (Carr 2000).

The most frequent pathogens involved in acute appendicitis are the aerobe *Escherichia Coli* and the anaerobe *Bacteroides fragilis*. Aerobic infection is common in early acute appendicitis while mixed aerobic and anaerobic infection is predominant in late acute appendicitis (Lau et al. 1984).

Last but not least, a new etiology of pain from appendiceal origin has also been recently been suggested also: the so-called "neuroimmune appendicitis". This entity is based on the observation of neuroproliferation in the appendix in association with an increase in neurotransmitters substance P and vasoactive intestinal peptide in patients with acute right acute abdominal pain suggestive of acute appendicitis but with a histologically normal appendix (Bouchard et al. 2001; Di Sebastiano et al. 1999). This observation could explain why the pain disappears after appendectomy in some patients with acute right abdominal pain while their appendix is histologically normal.

4 Conclusion

Appendix and acute appendicitis are respectively, an organ and a disease that are the subjects of numerous publications, the number of which results from the important controversies and unsolved questions related to them. These controversies and questions address the physiological role of the appendix, the etiology of acute appendicitis, its histological definition, and its diagnosis—diagnosis by imaging will be extensively discussed in this book—as well as its treatment.

References

Addiss DG, Shaffer N, Fowler BS, Tauxe RV (1990) The epidemiology of appendicitis and appendectomy in the United States. Am J Epidemiol 132:910–925

Ahmed I, Asgeirsson KS, Beckingham IJ, Lobo DN (2007) The position of the vermiform appendix at laparoscopy. Surg Radiol Anat 29:165–168

Alvarado A (1986) A practical score for the early diagnosis of acute appendicitis. Ann Emerg Med 15:557–564

Andersson N, Griffiths H, Murphy J et al (1979) Is appendicitis familial? Br Med J 2:697–698

Andersson RE, Olaison G, Tysk C, Ekbom A (2001) Appendectomy and protection against ulcerative colitis. N Engl J Med 344:808–814

Andreou P, Blain S, Du Boulay CE (1990) A histopathological study of the appendix at autopsy and after surgical resection. Histopathology 17:427–431

Arnbjornsson E, Bengmark S (1984) Role of obstruction in the pathogenesis of acute appendicitis. Am J Surg 147: 390–392

Balthazar EJ (2000) Diseases of the appendix. In: Gore RM, Levine MS (eds) Textbook of gastrointestinal radiology. WB Saunders, Philadelphia, pp 1128–1129

Basta M, Morton NE, Mulvihill JJ, Radovanovic Z, Radojicic C, Marinkovic D (1990) Inheritance of acute appendicitis: familial aggregation and evidence of polygenic transmission. Am J Hum Genet 46:377–382

Bouchard S, Russo P, Radu AP, Adzick NS (2001) Expression of neuropeptides in normal and abnormal appendices. J Pediatr Surg 36:1222–1226

Butler C (1981) Surgical pathology of acute appendicitis. Hum Pathol 12:870–878

Carmichael DH (1985) Reginald fitz and appendicitis. South Med J 78:725–730

Carr NJ (2000) The pathology of acute appendicitis. Ann Diagn Pathol 4:46–58

Colombel JF, Watson AJ, Neurath MF (2008) The 10 remaining mysteries of inflammatory bowel disease. Gut 57:429–433

Dachman AH, Nichols JB, Patrick DH, Lichtenstein JE (1987) Natural history of the obstructed rabbit appendix: observations with radiography, sonography, and CT. AJR Am J Roentgenol 148:281–284

Dasso JF, Obiakor H, Bach H, Anderson AO, Mage RG (2000) A morphological and immunohistological study of the human and rabbit appendix for comparison with the avian bursa. Dev Comp Immunol 24:797–814

De Frances CJ, Lucas CA, Buie VC, Golosinskiy A (2006) National Hospital Discharge Survey. National health statistics reports; n°5. Hyattsville, MD: National Center for Health Statistics. 2008. www.cdc.gov/nchs/data/nhsr/nhsr005.pdf. Accessed 26 June 2009

Di Sebastiano P, Fink T, di Mola FF et al (1999) Neuroimmune appendicitis. Lancet 354:461–466

Fisher RE (2000) The primate appendix: a reassessment. Anat Rec 261:228–236

Fitz RH (1886) Perforating inflammation of the vermiform appendix with special reference to its early diagnosis and treatment. Am J Med Sci 92:321–346

Flum DR, Morris A, Koepsell T, Dellinger EP (2001) Has misdiagnosis of appendicitis decreased over time? A population-based analysis. JAMA 286:1748–1753

Hale DA, Molloy M, Pearl RH, Schutt DC, Jaques DP (1997) Appendectomy: a contemporary appraisal. Ann Surg 225: 252–261

Jones BA, Demetriades D, Segal I, Burkitt DP (1985) The prevalence of appendiceal fecaliths in patients with and without appendicitis. A comparative study from Canada and South Africa. Ann Surg 202:80–82

Körner H, Söndenaa K, Söreide JA et al (1997) Incidence of acute nonperforated and perforated appendicitis: age-specific and sex-specific analysis. World J Surg 21:313–317

Lau WY, Teoh-Chan CH, Fan ST, Yam WC, Lau KF, Wong SH (1984) The bacteriology and septic complication of patients with appendicitis. Ann Surg 200:576–581

Livingston EH, Woodward WA, Sarosi GA, Haley RW (2007) Disconnect between incidence of nonperforated and perforated appendicitis: implications for pathophysiology and management. Ann Surg 245:886–892

McBurney C II (1891) The indications for early laparotomy in appendicitis. Ann Surg 13:233–254

McBurney C IV (1894) The incision made in the abdominal wall in cases of appendicitis, with a description of a new method of operating. Ann Surg 20:38–43

Papadopoulos AA, Polymeros D, Kateri M, Tzathas C, Koutras M, Ladas SD (2008) Dramatic decline of acute appendicitis in Greece over 30 years: index of improvement of socioeconomic conditions or diagnostic aids? Dig Dis 26: 80–84

Peddu P, Sidhu PS (2004) Appearance of a type B duplex appendix on barium enema. Br J Radiol 77:248–249

Prenant A (1912) Développement de l'intestin digestif. In: Poirier P, Charpy A (eds) Traité d'anatomie humaine. Masson et Cie, Paris, pp 34–35

Prystowsky JB, Pugh CM, Nagle AP (2005) Current problems in surgery. Appendicitis. Curr Probl Surg 42:694–742

Wagner JM, McKinney WP, Carpenter JL (1996) Does this patient have appendicitis? JAMA 276:1589–1594

Wakeley C, Childs P (1950) Appendicitis. Br Med J 2: 1347–1352

Walker AR, Segal I (1995) Appendicitis: an African perspective. J R Soc Med 88:616–619

Wallbridge PH (1962) Double appendix. Br J Surg 50:346–347
Wangensteen OH, Dennis C (1939) Experimental proof of the obstructive origin of appendicitis in man. Ann Surg 110:629–647
Williams GR (1983) Presidential address: a history of appendicitis with anecdotes illustrating its importance. Ann Surg 197:495–506
Williams RA (1994) Development, structure and function of the appendix. In: Williams RA, Myers P (eds) Pathology of the appendix and its surgical treatment. Chapman and Hall, London, pp 9–30
Williams NM, Jackson D, Everson NW, Johnstone JM (1998) Is the incidence of acute appendicitis really falling? Ann R Coll Surg Engl 80:122–124

Part II

Treatment Approaches and Issues in Patients with Suspected Acute Appendicitis

Clinical Presentation of Acute Appendicitis: Clinical Signs—Laboratory Findings—Clinical Scores, Alvarado Score and Derivate Scores

David J. Humes and John Simpson

Contents

D. J. Humes (✉) · J. Simpson
Department of Surgery, NIHR Nottingham Digestive Disease Centre and Biomedical Research Unit, Nottingham University Hospital NHS Trust, QMC Campus, E Floor, West Block, Derby Road, Nottingham, NG7 2UH, UK
e-mail: david.humes@nottingham.ac.uk

Abstract

Appendicectomy is the most commonly performed emergency operation worldwide with a lifetime risk of appendicitis of 8.6% in males and 6.7% in females (Flum and Koepsell 2002; Addiss et al. 1990). The diagnosis of acute appendicitis is predominantly based on clinical findings (Humes and Simpson 2006). Whilst a clinical diagnosis can often be made there are groups of patients in whom the clinical diagnosis is difficult and these patients provide a degree of diagnostic uncertainty. Studies reporting the mortality associated with appendicitis have demonstrated a significant increase in mortality associated with perforation (Blomqvist et al. 2001). The rate of perforation is reported to increase by 5% per 12 h period 36 h after the onset of symptoms, therefore, expedient diagnosis and treatment are required (Bickell et al. 2006). High rates of negative appendicectomy (operation without histological confirmation of appendicitis) have been reported with some groups such as females of reproductive age having rates of up to 26% (Flum et al. 2001). Delayed or incorrect diagnosis therefore has both clinical and economic consequences (Flum and Koepsell 2002) and this has resulted in considerable research to identify clinical, laboratory and radiological findings that are diagnostic of appendicitis and the development of clinical scoring systems (some computer aided) to guide the clinician in making the correct diagnosis. Thus reducing the delay in diagnosis and decreasing the rates of negative appendicectomy. There is evidence that despite the introduction of new specialist tests that the diagnosis of appendicitis has not improved on a

C. Keyzer and P. A. Gevenois (eds.), *Imaging of Acute Appendicitis in Adults and Children*, Medical Radiology. Diagnostic Imaging, DOI: 10.1007/174_2011_211, © Springer-Verlag Berlin Heidelberg 2011

population level (Flum et al. 2001). This chapter aims to outline the presentation, investigation and diagnosis of acute appendicitis.

1 Clinical Presentation

The clinical diagnosis of acute appendicitis relies upon a detailed history and thorough physical examination. The differential diagnosis is that of the acute abdomen as it can mimic the presentation of most abdominal emergencies (Box 1).

1.1 History

The principal presenting complaint of patients with acute appendicitis is abdominal pain. Murphy was the first to describe the sequence of colicky central abdominal pain followed by vomiting and migration of the pain to the right iliac fossa (Murphy 1904). This classical presentation is only seen in approximately 50% of patients. The history of pain is usually 24 h of colicky peri-umbilical pain followed by migration of the pain to the right iliac fossa with a progression to a more constant severe pain (Wagner et al. 1996). This progression results from the initial pain being referred from the visceral innervation of the midgut followed by more defined localization of the pain when the parietal peritoneum is involved by the inflammatory process. Associated symptoms include loss of appetite and nausea but profuse vomiting is rarely a feature of simple appendicitis and may well represent the development of diffuse peritonitis following perforation. Patients will often have a low grade fever. It is common for patients to report no change in bowel habit but a range of bowel habit disturbances may be associated with the onset of pain. Cope reported that patients may feel constipated and anticipate relief of pain with defecation but this does not occur (Cope 2000).

The appendix can take a variety of anatomical positions and as a result the clinical presentation is influenced by the surrounding structures that become involved in the inflammatory process (Box 2). Those at the extremes of age often present a significant diagnostic challenge as they may present with atypical signs and symptoms (Paulson et al. 2003). Infants may appear listless whilst the elderly may present with

Box 1 Differential diagnosis of acute appendicitis

Surgical

Acute cholecystitis

Perforated peptic ulcer

Intestinal obstruction

Pancreatitis

Intussusception

Mesenteric adenitis

Meckel's diverticulitis

Colonic/appendicular diverticulitis

Rectus sheath haematoma

Urological

Right ureteric colic

Urinary tract infection

Right pyelonephritis

Gynaecological

Ectopic pregnancy

Salpingitis/pelvic inflammatory disease

Ruptured ovarian follicle

Torted ovarian cyst

Medical

Pneumonia

Gastroenteritis

Diabetic ketoacidosis

Terminal ileitis

Porphyria

Preherpetic pain on the right 10th and 11th dorsal nerves

Box 2 Anatomical position of the appendix and possible changes in clinical presentation

Retrocaecal/Retrocolic (75%)—Right loin pain is often present with tenderness on examination. Muscular rigidity and tenderness to deep palpation are often absent due to protection from the overlying caecum. The psoas muscle may be irritated in this position leading to hip flexion and exacerbation of the pain on hip extension (psoas stretch sign).

Subcaecal and Pelvic appendix (20%)—Suprapubic pain and urinary frequency may predominate. Diarrhoea may be present due to irritation of the rectum. Abdominal tenderness may be lacking but rectal or vaginal tenderness may be present on the right. Microscopic haematuria and leucocytes may be present on urinalysis.

Pre and Post-ileal (5%)—Signs and symptoms may be lacking. Vomiting may be more prominent and diarrhoea due to irritation of the distal ileum.

confusion. A high index of suspicion is therefore required to make the diagnosis in such cases.

A systematic review of the symptoms which are associated with acute appendicitis has revealed that two symptoms have a high positive likelihood ratio (LR+) when present for diagnosing acute appendicitis; a history of right lower quadrant pain (LR += 8.0, 95% CI 7.3–8.5) and migration of initial periumbilical pain to the right lower quadrant (LR += 3.1, 95% CI 2.4–4.2) (Wagner et al. 1996). A further systematic review and meta-analysis of studies of patients admitted to hospital with suspected appendicitis concluded that individual elements of the history were of weak predictive value in the diagnosis of acute appendicitis. Pain migration was the best individual predictor of acute appendicitis (LR + 2.1, 95% CI 1.6–2.6) (Andersson 2004). Anorexia, nausea and vomiting were found in both reviews not to alter the likelihood of acute appendicitis. The likelihood of acute appendicitis also decreased with a history of similar previous pain (LR −= 0.3, 95% CI 0.2–0.4) and with the absence of right lower quadrant pain (LR −= 0.2, 95% CI 0.0–0.3). A synthesis of information based on clinical and laboratory findings was reported as the most useful mechanism of diagnosing acute appendicitis.

1.2 Examination

The patient presents with systemic features of an inflammatory response. They usually have a low grade fever (<38°C) with associated tachycardia, and appear flushed and a fetor oris may be present. The patient will often lie still as movement and coughing exacerbate the pain. In children the hop test has been advocated as a test to confirm appendicitis. The child is asked to hop but refuses as this causes pain. On abdominal palpation the maximal site of tenderness is said to lie over McBurney's point, which lies two-thirds of a way along a line drawn from the umbilicus to the anterior superior iliac spine (McBurney 1889). The patient will be tender and may display signs of peritoneal irritation with localized guarding and muscular rigidity. Rebound tenderness should not be elicited to avoid distressing the patient. The signs found on clinical examination which are associated with a high positive likelihood ratio are signs of peritoneal irritation (rebound and percussion tenderness, guarding and rigidity) (Andersson 2004) these were confirmed in a further systematic review which demonstrated a LR += 4.0 for the presence of rigidity (Wagner et al. 1996).

Findings on rectal or vaginal examination may be normal although pain on the right on rectal examination may indicate a pelvic appendix. A rectal examination is part of a thorough assessment of the patient with acute abdominal pain, however, the value of rectal examination in the diagnosis of appendicitis is debatable. In the presence of tenderness and guarding in the right iliac fossa in a study of 1,204 patients admitted to hospital with right lower quadrant pain little extra information was gained. The presence of right sided pain on rectal examination was more common in those with appendicitis (Odds Ratio [OR] 1.3) but this gave little diagnostic information (Dixon et al. 1991). These findings were confirmed in a further study of 477 patients with acute appendicitis and a systematic review and meta-analysis which concluded that the opinion that rectal examination is indispensible in the diagnosis of appendicitis cannot be supported (Andersson 2004; Kremer et al. 1998).

It has been suggested that opiate analgesia should be withheld from patients with suspected acute appendicitis as its administration masks clinical signs (Rusnak and Borer JM 1994). Two small randomized controlled studies in adult and paediatric cohorts have concluded that analgesia does not alter the clinician's ability to accurately diagnose acute appendicitis, and therefore, appropriate analgesia should be given to all patients on admission (Attard et al. 1992; Green et al. 2005).

Further examination findings have been suggested to aid in the diagnosis of appendicitis. Rovsing's sign is named after Danish surgeon Niels Rovsing and is said to be present when palpation in the left iliac fossa results in pain in the right iliac fossa (Wagner et al. 1996). The psoas muscle can be irritated by an inflamed appendix and movement of the muscle can result in pain. The patient may lie in the supine position with the hip flexed. This can be tested by asking the supine patient to lift the thigh whilst applying pressure just above the knee or by extending the right leg at the hip with the patient in the left lateral decubitus position. Pain with either maneuver confirms psoas irritation and is regarded as a positive psoas sign (Wagner et al. 1996). Lastly the obturator sign results from irritation of the obturator muscle. This can be elicited by passively flexing the right hip and knee and internally rotating the leg at the hip which stretches the obturator muscle and causes pain in the right side of the abdomen (Wagner et al. 1996).

2 Laboratory Investigations

Specialist investigations are rarely needed to make the diagnosis of appendicitis as the diagnosis is predominantly clinical. The judicious use of simple bedside tests and laboratory markers of inflammation can provide additional evidence to support the diagnosis of acute appendicitis and exclude important differentials. The majority of patients presenting with abdominal pain will have blood drawn for a full blood count and urea and electrolyte analysis. Urine analysis and microscopy can exclude urinary tract infection but may be abnormal in up to 48% of patients undergoing appendicectomy (Puskar et al. 1995). The cause for abnormalities often leukocytosis and microscopic haematuria is the underlying inflammatory process irritating the renal tract along the line of the inflamed appendix (Puskar et al. 1995).

The most commonly used serological markers of inflammation in the diagnosis of acute appendicitis are the leukocyte count and C-reactive protein (CRP). Neither is diagnostic of acute appendicitis and studies have attempted to define potential thresholds values which are predictive of a diagnosis and disease severity (Coleman et al. 1998; Korner et al. 1999; Hallan et al. 1997; Gurleyik et al. 1995). Repeated tests may also be useful in the context of patients in whom the diagnosis is unclear initially and are observed clinically with two studies suggesting other diagnoses or further tests should be considered if repeat measures are normal (Thompson et al. 1992; Eriksson et al. 1994). In the presence of normal inflammatory markers CRP, WBC and neutrophil count the diagnosis of acute appendicitis is unlikely (Andersson 2004; Grönroos and Grönroos 1999; Dueholm et al. 1989; Yang et al. 2006). The performance of these tests is clearly related to the population under study and a meta-analysis of studies of reporting results on patients admitted to hospital with acute abdominal pain and those selected for appendicectomy demonstrated that CRP performed better as a diagnostic test in those with an acute abdomen than in those selected already for surgery (Hallan et al. 1997). A further meta-analysis of studies reporting on patients with a clinical suspicion of appendicitis concluded that the diagnosis of acute appendicitis was more likely when two or more inflammatory variables [granulocyte count, proportion of polymorphonuclear blood cells, white blood cell count (WBC) and CRP] were elevated (Andersson 2004). Studies of inflammatory markers in children notably of CRP and WBC count have concluded that an elevation of both parameters can support the diagnosis of acute appendicitis (Sack et al. 2006; Beltrán et al. 2007; Kwan and Nager 2010). These studies have all used different cut off levels to determine abnormal results and have generally been small single centre studies. The authors, therefore, suggest that the use of inflammatory variables should be used to support a clinical diagnosis of acute appendicitis and to exclude other pathologies. All women of child bearing age should have a serum or urine beta HCG requested to confirm pregnancy status. Given the differential diagnosis of acute appendicitis other blood tests including amylase, lipase, liver function tests, and clotting studies may be required to confirm or exclude other diagnoses.

Given the limitations of the current inflammatory markers there has been considerable research interest in identifying other potential biomarkers for the diagnosis of acute appendicitis and for predicting perforation. Hyper-bilirubinaemia has been shown to correlate with a diagnosis of perforated appendicitis (Estrada et al. 2007) but a stronger correlation has been recently reported for CRP (Käser et al. 2010). Interleukin-6 serum levels have not been shown to aid the diagnosis of appendicitis or reduce negative laparotomy rates (Gurleyik et al. 2002; Paajanen et al. 2002; Goodwin et al. 1997). The use of plasma D-lactate levels in the diagnosis of appendicitis is unclear with some studies suggesting it may (Demircan et al. 2004; Duzgun et al. 2007) or may not be a useful adjunct (Caglayan et al. 2003). A recent study of 51 patients with appendicitis suggested plasma concentration of lactoferrin and calprotectin are elevated in those with appendicitis but their role in diagnosis is unclear (Thuijls et al. 2011). Clearly the use of these markers in routine clinical practice will require much larger validation studies in defined cohorts of patients.

Laboratory tests have also been used to try and determine the need for further investigation in patients presenting with abdominal pain. Due to the non specific nature of most inflammatory variables, however, no single specific test has been able to predict the need for further radiological investigation (Scheinfeld et al. 2010).

3 Scoring Systems

The diagnosis of acute appendicitis can be difficult and any delay in definitive treatment with surgery can lead to an increase in mortality and morbidity as the disease progresses to appendiceal perforation. This increase in morbidity and mortality has been used to justify the high rates of negative appendicectomy which range from 14 to 75% (Alvarado 1986). A drive, therefore, has been to improve the diagnosis of appendicitis using clinical scoring systems. These systems have been based on symptoms, signs and laboratory findings. In some instances they have been part of a computer-aided diagnostic algorithm. The most widely cited score in the diagnosis of adults with acute appendicitis is the Alvarado score (Alvarado 1986). Whereas, in children the pediatric appendicitis score or Samuel score is most widely used (Samuel 2002). The scores have now been validated in a wide variety of populations, however, they have not made it into routine clinical practice in all settings. A number of studies have also used computer aided diagnosis in patients with acute abdominal pain in an attempt to improve the management of patients presenting with acute abdominal pain (De Dombal et al. 1974; Wellwood et al. 1992; Scarlett et al. 1986). These systems have reported a diagnostic accuracy of 97.2% in acute appendicitis (De Dombal et al. 1974), improvement in time to surgery, with a reduction in the number of perforations over a 2 year period (Scarlett et al. 1986). They have, however, not been introduced into routine clinical practice. In an aid to further improve diagnosis artificial neural networks have been suggested as adjuncts to diagnosis but this remains an area of research with only a small number of patients having had diagnoses made in this way (Prabhudesai et al. 2008; Hsieh et al. 2011).

3.1 Alvarado Score or MANTRELS Score

The score was originally developed by Alfredo Alvarado in 1986 as an aid to the diagnosis of patients with appendicitis. The score was based on a cohort of 305 patients based at the Nazareth Hospital in Philadelphia in the United States of America who presented with suspected appendicitis. The charts of these patients were reviewed retrospectively and the sensitivity and specificity of a number of symptoms, signs and laboratory variables were assessed with those with the greatest diagnostic value being used to form a scoring system. This resulted in the formation of a simple score consisting of three symptoms, three signs and two laboratory markers of inflammation weighted as either one or two based on their importance in diagnosis (Table 1). These variables could be recalled using the pneumonic MANTRELS. The maximum total score achievable is, therefore, 10. A score of 5 or 6 is compatible with a diagnosis of acute appendicitis, with a score of 7 or 8 indicating probable appendicitis and a score of 9 or 10 indicating a very probable acute appendicitis. It has been suggested that score can used as a guide to determine which patients require further observation and which patients require surgery. Those with a score of 5 or 6 required observation while those with a score of 7 or above needed to proceed to surgery as it was likely that they had appendicitis.

Table 1 Alvarado score

	Variable	Value
Symptoms	Migration	1
	Anorexia-acetone	1
	Nausea-vomiting	1
Signs	Tenderness in right lower quadrant	2
	Rebound pain	1
	Elevation of temperature >37.3°C	1
Laboratory	Leukocytosis $>10.0 \times 10^9$/L	2
	Shift to the left >75%	1

The Alvarado score is the best performing of the clinical scoring systems in current use (Ohmann et al. 1995). The score, however, is not based on a formal mathematical model which has accounted for the variables independent ability to predict a diagnosis. It was also based on retrospective data. These factors have resulted in a number of authors proposing multiple other scoring systems including a variety of other clinical, laboratory and imaging findings.

3.2 Other Scoring Systems

All of the described clinical scoring systems have attempted to aid the clinician in the diagnosis of the patient with acute appendicitis. The systems use a variety of signs, symptoms and investigations to form their respective scores. None has been adopted into wide spread clinical practice. They remain only as an aid to clinical diagnosis but do alert the clinician to all probable variables that should be considered in making a diagnosis of appendicitis.

The Tzanakis scoring system incorporated ultrasound scanning along with clinical and laboratory findings to predict the diagnosis of appendicitis. Following a multivariate logistic regression analysis four variables formed the scoring system (Ultrasound positive for acute appendicitis, tenderness in the right lower quadrant, rebound tenderness and a leukocyte count >12,000/μL) (Tzanakis et al. 2005).

The Appendicitis Inflammatory Response Score was constructed from eight independent predictive variables (right lower quadrant pain, rebound tenderness, muscular defense, WBC count, proportion of neutrophils, CRP, body temperature and vomiting) and performed better than the Alvarado score in a sample of 229 patients suspected of appendicitis (Sensitivity 0.97 vs. 0.92, $p = 0.0027$ and Specificity 0.93 vs. 0.88, $p = 0.0007$) (Andersson and Andersson 2008).

The Ohmann score was developed in Germany and was subject to a before and after intervention study and used computer – aided diagnosis. The variables completing the score are tenderness in the right lower quadrant, rebound tenderness, no micturition difficulties, steady pain, leukocyte count $>10.0 \times 10^9$/L, age <50 years, relocation of the pain to right lower quadrant and rigidity (Ohmann et al. 1995). The score was developed using stepwise logistic regression analysis of a German database and confirmed on a Dutch database. Following introduction of the score over a 4 month period the rates of delayed appendicectomy (2 vs. 8%) and delayed discharge (11 vs. 22%) decreased significantly ($p < 0.02$), however, there were no changes in the number of perforations or complications.

The Lintula score was developed from 35 symptoms and signs recorded for 131 Finnish children with abdominal pain which were modeled using logistic regression for their predictive value for a diagnosis of acute appendicitis. The score was then validated on a cohort of prospectively collected children with abdominal pain. The score uses gender, intensity of pain, relocation of pain, vomiting, pain in the right lower quadrant, fever, guarding, bowel sounds and rebound tenderness to form a score which if greater than 21 appendicectomy was advocated (Lintula et al. 2005). The Lintula score was developed for use in children but has subsequently been validated in adults (Lintula 2010). The Fenyo-Lindberg scoring system was developed using a prospectively collected sample of 1,167 patients with suspected appendicitis. The system uses nine clinical and one laboratory variable to form a score. Each variable is given a weight between −15 and +15 (Fenyo et al. 1997). The authors initially reported a reduction in the rate of negative laparotomies associated with the use of the score.

3.3 Pediatric Appendicitis Score (Samuel Score)

The Pediatric Appendicitis Score (PAS) was first described by Madan Samuel in 2002. It was based on an analysis of a prospectively collected cohort of 1,170 children aged 4–15 years (Samuel 2002). The symptoms, signs and laboratory findings were evaluated for sensitivity, specificity, predictive value and joint probability. A diagnostic index/weight for each clinical feature and investigation was calculated. A stepwise multiple linear regression analysis was then performed on the best independent predictors to develop a scoring system based on eight variables. The variables were given a score of one except for physical signs which were assigned a score of 2 to give a total score of 10. The variables in order of diagnostic index are, cough/percussion/hoping tenderness in the right lower quadrant of the abdomen, anorexia, pyrexia, nausea and emesis, tenderness over the right iliac fossa, leukocytosis, polymorphonuclear neutrophilia and migration of pain. The score was then validated on the cases and was found to have a sensitivity of 1, specificity of 0.92, positive predicted value of 0.96 and negative predictive value of 0.99.

The PAS has been evaluated in other cohorts of paediatric patients. It has been suggested that it is useful in stratifying the clinical risk of acute appendicitis in those children presenting to the emergency department with abdominal pain and classifying them as low, medium and high risk of acute appendicitis (Goldman et al. 2008). A score of less than or equal to 2 was found to have a high validity of ruling out acute appendicitis while a score greater than or equal to 7 was found to have a high validity of predicting acute appendicitis. In two prospectively collected cohorts of 588 and 287 paediatric patients evaluated for acute appendicitis a PAS score of 6 or more had a sensitivity of 77–88% and a specificity of 65–50%, respectively (Schneider et al. 2007; Mandeville et al. 2010). Following both evaluations the authors concluded that neither the Alvarado nor PAS could be used in isolation to diagnose acute appendicitis.

3.4 Scoring Systems and the Use of Radiological Investigations

None of the scoring systems described have been able to replace the clinical diagnosis of acute appendicitis, however, they do act as an adjunct to diagnosis. Several studies have detailed their possible use in determining the need for further investigation in patients with abdominal pain. The authors of a prospective evaluation of 849 children with abdominal pain suggested that those with a PAS score of between 3 and 6 should go on to have further investigation such as ultrasound or computed tomography or a period of further evaluation (Goldman et al. 2008). A second prospective review of 246 children concluded that a PAS score of 5–7 may indicate the need for further investigation (Bhatt et al. 2009). A further retrospective review of 150 patients aged over 7 years presenting with abdominal pain concluded that those with an Alvarado score between 3 and 6 should undergo a CT scan of the abdomen with a sensitivity of CT of 90.4% and specificity of 95% (McKay and Shepherd 2007). A randomized controlled trial of graded ultrasonography and Alvarado scoring compared to standard clinical diagnosis demonstrated a significant decrease in time to surgery in the intervention group without a decrease in hospital stay or perforation rates (Douglas et al. 2000) The scoring, however, was carried out by just one observer and the intervention arm had three non-diagnosed cases of perforation which was worse than the control arm of the study.

The evidence, therefore, suggests that these scoring systems when equivocal may indicate the need for further investigation or a period of observation with serial physical examinations (Pouget-Baudry et al. 2010). None of the systems allow a definitive diagnosis of acute appendicitis or have the ability to accurately predict the need for further investigation. Therefore, clinical diagnosis and clinical judgment should still be the main guides to further investigation in those patients in whom the diagnosis of appendicitis is unclear.

4 Difficult Diagnostic Areas

4.1 Abscess

Patients with an appendix abscess present with a swinging pyrexia associated with a tender mass in the right lower quadrant and a leucocytosis. The abscess is most often located in the lateral aspect of the right iliac fossa although a pelvic abscess may be palpable per rectum. The diagnosis is often confirmed on ultrasound or using computed tomography. The abscess can be drained percutaneously but open drainage allows appendicectomy to be performed (Humes and Simpson 2006).

4.2 Mass

Delayed presentation of appendicitis can be associated with presentation with a tender mass in the right iliac fossa. The mass can be confirmed using radiological imaging and patients who are clinically well are treated with intravenous antibiotics. In the majority of cases the mass will resolve and if indicated an interval appendicectomy can be performed. In elderly patients, the possibility of an underlying malignancy must be excluded. Careful clinical review is required to ensure resolution of the inflammatory process.

4.3 Pregnancy

Displacement of the appendix by the gravid uterus results in an atypical presentation of appendicitis in this group of patients. Nausea and vomiting may be present with tenderness located at any point on the right side of the abdomen. Acute appendicitis is the most common non-obstetric emergency requiring surgery in pregnancy with an incidence of 0.15–2.1 per 1,000 pregnancies (Guttman et al. 2004). The diagnosis may require specialist investigation with magnetic resonance imaging or ultrasound. A high index of suspicion is required as a delay in diagnosis results in an increase in both maternal (<1–4%) and fetal (1.5–35%) mortality associated with perforation (Guttman et al. 2004).

4.4 Chronic or Neuroimmune Appendicitis

A small number of patients present with recurrent episodes of right lower quadrant abdominal pain with no associated inflammatory changes (Barber et al. 1997). These patients are often difficult to diagnose and treat. Due to their small numbers only a few studies have attempted to define these cases in more detail. There appears to be two distinct groups of patients those with recurrent episodes of abdominal pain who ultimately have a chronically inflamed appendix removed reported as 6.5% of patients presenting with appendicitis in one study (Barber et al. 1997) and those in whom a histologically normal appendix is removed. Characteristics of these patients with recurrent episodes of pain are the presence of chronic inflammatory changes at the time of appendicectomy (Mattei et al. 1994), and the presence of appendicolith on CT scan with a thickened appendix greater than 9 mm in width (Giuliano et al. 2006). In those with a normal appendix neuroimmune changes with an increased expression of substance P and vasoactive intestinal peptide (VIP) containing nerves have been demonstrated suggesting a possible neuroimmune explanation for symptoms other than acute inflammation (Di Sebastiano et al. 1999). There is no current standardized strategy for the management of these patients who must be dealt with on an individual basis. "Spontaneously Resolving and Chronic Appendicitis" is further discussed by LP Cobben.

5 Conclusion

The diagnosis of acute appendicitis is clinical and specialist investigations should only be requested in those patients in whom the clinical diagnosis is uncertain. The Alvarado and other scoring systems are still only an aid to clinical diagnosis and may aid in the clinicians judgment of how to manage patients.

References

Addiss D et al (1990) The epidemiology of appendicitis and appendectomy in the United States. Am J Epidemiol 132(5):910–925

Alvarado A (1986) A practical score for the early diagnosis of acute appendicitis. Ann Emerg Med 15(5):557–564

Andersson R (2004) Meta-analysis of the clinical and laboratory diagnosis of appendicitis. Br J Surg 91(1):28–37

Andersson M, Andersson R (2008) The appendicitis inflammatory response score: a tool for the diagnosis of acute appendicitis that outperforms the Alvarado score. World J Surg 32(8):1843–1849

Attard AR et al (1992) Safety of early pain relief for acute abdominal pain. BMJ 305(6853):554–556

Barber MD, McLaren J, Rainey JB (1997) Recurrent appendicitis. Br J Surg 84(1):110–112

Beltrán MA et al (2007) Predictive value of white blood cell count and C-reactive protein in children with appendicitis. J Pediatr Surg 42(7):1208–1214

Bhatt M et al (2009) Prospective validation of the pediatric appendicitis score in a canadian pediatric emergency department. Acad Emerg Med 16(7):591–596

Bickell NA et al (2006) How time affects the risk of rupture in appendicitis. J Am Coll Surg 202(3):401–406

Blomqvist PG et al (2001) Mortality after appendectomy in Sweden, 1987–1996. Ann Surg 233(4):455–460

Caglayan F et al (2003) Plasma D-lactate levels in diagnosis of appendicitis. J Invest Surg 16(4):233–237

Coleman C et al (1998) White blood cell count is a poor predictor of severity of disease in the diagnosis of appendicitis. Am Surg 64(10):983–985

Cope Z (2000) Early diagnosis of the acute abdomen. 20th Edn. Oxford University Press

De Dombal FT et al (1974) Human and computer-aided diagnosis of abdominal pain: further report with emphasis on performance of clinicians. Br Med J 1(5904):376–380

Demircan M et al (2004) Plasma D-Lactic acid level: a useful marker to distinguish perforated from acute simple appendicitis. Asian J Surg 27(4):303–305

Di Sebastiano P et al (1999) Neuroimmune appendicitis. The Lancet 354(9177):p 461

Dixon JM et al (1991) Rectal examination in patients with pain in the right lower quadrant of the abdomen. BMJ 302(6773):386–388

Douglas CD et al (2000) Randomised controlled trial of ultrasonography in diagnosis of acute appendicitis, incorporating the Alvarado score. BMJ 321(7266):919

Dueholm S, Bagi P, and Bud M (1989) Laboratory aid in the diagnosis of acute appendicitis. A blinded, prospective trial concerning diagnostic value of leukocyte count, neutrophil differential count, and C-reactive protein. Dis Colon Rectum 32(10):855–859

Duzgun AP et al (2007) Serum D-lactate: a useful diagnostic marker for acute appendicitis. Hepatogastroenterology 54(77):1483–1486

Eriksson S, Granstrom L, Carlstrom A (1994) The diagnostic value of repetitive preoperative analyses of C-reactive protein and total leucocyte count in patients with suspected acute appendicitis. Scand J Gastroenterol 29(12):1145–1149

Estrada J et al (2007) Hyperbilirubinemia in appendicitis: a new predictor of perforation. J Gastrointest Surg 11(6):714–718

Fenyo G et al (1997) Diagnostic decision support in suspected acute appendicitis: validation of a simplified scoring system. Eur J Surg 163(11):831–838

Flum DR, Koepsell T (2002) The clinical and economic correlates of misdiagnosed appendicitis: Nationwide analysis. Arch Surg 137(7):799–804

Flum DR et al (2001) Has misdiagnosis of appendicitis decreased over time? A population-based analysis. JAMA 286(14):1748–1753

Giuliano V et al (2006) Chronic appendicitis "syndrome" manifested by an appendicolith and thickened appendix presenting as chronic right lower abdominal pain in adults. Emerg Radiol 12(3):96–98

Goldman RD et al (2008) Prospective validation of the pediatric appendicitis score. J Pediatr 153(2):278–282

Goodwin AT et al (1997) Can serum interleukin-6 levels predict the outcome of patients with right iliac fossa pain? Ann R Coll Surg Engl 79(2):130–133

Green R et al (2005) Early analgesia for children with acute abdominal pain. Pediatrics 116(4):978–983

Grönroos JM, Grönroos P (1999) Leucocyte count and C-reactive protein in the diagnosis of acute appendicitis. Br J Surg 86(4):501–504

Gurleyik E, Gurleyik G, Unalmiser S (1995) Accuracy of serum C-reactive protein measurements in diagnosis of acute appendicitis compared with surgeon's clinical impression. Dis Colon Rectum 38(12):1270–1274

Gurleyik G et al (2002) Serum interleukin-6 measurement in the diagnosis of acute appendicitis. ANZ J Surg 72:665–667

Guttman R, Goldman RD, Koren G (2004) Appendicitis during pregnancy. Can Fam Physician 50:355–357

Hallan S, Asberg A, Edna T (1997) Additional value of biochemical tests in suspected acute appendicitis. Eur J Surg 163:533–538

Hsieh C-H et al (2011) Novel solutions for an old disease: Diagnosis of acute appendicitis with random forest, support vector machines, and artificial neural networks. Surgery 149(1):87–93

Humes DJ, Simpson J (2006) Acute appendicitis. BMJ 333(7567):530–534

Käser SA et al (2010) C-reactive protein is superior to bilirubin for anticipation of perforation in acute appendicitis. Scand J Gastroenterol 45(7–8):885–892

Korner H, Soreide J, Sondenaa K (1999) Diagnostic accuracy of inflammatory markers in patients operated on for suspected acute appendicitis: a receiver operating characteristic curve analysis. Eur J Surg 165:679–685

Kremer K et al (1998) The diagnostic value of rectal examination of patients with acute appendicitis. Langenbecks Arch Chir Suppl Kongressbd 115:1120–1122

Kwan KY, Nager AL (2010) Diagnosing pediatric appendicitis: usefulness of laboratory markers. Am J Emerg Med 28(9):1009–1015

Lintula H (2010) Diagnostic score in acute appendicitis. Validation of a diagnostic score (Lintula score) for adults with suspected appendicitis. Langenbeck's Arch Surg 395(5):495–500

Lintula H et al (2005) A diagnostic score for children with suspected appendicitis. Langenbeck's Arch Surg 390(2):164–170

Mandeville K, Pottker T, and Bulloch B (2010) Using appendicitis scores in the pediatric ED. Am J Emerg Med. 2010 Jul 30, Epub ahead of print

Mattei P, Sola JE, Yeo CJ (1994) Chronic and recurrent appendicitis are uncommon entities often misdiagnosed. J Am Coll Surg 178(4):385–389

McBurney C (1889) Experiences with early operative interference in cases of diseases of the vermiform appendix. NY Med J 50:676–684

McKay R, Shepherd J (2007) The use of the clinical scoring system by Alvarado in the decision to perform computed tomography for acute appendicitis in the ED. Am J Emerg Med 25(5):489–493

Murphy J (1904) Two thousand operations for appendicitis with deductions from his personal experience. Am J Med Sci 128:187–211

Ohmann C, Yang Q, Franke C (1995) Diagnostic scores for acute appendicitis. Abdom Pain Study Group. Eur J Surg 161(4):273–281

Paajanen H et al (2002) Novel serum inflammatory markers in acute appendicitis. Scand J Clin Lab Invest 62:579–584

Paulson EK, Kalady MF, Pappas TN (2003) Suspected appendicitis. N Engl J Med 348(3):236–242

Pouget-Baudry Y et al (2010) The use of the Alvarado score in the management of right lower quadrant abdominal pain in the adult. Journal of Visceral Surgery 147(2):e40–e44

Prabhudesai S et al (2008) Artificial Neural Networks: Useful Aid in Diagnosing Acute Appendicitis. World J Surg 32(2):305–309

Puskar D et al (1995) Urinalysis, ultrasound analysis, and renal dynamic scintigraphy in acute appendicitis. Urology 45(1):108–112

Rusnak RA, Borer JM FJS (1994) Misdiagnosis of acute appendicitis: common features discovered in cases after litigation. Am J Emerg Med 12(4):397–402

Sack U et al (2006) Diagnostic value of blood inflammatory markers for detection of acute appendicitis in children. BMC Surgery 6(1):15

Samuel M (2002) Pediatric appendicitis score. J Pediatr Surg 37(6):877–881

Scarlett PY et al (1986) Computer aided diagnosis of acute abdominal pain at Middlesbrough General Hospital. Ann R Coll Surg Engl 68(4):179–181

Scheinfeld M et al (2010) Can lab data be used to reduce abdominal computed tomography (CT) usage in young adults presenting to the emergency department with nontraumatic abdominal pain? Emerg Radiol 17(5):353–360

Schneider C, Kharbanda A and Bachur R (2007) Evaluating Appendicitis Scoring Systems Using a Prospective Pediatric Cohort. Annals of Emergency Medicine 49(6):778–784.e1

Thompson MM et al (1992) Role of sequential leucocyte counts and C-reactive protein measurements in acute appendicitis. Br J Surg 79(8):822–824

Thuijls G et al (2011) A pilot study on potential new plasma markers for diagnosis of acute appendicitis. Am J Emerg Med Med 29(3):256–260

Tzanakis N et al (2005) A new approach to accurate diagnosis of acute appendicitis. World J Surg 29(9):1151–1156

Wagner JM, McKinney WP, Carpenter JL (1996) Does this patient have appendicitis? Jama 276(19):1589–1594

Wellwood J, Johannessen S, Spiegelhalter DJ (1992) How does computer-aided diagnosis improve the management of acute abdominal pain? Ann R Coll Surg Engl 74(1):40–46

Yang H-R et al (2006) Laboratory tests in patients with acute appendicitis. ANZ J Surg 76(1–2):71–74

Appendicitis Perforation Rates and Time Interval between Symptom Onset and Surgery

Tehillah S. Menes and Nina A. Bickell

Contents

Abstract

This chapter examines the evidence on the association between time to treatment and perforation rates. Time to treatment is divided into two components; patient time, which is the time from symptom onset to presentation to healthcare system and system time which includes time delays between presentation and definitive treatment. While patient time is associated with increased perforation rates and worse outcomes, poor effects of system delays are less consistently shown, likely because total time duration between symptom onset and treatment is not taken into account, timing has not been accurately documented, and possibly due to different disease processes for perforated and non-perforated appendicitis. The impact of increased use of CT for the diagnosis of appendicitis on delay and perforation rates is discussed.

1 Background

1.1 Historical Overview: Surgical Management of Suspected Appendicitis: From Early Intervention to Active Observation

One of the most vexing and important questions in the course of appendicitis is the role of time. Fitz's first descriptions of appendicitis in the late 1800s portrayed the progression from inflammation to peritonitis and abscess formation making it an easy leap to recommend early surgery (Berry and Malt 1984).

T. S. Menes
Department of Surgery, Tel Aviv Sourasky Medical Center, 6 Weizmann Street, 64239 Tel Aviv, Israel

N. A. Bickell (✉)
Departments of Health Evidence and Policy and Medicine, Mount Sinai Medical Center, One Gustave L. Levy Place, New York, NY 10029, USA
e-mail: nina.bickell@mssm.edu

C. Keyzer and P. A. Gevenois (eds.), *Imaging of Acute Appendicitis in Adults and Children*, Medical Radiology. Diagnostic Imaging, DOI: 10.1007/174_2011_209,

In 1900, Riddell advocated operation for patients with 'perforative appendicitis' arguing that without treatment there was no recovery, and therefore, surgery was the patient's only choice. Of course, this occurred in the pre-antibiotic era. The risk of ruptured appendicitis with its associated high rates of mortality led to the practice of early surgery, even for equivocal cases. This treatment approach was accompanied by high rates (20–30%) of negative appendectomies. Thus, for many years, it was widely understood that a proportion of normal appendices needed to be removed in order to avoid perforations (Berry and Malt 1984), and the more the time between symptom onset and definitive surgical treatment, the greater the chance of appendiceal perforation.

By the 1960s and early 1970s, large studies examining admissions for acute abdominal pain found that one-third of patients with suspected acute appendicitis on presentation recover without any treatment (Jones 2001). These findings prompted a change in the approach to patients presenting with acute abdominal pain: those clearly presenting with a clinical picture consistent with acute appendicitis were promptly taken to the operating room (OR). Others with a non-specific clinical picture were observed closely. This active observation included regular examination by physicians and nurses, nothing given by mouth, IV fluids, and serial blood tests (white blood cell count and C-reactive protein level). Patients who proceeded to develop findings more suggestive of acute appendicitis (or another surgical abdomen) were taken to the OR as were those who did not recover. The use of active observation lowered rates of negative appendectomies to 3–10% without a concomitant increase in rates of perforation (Jones 2001). The practice of active observation in equivocal cases became widely accepted. However, it was also accepted that rates of ruptured appendicitis are inversely associated with the rates of appendectomies for normal appendices and that delaying surgery in some patients may come at the cost of higher perforation rates and its associated morbidity (Von Titte et al. 1996). In more recent years, the approach to treat appendicitis is changing. Physicians start intravenous antibiotics immediately and in certain circumstances have safely delayed surgery from "off-hours" to "regular hours" when staffing and services are readily available (Surana et al. 1993; Yardeni et al. 2004). As some patients can be safely watched and monitored without serious consequence, these studies raise the question of the role of time in the risk of perforation (Ingraham et al. 2010; Hunter 2010).

1.2 Epidemiology of Appendicitis

Population-based studies allow for analysis of trends in the incidence of non-perforated and perforated appendicitis in the entire population at risk. Data from the National Hospital Discharge Survey (NHDS, a database representative of the US hospitalized population) between the years 1970–2004 show an initial reduction followed by a slight rise in the incidence rates of both non-perforated and perforated appendicitis in recent years. Negative appendectomies decreased over time with the increased use of CT imaging (Livingston et al. 2007).

1.3 Rates of Perforation and Associated Morbidity

Rates of ruptured appendicitis vary widely (15–35%) (Luckmann 1989; Braveman et al. 1994; Körner et al. 2001; Sicard et al. 2007). Perforated appendicitis is associated with increased morbidity and mortality. Complications include wound infection [17 vs. 9% in non-perforated appendicitis (Berry and Malt 1984)], intra-abdominal collection, small bowel obstruction, cutaneous fistulae, incisional hernia as well as non-specific complications such as pneumonia, pulmonary emboli, deep vein thrombosis, acute cardiac ischemia, urinary retention, and urinary tract infection (Berry and Malt 1984; Cacioppo et al. 1989). Complication rates increase from 6–10% in simple appendicitis to 20–36% in perforated appendicitis (Eldar et al. 1997; Savrin and Clatworthy 1979). Mortality rates increase as well from 0.05% in simple appendicitis to 0.3% in perforated appendicitis (Luckmann 1989). Mortality rates in patients with perforated appendicitis increase even more with age to a peak of 6% in patients older than 79 years (Luckmann 1989). This increased complication rate is associated with increased hospital length of stay and higher healthcare costs (Sicard et al. 2007). Long-term morbidity associated with perforated appendicitis includes small bowel obstruction and possibly tubal infertility (Webb and Holman 1992). These worse outcomes compel us to identify alterable risk factors for perforation and intervene to reduce the risk.

2 Risk Factors for Perforation

Several risk factors have been associated with higher rates of perforated appendicitis:

2.1 Age

The proportion of cases with perforation dramatically changes with age (Kraemer et al. 1999; Bratton et al. 2000; Pittman-Waller et al. 2000; Körner et al. 2001; Sicard et al. 2007). Highest rates of perforation are found in the very young and in the elderly. These rates peak in the 0–9 age group, drop and then gradually increase from age 20 upward to a peak of 75% in the 80 plus age group. However, a population-based study of discharges from all California hospitals in 1984, found that of 24,794 appendectomies, the incidence of non-perforated appendicitis peaked in the teens and then slowly declined for both sexes. Incidence rates of perforated appendicitis were fairly constant with age, with a small peak in the teens as well (Fig. 1): 30–40 cases/100,000 males; 20–25 cases/100,000 females (Luckmann 1989). Similarly, Korner reported incidence rates of perforated appendicitis in Stavanger, Norway. The rates did not change significantly in different age groups (Körner et al. 1997).

2.2 Sex

There are conflicting studies about the role of gender in perforation. Some studies report a higher rate of perforation in men (Kraemer et al. 1999; Pittman-Waller et al. 2000) while others do not find such an association (Körner et al. 1997; Redmond et al. 2002). Kraemer, with the Acute Abdominal Pain Study Group, conducted a prospective multicenter study in Germany and Austria in 1994–1995 (Kraemer et al. 1999). The study group included 2,280 patients with acute abdomen, excluding children under the age of six. Of the 519 appendectomies with histology proven acute appendicitis, 18% had perforated. Perforation rates were higher in males, with a ratio of 1.5:1,

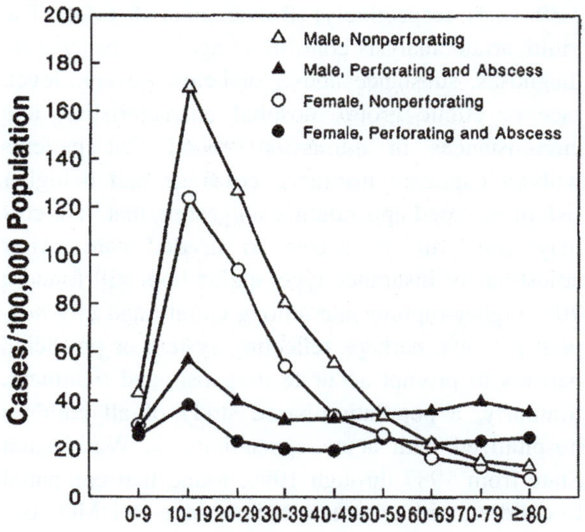

Fig. 1 Incidence of appendectomy and drainage of abscess for appendicitis by age, sex and type in California in 1984. Perforated appendicitis and appendicieal abscess are combined. Reprinted with permission from Luckmann (1989)

despite the fact that in the whole group male to female ratio was 1.

2.3 Type of Insurance

In countries without universal health care, type of insurance can affect access to care due to financial constraints by reducing access and increasing time to effective treatment. In the United States, several studies examined the association of perforated appendicitis with the type of or lack of health insurance. Braveman used statewide California hospital-discharge data to study differences in the rates of appendiceal perforation in adults, according to type of insurance coverage. Of all California residents patients in the age group of 18–64 years old that were hospitalized with a principal diagnosis of acute appendicitis from 1984 through 1989 ($N = 96,587$), 34% of uninsured, 34% of Medicaid, 29% of commercial fee-for-service, and 26% of private capitated-payment insurance patients experienced a perforated appendix. Patients with appendicitis who had Medicaid coverage or were uninsured were about 1.5 times more likely to have appendiceal rupture when compared to those with capitated private coverage (OR = 1.49 [95% confidence interval, 1.41–1.59] and 1.46 [95% confidence interval,

1.39–1.54], respectively) (Braveman et al. 1994). The multivariate analysis controlling age, sex, psychiatric diagnoses, substance abuse, diabetes, poverty level, race or ethnic group, hospital characteristics, and circumstances of admission, found that patients with*out* capitated insurance coverage had a higher risk of ruptured appendicitis suggesting that visit cost may affect timely access to needed care. After adjusting for insurance type, the authors still found a 70% higher-rupture rate among county and city hospital patients, perhaps reflecting system or physician barriers to prompt accurate diagnosis and treatment. Similarly, a population-based study of all children hospitalized with acute appendicitis in Washington State from 1987 through 1996, found that compared to children with commercial insurance or HMO coverage, children covered by Medicaid insurance had increased risk of complicated appendicitis (Bratton et al. 2000). Indeed, the effect of insurance was also found in Maryland. Data from Maryland Medicaid inpatient claims and the Maryland Health Services and Cost Review Commission (HSCRC) for hospital discharges of children <18 years, which included all payers, found a higher proportion of ruptured appendicitis occurred among Medicaid recipients, 36% compared to 29% among those privately insured. Interestingly, among Medicaid beneficiaries, there was an inverse association between the number of preventive care visits and the occurrence of ruptured appendicitis suggesting that preventive visits are a proxy for parental attentiveness to health care issues, and that these kids are more likely to have a relationship with a healthcare provider who can expedite care (Gadomski and Jenkins 2001). The challenge of using administrative data to assess factors associated with perforation is that it does not permit assessment of whether barriers to care were concentrated in the pre-hospital phase, caused by patients delaying calls due to reluctance to pay the out of pocket costs or not knowing whom to call, or whether the barriers were within the system, related to physicians' inability to get timely consultations, tests or treatments. In a study of childhood appendicitis, Brender found that parents encouraged to observe their children at home by the health professional first contacted, had the highest incidence of appendiceal rupture (67%) (Brender et al. 1985). These studies highlight the importance of insurance and access to care and their effects on perforation rates, both positively and negatively.

2.4 Daily and Seasonal Variation

Examining variability in rates of perforation with the day of the week, month, or season provides insight into external influences of different elements on the pathologic progression and outcome of appendicitis. For example, the Kids Inpatient Database (KID) Healthcare Cost and Utilization Project, a national database representative of 80% of pediatric admissions from 2,521 hospitals in 22 US states, described variation in the incidence of appendicitis in children by day of the week: Mondays had the highest rates for acute and perforated appendicitis, weekends had the lowest rates (Deng et al. 2010). Such findings may reflect parents' and patients' access to health care on weekends. However, they do not explain whether emergency services were less available or if parents prefer to wait for the weekend before contacting their pediatricians. A study from Montreal, found a non-significant increase in perforation rates on the weekends and holidays when compared to weekdays (Sicard et al. 2007).

Other studies examine seasonal variation which can indicate the effects of training (e.g., July/August, when residents are relatively inexperienced), or infectious etiologies resulting in lymphoid hyperplasia and subsequent appendiceal obstruction. A study analyzing the outcome of 4,325 patients with appendicitis by the month of the year found no difference in outcome of patients presenting in the beginning of the academic year and the rest of the year (Yaghoubian et al. 2010). In the KID study, the highest incidence of appendicitis was in the summer and the highest incidence of perforated appendicitis was found in the fall (Deng et al. 2010).

2.5 Hospital Organization Model

Hospital organization may also impact the outcome of patients with acute appendicitis as access to dedicated emergency imaging and surgery can affect time to care. Sicard examined outcomes of patients with acute appendicitis in different hospitals in Montreal. Twelve hospitals, each performing over 50 appendectomies a year, were included. A wide variation (19–35%) was found in the rates of complicated appendicitis across different hospitals. Hospitals with a high volume of patients (as measured by total annual volume of patients admitted to the hospital and annual volume of surgery), with readily available imaging, presence of surgical specialties, and a dedicated emergency OR had lower rates of ruptured appendicitis than hospitals without these organizational features (Sicard et al. 2007).

2.6 Time Delay

2.6.1 Delay in Presentation versus Delay in Evaluation:

Given the pathologic progression that results in rupture with its associated worse morbidity and mortality (Luckmann 1989), assessing the effect of time on outcome is key. Once the effect of time is ascertained, identifying the source of delays may provide remediable points to intervene. A study evaluating the changing risk of perforation with time from symptom onset to treatment found a steady rise in risk with passing hours up to 36 h following which, the risk of perforation in each subsequent 12 h period remained at a steady high level (Bickell et al. 2006). Similarly, Ditillo described pathologic worsening with passing time. In this large study of over 1,000 patients, appendicitis was graded according to the pathological findings: G1 for uncomplicated appendicitis, G2 for gangrenous, G3 for perforated or phlegmonous, and G4 for periappendiceal abscess. As the total time between symptom onset and treatment increased from less than 12 h to over 71 h, the rates of G1 decreased from 94 to 54% while G4 increased from 3 to 13% (Ditillo et al. 2006).

Identifying where and why patients experience delays provides points to intervene to speed processes and in turn, reduce perforation rates and poorer outcomes (Bickell and Siu 2001). The time between symptom onset and treatment (appendectomy) consists of various components (Fig. 2):

A. Patient-Time the time between start of symptoms and presentation to health care, e.g., physician, nurse practitioner, and emergency department. This period requires correct recognition of symptoms and ability to present to health care. It lies within the patient domain and is perceived as more difficult to alter. (Rosenstock 1966; Ting et al. 2008).
B. System time: the time between presentation to care and definitive treatment. This period encompasses initial examination, diagnostic assessments, and treatment. It requires clinical acumen and availability of needed services and personnel. This component of time is perceived to be more easily altered than patient-time as it lies within the system's domain.

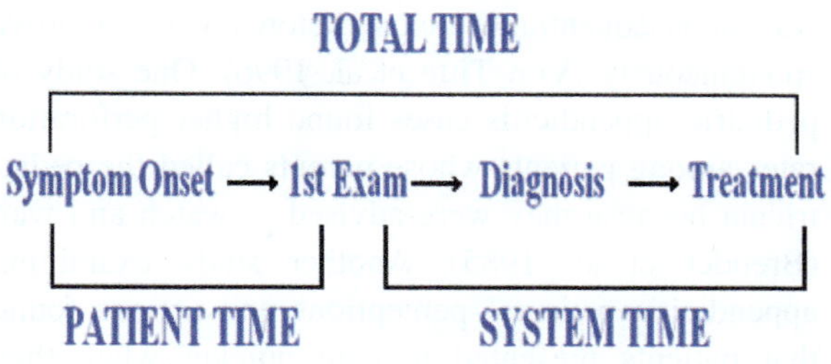

Fig. 2 Components of time delay between symptom onset and treatment

Patient factors that can affect patient-time include elements of the health belief model [perceived vulnerability, severity, curability, and coping strategies (Rosenstock 1974; Kirscht 1974; Kasl 1975; Safer et al. 1979)], knowledge of disease symptoms, and skill in negotiating their health care system, insurance type, and competing demands. Physician factors that may contribute to delay include: physician availability (initial contact and specialist consultation), referral practices, and diagnostic and treatment acumen. Health system organizational factors include: availability of urgent contact, pre-authorization demands, availability of diagnostic tests or treatment facilities, and the technical quality of care. Each group of factors affects the amount of time between patient recognition of symptoms, their contact with the health care system, determination of the correct diagnosis, and institution of effective treatment.

Numerous studies examine the time between symptom onset and presentation to care (Temple et al. 1995; Körner et al. 2001; Pittman-Waller et al. 2000; Bickell et al. 2006; Sicard et al. 2007) with most finding higher rates of perforation among patients who present to care later rather than earlier (Eldar et al. 1997; Kraemer et al. 1999; Pittman-Waller et al. 2000; Cappendijk and Hazebroek 2000; Bickell et al. 2006). Von Titte found that patients with >72 h time lapse between symptom onset and treatment experienced a very high rate of perforation (90%). In 38% of these patients, the delay was fully attributed to patients' delay with patients thinking that the pain was inconsequential or that symptoms would improve spontaneously (Von Titte et al. 1996). One study of pediatric appendicitis cases found higher perforation rates among patients whose parents called the pediatrician because they were advised to watch and wait (Brender et al. 1985). Another study examining appendicitis patients' perceptions and actions found that patients presented to care quicker when they perceived the condition to be serious and their prior health status was good; thus, it appears that the abrupt change in their health and acuity of pain hastened action. Appendicitis patients' beliefs about the health system, having a regular doctor and knowing whom to call, coping strategies, insurance, education, and clinical severity did not appear to affect the amount of time between symptom onset and presenting to care (Bickell et al. 2004).

2.6.2 Delay between Presentation and Treatment:

Reports examining the association between delays in treatment (i.e., time elapsed from presentation to treatment) and ruptured appendicitis are less consistent. Some of the discrepancy is likely due to diagnostic uncertainty and protocols in place to assess patients presenting with acute abdominal pain. For example, patients presenting with classic appendicitis symptoms are treated more quickly and have lower perforation rates (Cappendijk and Hazebroek 2000; Omundsen and Dennett 2006). Many studies find an association between delays to treatment and rupture rate (Berry and Malt 1984; Cacioppo et al. 1989; Linz et al. 1993; Walker et al. 1995; Cappendijk and Hazebroek 2000; Ditillo et al. 2006; Omundsen and Dennett 2006; Bickell et al. 2006). Studies that examine this question divide the patient groups according to time elapsed between admission and surgery, and compare the proportion of patients with perforated appendicitis in both groups (Walker et al. 1995; Cappendijk and Hazebroek 2000; Bickell et al. 2006; Ditillo et al. 2006). In patients followed prospectively during a 12 month period, there was a non-significant increase in the proportion of perforated appendicitis in patients with longer delays between admission and surgery: 18% among those operated within 6 h versus 33% in those operated after 24 h (Walker et al. 1995). Similarly, a higher rate of perforation was found in patients operated on or after 24 h when compared to less than 24 h. Those operated on after 24 h from presentation tended to be older, female and their outcomes, length of stay, use of antibiotics, and perforation rates, were worse when compared to the group operated within 24 h. The authors conclude that these are different patients with diagnostically challenging appendicitis (Omundsen and Dennett 2006). Similarly, a study of 129 children with acute appendicitis evaluated diagnostic delay. Diagnostic delay was divided into early, less than 48 h, and late, greater than 48 h. Patients in the "early" group presented more often with classic symptoms whereas those in the "later" group had more non-specific abdominal pain or diarrhea. Perforation was more common in the latter group (71 vs. 24%) (Cappendijk and Hazebroek 2000). Delay in surgeon consultation and time to OR were associated with complicated appendicitis in the pediatric community (Linz et al. 1993). Delays in surgical consultation were found in a study examining referral to surgeons in two time periods (1980 vs. 1986 and 1987) and outcome of patients with acute appendicitis. In the later periods there were longer delays to treatment, with more patients treated by non-surgical personnel in the pre-hospital setting, and delays in surgeon consultation, possibly related to changes in the healthcare system, with increased gatekeeper activity. These delays in turn were associated with an increase in the rates of complicated appendicitis and its associated morbidity (Cacioppo et al. 1989).

Others did not find an association between delay in treatment and rupture: multiple studies comparing time from presentation to surgery in patients with perforated and non-perforated appendicitis, did not find a significant difference (McLean et al. 1993; Eldar et al. 1997; Kraemer et al. 1999; Pittman-Waller et al. 2000; Sicard et al. 2007; Lee et al. 2001).

The retrospective nature and different methodology used may explain these conflicting results. In retrospective studies it is difficult to ascertain the exact time of symptom onset, which is subject to recall bias. The outcome, perforated appendicitis, can be determined using diagnostic or billing codes, chart notes, imaging findings, operative reports, positive peritoneal cultures, or the pathology report, and therefore misclassifications are a concern. Most studies compare proportions of perforated appendicitis, which are determined by the total number of appendectomies and will change with the number of negative appendectomies. Negative appendectomy rates are influenced by local practice and have been decreasing over time. Moreover, if perforated appendicitis is suspected on presentation, it can influence the delays, either by shortening time to the operating room because of the perceived urgency (Van Breda Vriesman et al. 2003; Temple et al. 1995), or by increasing delays if abscess formation is suspected, as further workup maybe requested. Finally, the use of antibiotics may also alter the natural history of the disease.

2.6.3 Recent Trends in Management of Non-Complicated Appendicitis in the Era of IV Antibiotics:

Anecdotal episodes describe individuals with presumed appendicitis aboard submarines, and merchant ships who were treated with intravenous antibiotics without progression to rupture (Groetsch and Shaughnessy 2001; Mason 2008). Although this is not universally accepted as standard of care, several studies report that for patients who have not perforated at presentation, it is safe to treat with intravenous antibiotics and wait until regular work hours to perform an appendectomy (Surana et al. 1993; Yardeni et al. 2004; Ingraham et al. 2010; Hunter 2010). In Our Lady's Hospital for Sick Children in Dublin, Ireland a policy of delaying surgery to morning was instituted in the late 1980s. Surana compared the outcome of patients presenting during the day and operated on or before midnight, with a group of patients who presented or were diagnosed during the night hours and were placed on antibiotics and operated on the next morning. There were 695 patients in total. No significant difference in rates of perforation (18 vs. 21%) was found (Surana et al. 1993). A similar report from the Pediatric Department of Surgery at the University of Michigan Health System in Ann Arbor, Michigan, examined the outcome of patients treated under a new protocol. Children presenting in the evening or early morning hours with non-perforated appendicitis were given antibiotics and operated on within 24 h of admission. These patients were compared to patients who were operated within 6 h of presentation. Patients who were operated after 24 h were excluded, assuming that an inconclusive diagnosis contributed to the delay in surgery. They did not find a difference in the perforation rates between the two groups. Based on their results they recommend a semi-elective approach to these patients, arguing that antibiotics can halt or slow the disease process and allow a planned delay in treatment. Delay was associated with a slight increase in cost as well as length of stay (Yardeni et al. 2004). Both these studies may lack power to show significant differences in perforation rates, and suffer from selection bias. However, a recent retrospective cohort study of 32,782 patients reporting data to the American College of Surgeons' National Surgical Quality Improvement Program found that 75% of patients were operated within 6 h of surgical admission, 15% between 6 and 12 h, and 10% more than 12 h after admission. Although there was a higher rate of perforation in the patients operated on after 12 h from admission, there was no significant difference among these groups in post-operative stay, morbidity, or mortality (Ingraham et al. 2010). These studies did not assess the effect of total time between symptom onset and treatment but they do raise the tantalizing possibility that not all appendicitis cases require immediate surgical intervention.

3 Is Perforated Appendicitis a Separate Disease?

While the classic teaching is of a progressive disease that needs to be surgically treated urgently in order to prevent rupture and complication, the theory of progression of acute appendicitis through the four pathologic steps previously described (Ditillo et al. 2006) has been questioned by several reports. Population-based studies show a disconnect between the age-related incidence rates of perforated and non-perforated appendicitis (Luckmann 1989; Andersson et al. 1994). Age-adjusted incidence rates of appendicitis were calculated for the county of Jonkoping in Sweden during 1984–1989. The incidence of perforated appendicitis was fairly stable for the different age groups, whereas the incidence of non-perforated appendicitis peaked in the 10–14 age group. To examine temporal trends in appendicitis, and appendectomies, the authors examined all appendectomies done in the town of Jonkoping between 1970 and 1989. They found a decrease of 29% in the rates of appendectomies over the years studied. There was a similar decrease in the rates of appendicitis by 24%. This was associated with a 40% decrease in the rates of appendectomies done for normal appendices. The incidence of non-perforated appendicitis fell by 27% from 152 cases to 111 per 100,000/year. This was in contrast to the incidence of perforated appendicitis which remained stable at 21 per 100,000 (Andersson et al. 1994). In order to examine the association between the laparotomy rate and incidence of perforated and non-perforated appendicitis, the same authors reviewed six published reports of series of appendectomies from different countries. Diagnostic accuracy and rates of negative laparotomies were used as indicators of a surgeon's attitude toward exploring in equivocal cases. These studies included over 53,000 patients. There was a wide variation in the incidence of appendectomies in the different series. However, the variance was seen mainly for non-perforated appendicitis and for negative appendectomies and much less so for perforated appendicitis. These authors conclude that differences in management of non-perforated appendicitis influence the reported incidence of the disease, e.g., an aggressive approach with early exploration of equivocal cases will increase the reported or observed incidence rates of non-perforated appendicitis, suggesting that some forms of appendicitis may resolve without surgery. Similarly in studies that randomized patients with equivocal findings to CT versus expectant management, or laparoscopy compared to expectant management, higher rates of appendectomy and appendicitis were found in the patients undergoing CT or laparoscopy versus those who were followed. These reports suggest that some of these cases would have resolved without surgery (Mason 2008).

Perforation rates are inversely associated with the number of total appendectomies as well as the number of negative appendectomies. These authors reject the premise that early exploration will reduce the number of cases with perforated appendicitis, and criticize the use of rates of perforated appendicitis as a proxy of quality of care (Andersson et al. 1994). However, at this point in time, there are no established clinical prediction rules to validly and safely distinguish which appendicitis cases will resolve with antibiotics only and which will perforate.

4 Effect of CT Imaging on System Time and Perforation Rates

The introduction of CT has revolutionized the management of patients with acute abdomen. However, the increased use of CT for the diagnosis of acute appendicitis can contribute to delays particularly if oral contrast is used to opacify the cecum. On the other hand, routine use of imaging may lead to rapid diagnosis in equivocal cases and actually decrease delays in treatment and thereby, reduce the rates of perforation. Several studies showed that patients undergoing CT had a higher rate of perforation (Pittman-Waller et al. 2000; Bendeck et al. 2002; Bickell et al. 2006; Musunuru et al. 2007; Augustin et al. 2009). Other studies did not show a significant association (Applegate et al. 2001; McDonald et al. 2001; Weyant et al. 2001; Perez et al. 2003; Mathis et al. 2005; Wong et al. 2008), although some lacked power to detect differences (McDonald et al. 2001; Weyant et al. 2001).

Numerous studies examined the impact of increased use of imaging on the outcome of patients. These studies can be divided according to their methodology. Descriptive observational studies showed that patients undergoing CT for the evaluation of acute appendicitis had longer delays when compared to patients who were operated on without imaging (Lee et al. 2001; McDonald et al. 2001; Perez et al. 2003; Menes et al. 2006; Bickell et al. 2006; Musunuru et al. 2007; Riesenman et al. 2008). Bickell found an association between use of CT and longer delays. However, use of CT was also associated with unclear diagnosis at presentation, according to doctors' notes. In general, patients who waited longer prior to presentation, more often had uncertain diagnoses and thus, more use of imaging studies, and subsequent longer times to treatment. Others did not find delays associated with CT (Mathis et al. 2005). Augustin compared the outcome of patients undergoing CT prior to appendectomy with those who did not. The rate of perforated appendicitis was significantly higher in patients who underwent CT scans. In order to check if the difference in perforation rate between the two groups was due to patients presenting with perforated appendicitis on admission receiving CT scans, they excluded patients with perforated appendicitis on initial CT scans and repeated the analyses. The difference in perforation rates continued to remain significant ($P = 0.037$) (Augustin et al. 2009). Menes examined the delay associated with use of CT, and found that while use of CT was associated with delay, there appeared to be a learning curve. Over time, as use of CT increased, access to CT was quicker and readings were more accurate (Menes et al. 2006), a common finding among innovations adopted in medicine (Ascheim et al. 2009).

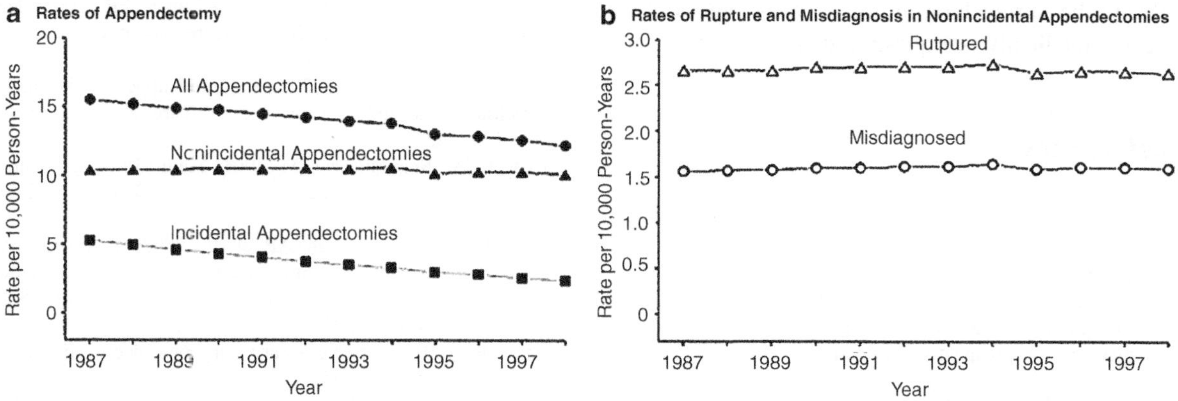

Fig. 3 Population-Adjusted Rates of Total, Incidental, and Nonincidental Appendectomy and Misdiagnosis and Rupture in Nonincidental Appendectomy (**a**), in Washington State, the population-based rate of nonincidental appendectomy remained stable over time, with a decrease in the rate of all appendectomies related to a 7.3% yearly decrease in the rate of incidental appendectomy (**b**), among patients undergoing nonincidental appendectomy, the population-adjusted rates of misdiagnosis and perforation remained unchanged from 1987 through 1998. (from Flum et al. (2001) Copyright © American Medical Association 2001. All rights reserved. Reprinted with permission)

Population-based studies enable us to examine trends in use of CT and its overall impact on rates of negative appendectomies and perforated appendicitis. In Washington State, among 15 hospitals performing over 50 appendectomies a year, there was an increasing rate of use of CT but no associated change in the perforation rate (SCOAP Collaborative et al. 2008). Similarly, a population-based study of 85,790 patients operated on for appendicitis during 1987–1998 found that the incidence of perforated appendicitis did not change over time. However, it is possible that assessing this question with data ending in 1998 was too early to capture the true impact of CT (Fig. 3) (Flum et al. 2001).

In a randomized trial of CT versus clinical assessment, Hong compared the outcome of 182 patients with an intermediate probability of having appendicitis, half of whom received a CT scan and the other half, received clinical assessment only. The CT group experienced longer delays to treatment (19 h vs. 11, $P < 0.01$). Perforation rates were higher among scanned patients (9 vs. 6%, $P = 0.4$), however, the trend was not statistically significant. This is a small study that lacked power to show a significant difference (Hong et al. 2003).

The classic teaching of a progressive disease that ultimately results in perforation has been questioned by studies suggesting the possibility of different disease processes for perforated and non-perforated appendicitis, with resolution of symptoms without surgery in some cases (Andersson et al. 1994). These theories question the ability of better patient management to decrease perforation rates and affect outcome and healthcare costs. However, several studies show that using standardized protocols to evaluate patients presenting with acute abdominal pain, limiting imaging to equivocal cases and older patients, can decrease time to surgery (Torbati and Guss 2003), negative appendectomy rates (Naoum et al. 2002; Antevil et al. 2006), and perforation rates (Peña et al. 2002).

In summary, delays between symptoms onset and treatment have been associated with higher perforation rates and increased morbidity and mortality in multiple studies. While patient delays are clearly associated with higher perforation rates, the reports on system delays and perforation are conflicting. With the standard use of antibiotics, the need for urgent surgery in night hours has been questioned. Several studies examining this question, although retrospective and somewhat underpowered, have reached the conclusion that delaying surgery to regular working hours does not negatively impact the outcome of these patients. The possibility of a different disease process for perforated versus non-perforated appendicitis questions the importance of time. However, in the absence of definitive, validated clinical prediction rules, it remains prudent to treat appendicitis in a timely fashion as perforation clearly causes worse morbidity and mortality. Whether treatment must always be surgical or in some cases can safely be treated medically is a question demanding an answer.

References

Andersson R, Hugander A, Thulin A et al (1994) Indications for operation in suspected appendicitis and incidence of perforation. BMJ 308:107–110

Antevil JL, Rivera L, Langenberg BJ et al (2006) Computed tomography-based clinical diagnostic pathway for acute appendicitis: prospective validation. J Am Coll Surg 203: 849–856

Applegate KE, Sivit CJ, Salvator AE et al (2001) Effect of cross-sectional imaging on negative appendectomy and perforation rates in children. Radiology 220:103–107

Ascheim DD, Gelijns AC, Rose EA (2009) Innovation with experience using implantable left ventricular assist devices. Circ Heart Fail 2:1–2

Augustin T, Bhende S, Chavda K et al (2009) CT scans and acute appendicitis: a five-year analysis from a rural teaching hospital. J Gastrointest Surg 13:1306–1312

Bendeck SE, Nino-Murcia M, Berry GJ, Jeffrey RB Jr (2002) Imaging for suspected appendicitis: negative appendectomy and perforation rates. Radiology 225:131–136

Berry J Jr, Malt RA (1984) Appendicitis near its centenary. Ann Surg 200:567–575

Bickell NA, Siu AL (2001) Why do delays in treatment occur? Lessons learned from ruptured appendicitis. Health Serv Res 36:1–5

Bickell NA, Rojas M, Anderson RM, Chatterjee S, Leventhal H (2004) What takes so long for my patient to get treated? JGIM 19(1):217

Bickell NA, Aufses AH Jr, Rojas M, Bodian C (2006) How time affects the risk of rupture in appendicitis. J Am Coll Surg 202:401–406

Bratton SL, Haberkern CM, Waldhausen JH (2000) Acute appendicitis risks of complications: age and medicaid insurance. Pediatrics 106:75–78

Braveman P, Schaaf VM, Egerter S et al (1994) Insurance-related differences in the risk of ruptured appendix. N Engl J Med 331:444–449

Brender JD, Marcuse EK, Koepsell TD, Hatch EI (1985) Childhood appendicitis: factors associated with perforation. Pediatrics 76:301–306

Cacioppo JC, Diettrich NA, Kaplan G, Nora PF (1989) The consequences of current constraints on surgical treatment of appendicitis. Am J Surg 157:276–281

Cappendijk VC, Hazebroek FW (2000) The impact of diagnostic delay on the course of acute appendicitis. Arch Dis Child 83:64–66

Deng Y, Chang DC, Zhang Y et al (2010) Seasonal and day of the week variations of perforated appendicitis in US children. Pediatr Surg Int 26:691–696

Ditillo MF, Dziura JD, Rabinovici R (2006) Is it safe to delay appendectomy in adults with acute appendicitis? Ann Surg 244:656–660

Eldar S, Nash E, Sabo E et al (1997) Delay of surgery in acute appendicitis. Am J Surg 173:194–198

Flum DR, Morris A, Koepsell T, Dellinger EP (2001) Has misdiagnosis of appendicitis decreased over time? A population-based analysis. JAMA 286:1748–1753

Gadomski A, Jenkins P (2001) Ruptured appendicitis among children as an indicator of access to care. Health Serv Res 36:129–142

Groetsch SM, Shaughnessy JM (2001) Medical management of acute appendicitis: a case report. J Am Board Fam Pract 14:225–226

Hong JJ, Cohn SM, Ekeh AP et al (2003) A prospective randomized study of clinical assessment versus computed tomography for the diagnosis of acute appendicitis. Surg Infect (Larchmt) 4:231–239

Hunter JG (2010) Letting weary surgeons sleep and saving money. Arch Surg 145:892

Ingraham AM, Cohen ME, Bilimoria KY et al (2010) Effect of delay to operation on outcomes in adults with acute appendicitis. Arch Surg 145:886–892

Jones PF (2001) Suspected acute appendicitis: trends in management over 30 years. Br J Surg 88:1570–1577

Kasl SV (1975) Social-psychological characteristics associate with behaviors which reduce cardiovascular risk. Applying behavioral science to cardiovascular risk: proceedings of a conference (Edited by Enelow AJ and Henderson JB. Seattle, WA. American Heart Association, Dallas (TX), 173–190

Kirscht JP (1974) The health belief model and illness behavior. Health Educ Monogr 2:387–408

Körner H, Söndenaa K, Söreide JA et al (1997) Incidence of acute nonperforated and perforated appendicitis: age-specific and sex-specific analysis. World J Surg 21:313–317

Körner H, Söndenaa K, Söreide JA (2001) Perforated and non-perforated acute appendicitis–one disease or two entities? Eur J Surg 167:525–530

Kraemer M, Kremer K, Leppert R et al (1999) Perforating appendicitis: is it a separate disease? Acute abdominal pain study group. Eur J Surg 165:473–480

Lee SL, Walsh AJ, Ho HS (2001) Computed tomography and ultrasonography do not improve and may delay the diagnosis and treatment of acute appendicitis. Arch Surg 136:556–562

Linz DN, Hrabovsky EE, Franceschi D, Gauderer MW (1993) Does the current health care environment contribute to increased morbidity and mortality of acute appendicitis in children? J Pediatr Surg 28:321–326

Livingston EH, Woodward WA, Sarosi GA, Haley RW (2007) Disconnect between incidence of nonperforated and perforated appendicitis: implications for pathophysiology and management. Ann Surg 245:886–892

Luckmann R (1989) Incidence and case fatality rates for acute appendicitis in California. A population-based study of the effects of age. Am J Epidemiol 129:905–918

Mason RJ (2008) Surgery for appendicitis: is it necessary? Surg Infect (Larchmt) 9:481–488

Mathis RD, Chiumento AB, Yeh B, Dollieslager N (2005) An outcome study of the use of computed tomography for the diagnosis of appendicitis in a community-based emergency department. South Med J 98:1169–1172

McDonald GP, Pendarvis DP, Wilmoth R, Daley BJ (2001) Influence of preoperative computed tomography on patients undergoing appendectomy. Am Surg 67:1017–1021

McLean AD, Stonebridge PA, Bradbury AW et al (1993) Time of presentation, time of operation, and unnecessary appendicectomy. BMJ 306:307
Menes TS, Aufses AH Jr, Rojas M, Bickell NA (2006) Increased use of computed tomography does not harm patients with acute appendicitis. Am Surg 72:326–329
Musunuru S, Chen H, Rikkers LF, Weber SM (2007) Computed tomography in the diagnosis of acute appendicitis: definitive or detrimental? J Gastrointest Surg 11:1417–1421
Naoum JJ, Mileski WJ, Daller JA et al (2002) The use of abdominal computed tomography scan decreases the frequency of misdiagnosis in cases of suspected appendicitis. Am J Surg 184:587–589
Omundsen M, Dennett E (2006) Delay to appendicectomy and associated morbidity: a retrospective review. ANZ J Surg 76:153–155
Peña BM, Taylor GA, Fishman SJ, Mandl KD (2002) Effect of an imaging protocol on clinical outcomes among pediatric patients with appendicitis. Pediatrics 110:1088–1093
Perez J, Barone JE, Wilbanks TO et al (2003) Liberal use of computed tomography scanning does not improve diagnostic accuracy in appendicitis. Am J Surg 185:194–197
Pittman-Waller VA, Myers JG, Stewart RM et al (2000) Appendicitis: why so complicated? Analysis of 5755 consecutive appendectomies. Am Surg 66:548–554
Redmond JM, Smith GW, Wilasrusmee C, Kittur DS (2002) A new perspective in appendicitis: calculation of half time (T (1/2)) for perforation. Am Surg 68:593–597
Riesenman PJ, Riesenman KP, Stone TJ et al (2008) Nonfocused enhanced CT evaluation of acute appendicitis increases length of stay in the emergency department but does not increase perforation rate. Am Surg 74:488–492
Rosenstock IM (1966) Why people use health services. Millbank Mem Fund Q 44:94–127
Rosenstock IM (1974) Historical origins of the health belief model. Health Educ Monogr 2:328–335
Safer MA, Tharps QJ, Jackson TC, Leventhal H (1979) Determinants of three stages of delay in seeking care at a medical clinic. Med Care 17:11–29
Savrin RA, Clatworthy HW Jr (1979) Appendiceal rupture: a continuing diagnostic problem. Pediatrics 63:36–43
SCOAP Collaborative, Cuschieri J, Florence M, Flum DR et al (2008) Negative appendectomy and imaging accuracy in the Washington state surgical care and outcomes assessment program. Ann Surg 248:557–563
Sicard N, Tousignant P, Pineault R, Dubé S (2007) Non-patient factors related to rates of ruptured appendicitis. Br J Surg 94:214–221
Surana R, Quinn F, Puri P (1993) Is it necessary to perform appendicectomy in the middle of the night in children? BMJ 306:1168
Temple CL, Huchcroft SA, Temple WJ (1995) The natural history of appendicitis in adults. A prospective study. Ann Surg 221:278–281
Ting HH, Bradley EH, Wang Y et al (2008) Delay in presentation and reperfusion therapy in ST-elevation myocardial infarction. Am J Med 121:316–323
Torbati SS, Guss DA (2003) Impact of helical computed tomography on the outcomes of emergency department patients with suspected appendicitis. Acad Emerg Med 10:823–829
van Breda Vriesman AC, Kole BJ, Puylaert JB (2003) Effect of ultrasonography and optional computed tomography on the outcome of appendectomy. Eur Radiol 13:2278–2282
Von Titte S, McCabe CJ, Ottinger LW (1996) Delayed appendectomy for appendicitis: causes and consequences. Am J Emerg Med 14:620–622
Walker SJ, West CR, Colmer MR (1995) Acute appendicitis: does removal of a normal appendix matter, what is the value of diagnostic accuracy and is surgical delay important? Ann R Coll Surg Engl 77:358–363
Webb S, Holman D (1992) A survey of infertility, surgical sterility and associated reproductive disability in Perth, Western Australia. Aust J Public Health 16:376–381
Weyant MJ, Eachempati SR, Maluccio MA et al (2001) The use of computed tomography for the diagnosis of acute appendicitis in children does not influence the overall rate of negative appendectomy or perforation. Surg Infect (Larchmt) 2:19–23
Wong KK, Cheung TW, Tam PK (2008) Diagnosing acute appendicitis: are we overusing radiologic investigations? J Pediatr Surg 43:2239–2241
Yaghoubian A, de Virgilio C, Chiu V, Lee SL (2010) "July effect" and appendicitis. J Surg Educ 67:157–160
Yardeni D, Hirschl RB, Drongowski RA et al (2004) Delayed versus immediate surgery in acute appendicitis: do we need to operate during the night? J Pediatr Surg 39:464–469

Negative Appendectomy Rate and Implications of Removing a Normal Appendix

Wim T. van den Broek

Contents

Abstract

New diagnostic tools are used to lower the negative appendectomy rate. The human appendix can be safely removed because it has lost its function of cellulose digestion as found in the herbivorous cecum of our primate ancestors. A negative appendectomy should be avoided though because the removal of a normal appendix is accompanied with considerable morbidity and costs. Further diagnostic tools are, therefore, needed if on clinical grounds there is doubt about the diagnosis appendicitis. There is much debate about what to do with a normal appendix found during diagnostic laparoscopy. Because in the large clinical studies false-negative laparoscopies are rare, it is safe to leave a normal appendix in place to avoid added morbidity and costs associated with the removal of normal appendix. Symptoms mimicking appendicitis are probably due to self-limiting diseases. Care should be taken to not miss a diagnosis that needs further therapy such as carcinoid tumors which appear in 0.5% of the non-inflamed appendices. During long-term follow the chance of developing appendicitis appears to be no higher than in a normal population. So there can be no rational reason for a "prophylactic appendectomy".

1 Introduction

Many diagnostic tools have been introduced for patients with suspected acute appendicitis, in an attempt to lower the negative appendectomy rate.

W. T. van den Broek (✉)
Department of Surgery, Sint Anna Hospital,
P.O. Box 90, 5660 AB Geldrop, The Netherlands
e-mail: w.vd.broek@st-anna.nl

C. Keyzer and P. A. Gevenois (eds.), *Imaging of Acute Appendicitis in Adults and Children*,
Medical Radiology. Diagnostic Imaging, DOI: 10.1007/174_2011_213,

However, these diagnostic tools can be time consuming, expensive, expose patients to radiation or are even invasive procedures with their own morbidity. Therefore, we should consider whether it is worthwhile to lower the negative appendectomy rate and to what expense it should be attempted.

To answer these questions we should verify what are the costs and morbidity of these diagnostic procedures and weigh them against the morbidity and costs of performing a negative appendectomy. We should also consider that performing fewer appendectomies must not lead to more perforated appendectomies. We also have to define a normal appendix. Is it an appendix with no histological signs of inflammation or is it just an appendix, which causes no clinical signs? But first we should consider the possible function of the appendix and whether it is safe to remove the appendix or is it worthwhile to spare this organ?

2 Can We Remove a Normal Appendix or Should We Try to Preserve it?

In humans, the vermiform appendix is derived from the cecal diverticulum, which is formed in the sixth week after conception. It appears on the antimesenteric border of the caudal limb of the midgut loop as a conical pouch. The apex of this blind sac does not grow rapidly and forms the appendix. When the proximal part of the colon elongates, the cecum and appendix are displaced downward into the right iliac fossa. During this process, the appendix may pass posterior to the cecum (retrocecal), or it may descend over the brim of the pelvis (pelvic location). The appendix is located retrocecally in about 64% of the people, is longest in childhood and gradually shrinks throughout adult life (Moore 1982).

In most vertebrates, the cecum is a large, complex gastrointestinal organ, enriched in mucosal lymphatic tissue and specialized in digestion of plants (Kardong 2002). The cecum in herbivores is much larger than in humans. The human appendix is a derivative of the end of the more primitive herbivorous cecum found in our primate ancestors (Goodman et al. 1998; Shoshani et al. 1996). A few other mammals appear to have a structure similar to the human vermiform appendix, including the wombat, South American opossum (both marsupials), some rodents, and the rabbit. However, extensive comparative analyses have shown that the cecal appendixes of humans and these other mammals were derived from the cecum independently. So these structures are not homologous as appendixes and may have other functions (Shoshani and McKenna 1998). Originally, the appendix was specifically adapted for housing bacteria and extending the time course of digestion. The human appendix has lost this previously essential function, namely cellulose digestion. Even though humans eat cellulose, the contribution to cellulose digestion by both the human cecum and its associated appendix is negligible. Therefore, during primate evolution it has decreased in size to a mere rudiment (Douglas 2007).

So, the appendix does not have an essential function in humans anymore and can, therefore, be safely removed as over a century of medical evidence has firmly shown that the removal of the human appendix does not lead to any obvious ill effects, apart from surgical complications.

Recent studies even show that the removal of an appendix might protect against the development of ulcerative colitis and reduces its recurrence (Naganuma et al. 2001; Sandler 1998; Russel et al. 1997). It appears that appendectomy is three to five times more common in the groups without than in those with ulcerative colitis. Whereas studies investigating an association between ulcerative colitis and other operations such as tonsillectomy and cholecystectomy have found no relation between these interventions and the development of ulcerative colitis. The investigators speculated that antigen-processing lymphoid tissue in the appendix might mediate disease that is related to enteric bacteria.

In conclusion, there are no advantages in sparing the appendix because it has lost its function of cellulose digestion as found in the herbivorous cecum of our primate ancestors. Though, complications and costs due to the unnecessary appendectomy should be taken into account. A possible advantage of appendectomy might be the protection against the development of ulcerative colitis.

3 Negative Appendectomy Rates and Diagnostic Accuracy

Acute appendicitis is a common disease which occurs for 8.6% in men and for 6.7% in women (Addis et al. 1990). Because other diseases such as gynecological conditions, mesenteric lymfadenopathy and gastroenteritis can mimic the signs of acute appendicitis, its diagnosis remains difficult. A false positive diagnosis will lead to an unnecessary appendectomy and a false negative diagnosis may lead to a delayed operation, which could cause a perforation of the appendix in the delayed time to operation. The old school adagio "When in doubt, cut it out", where the diagnosis of acute appendicitis was based on clinical findings only, leads to 15–30 percent negative appendectomies (Pieper and Kager 1982; Anderson et al. 1992). It is considered that these patients with right lower abdominal pain undergo an unnecessary operation with all the accompanied costs, morbidity and even mortality. Strangely though, most patients recover well after a negative appendectomy and are relieved of their symptoms mimicking appendicitis.

Today, ultrasound, (helical) CT-scan and diagnostic laparoscopy are used in patients with suspected acute appendicitis.

Ultrasound (US) is an examination, which has been used in the diagnosis of acute appendicitis, since 1981. The advantages are the lack of ionizing radiation, relatively low costs, widespread availability and the ability to identify many alternative causes of acute right lower quadrant pain as ovarian cysts and urethral stone disease (Anderson et al. 1992; Rao and Boland 1998). Sensitivity rates vary from 0.75 to 0.90, specificity rates vary from 0.73 to 1 and accuracy rates vary from 0.76 to 0.96 (Wilson and SR 2000; Puylaert et al. 1987; Schwerk et al. 1990; Siegel et al. 1991; Wade et al. 1993; John et al. 1993; Ramachandran et al. 1996; Zielke et al. 1998; Lessin et al. 1999). It is reported that negative appendectomy rates are reduced from 28 to 8% by using ultrasound on a selective group of patients with suspected appendicitis (Bendeck et al. 2002; Puig et al. 2003). One should realize that the above-mentioned results are obtained by ultrasound dedicated radiologists. It remains doubtful if these rates can also be obtained in less specialized centers because the accuracy of US is thought to be observer dependent. The relatively low sensitivity rates of US indicate that US is not useful in ruling out appendicitis and can lead to an unacceptable delay in operation as reported in 11.3% of the patients (Verroken et al. 1996).

The first appendicitis seen on Computed Tomography (CT) scan was reported by Balthazar et al. (1986). The advantage of CT-scan is that high sensitivity (0.87–1), specificity (0.83–1) and accuracy (0.90–0.94) rates can be obtained (Balthazar et al. 1991; Malone et al. 1993; Rao et al. 1997; Lane et al. 1996; Schuler et al. 1998; Stroman et al. 1999; Kamel et al. 2000; Sivit et al. 2000). CT-scan is, therefore, useful in both ruling out and in diagnosing appendicitis and so preventing unnecessary appendectomies and also preventing patients from further delay in surgery. Increasing the use of CT-scan on patients with suspected appendicitis lowered the negative appendectomy rate from 20 to 3% in a recent study and prevented further delay in the treatment of appendicitis from 7.8 to 3.0%, reducing the complication rate from 33.3 to 21.3% in another study and is confirmed by others (Rhea et al. 2005; Frei et al. 2008; Kim et al. 2008). The impact of imaging on negative appendectomy rate will be further discussed in "Impact of Imaging on Negative Appendectomy Rate" by CA Coursey. The disadvantages of CT scan are the possible unavailability on a 24 hour base, the exposure to radiation (especially in fertile women) and allergic reactions and renal function disorders due to IV contrast material.

Diagnostic laparoscopy has been used for many years by gynecologists in women with acute and chronic abdominal pain (Semm and Mettler 1980). Since, the interest of general surgeons for laparoscopic surgery, diagnostic laparoscopy is also being used for suspected acute appendicitis. The excellent overview of the peritoneal cavity gives both information of the appendix as well as of other organs, in particular the internal genital organs in women. In case of acute appendicitis, one can proceed with laparoscopic appendectomy. Diagnostic laparoscopy offers also the possibility of leaving the normal appearing appendix in place. Nevertheless, diagnostic laparoscopy is an invasive procedure, which requires general anesthesia and usually hospital admission with additional costs and added morbidity. Specificity rates of diagnostic laparoscopy range from 0.73 to 1, achieving negative appendectomy rates from 0 to 13% (Kum et al. 1993; Jadallah et al. 1994; Borgstein et al. 1997; Tijtgat et al. 1998; Moberg et al. 1998; Barrat et al. 1999; Van den Broek et al. 2000). The reasons for the relative high negative appendectomy rates in some studies could be the difference in patient selection, no visualization of the appendix, failure of laparoscopic instruments and doubt or misinterpretation of the diagnosis appendicitis. In these studies no patient developed signs of appendicitis in the direct post-operative period: the sensitivity was, therefore, one (Kum et al. 1993; Jadallah et al. 1994; Borgstein et al. 1997; Tijtgat et al. 1998; Moberg et al. 1998; Barrat et al. 1999; Van den Broek et al. 2000; Ure et al. 2000; Thorell et al. 1999; Olsen et al. 1993; Mutter et al. 1996, 1998; Connor et al. 1995; Moberg and Montgomery 2000; Teh et al. 2000; Van den Broek et al. 2001). Complication rates varied from 0 to 2% and include pulmonary embolism, ileus, wound infections, lung complications and bleedings from trocart ports. No injuries due to introduction of the Veress needle were reported.

4 Lowering the Negative Appendectomy Rate, at What Cost?

To justify the use of these diagnostic tools, we should establish the cost and morbidity of removing a normal appendix and weight this against the costs and morbidity of these tools. The implications of removing a normal appendix was investigated in a Dutch study in 2003 (Bijnen et al. 2003). In 276 patients a normal appendix was removed by an open or laparoscopic procedure. The mean hospital stay was 4.4 days. Complications due to the unnecessary operation as wound infections, abscesses, ileus, hemorrhage and urine retention occurred in 6% of the patients and in 2% of the patients a re-operation was needed. This high complication rate is confirmed by others (Gough et al. 1983). Comparing these results to the patients in the same study who underwent a diagnostic laparoscopy without removing the normal appearing appendix shows that in these patients the mean hospital stay was only 2 days, the complication rate was 0.3% and the re-operation rate was 0%. No patients developed acute appendicitis in the direct post-operative period so there were no false negative patients. Thus the unnecessary removal of a normal appendix has considerable added morbidity and justifies the means of diagnostic tools to prevent this. Because morbidity rates of a diagnostic laparoscopy alone are much lower and there are no false negative patients reported, it is worthwhile to leave the normal appearing appendix in place during diagnostic laparoscopy.

Table 1 Hospital costs in 2003 of different procedures or interventions

Visit emergency ward:	€ 29
Consultation surgeon or resident:	€ 14
Routine laboratory examination:	€ 14
Ultrasound:	€ 63
CT-scan:	€ 88
Operation room costs diagnostic laparoscopy:	€ 267
Surgeon fee diagnostic laparoscopy:	€ 47
Anaesthesiologist fee diagnostic laparoscopy:	€ 30
One day admission:	€ 469
Operation room costs appendectomy:	€ 363
Surgeon fee appendectomy:	€ 163
Anaesthesiologist fee appendectomy:	€ 54
Extra costs laparoscopic appendectomy:	
Three Endoloop © EJ 10C:	€ 93
Endocatch©:	€ 108
Outpatient clinic control:	€ 44
Histopathologic examination:	€ 24

Costs in 2003 in Euro's, source (Bijnen et al. 2003)

But we should also consider the costs accompanying these diagnostic tools. Hospital costs in 2003 of different procedures or interventions derived from the 2003 Dutch study are shown in Table 1 (Bijnen et al. 2003). Apparently the removal of a normal appendix will cost € 2,712. According to the Dutch network and national database for Pathology (PALGA), 2,285 negative appendectomies are performed yearly in The Netherlands. Thus the negative appendectomies will cost the Dutch society € 6,196,920 per year. The economic loss due to sick leave after hospital discharge is more difficult to calculate but should be added to this amount.

So there are at least two important reasons to try to lower the number of negative appendectomies, namely preventing complications and reducing costs.

One way to reduce the percentage of negative appendectomies is to first observe all patients in whom the diagnosis is "not clinically evident" (Jones 2001a). This, however, could lead to delay in the diagnosis and treatment of acute appendicitis. Another solution could be the use of extra diagnostic tools. The cost-efficiency of the routine use of such diagnostic procedures depends upon their sensitivity, specificity and costs. For example, if we aim for budget neutrality and calculate € 2,712 as additional costs for the removal of a normal appendix, a maximum of 2712/63 (43) ultrasounds, 2712/88 (31) CT-scans or 2712/1282 (2) diagnostic laparoscopies could be used in order to prevent one negative appendectomy (Bijnen et al. 2003). These are of course theoretical estimates, as many other factors such as the potential consequences of a perforation due to delayed operation are not taken into account. It illustrates, however, that especially if one uses diagnostic laparoscopy without removing the appendix laparoscopically, the cost-efficiency could greatly gain by a selective application to a subset of patients in which the diagnosis is not clinically evident. Routine CT-scan for patients with suspected appendicitis though improves patient care and reduces the use of hospital resources and total costs in another study (Rao et al. 1998). It remains questionable, however, if it is justified to routinely impose a large group of women in the childbearing age to a radiation. The majority of negative appendectomies are performed in women of 15–50 years. This reflects the differential diagnostic difficulty in fertile women. For this reason, others advise to routinely perform a diagnostic laparoscopy in women of the childbearing age with suspected acute appendicitis but in men its use is not recommended (Borgstein et al. 1997; Mutter et al. 1996). However, a considerable number of normal appendices are also removed in pre-menarche children and in men. Also in these latter subsets the diagnosis is apparently not always obvious. The feasibility of identifying such subsets other than based on gender is demonstrated in other studies using scoring systems (van den Broek et al. 2002).

In the ideal situation, diagnostic tools should lower the negative appendectomy rate without increasing the delayed appendectomy rate. Considering the above aspects of our today's diagnostic tools I would recommend the following strategy for patients with suspected acute appendicitis. If on clinical grounds there is doubt about the diagnosis in a patient with right lower abdominal pain we should proceed with further diagnostic tools. When a skilled radiologist is available, ultrasound is the investigation of first choice because it is relatively cheap, non-invasive and not using ionizing radiation. If an inflamed appendix is found, one should proceed with appendectomy but if acute appendicitis could not be confirmed, one should continue with further investigations or careful observation. Helical CT-scan and diagnostic laparoscopy should be considered. When available, helical CT-scan can be performed for either ruling out or confirming acute appendicitis. The negative effects of the ionizing radiation of the CT-scan should be weighed against the negative effects of diagnostic laparoscopy, which is relatively expensive, invasive and needs hospital admission. Especially in fertile women, diagnostic laparoscopy is of value because gynecological disorders, mimicking acute appendicitis, can be recognized easily.

5 The Normal Appendix and What to Do with it?

Performing a diagnostic laparoscopy for suspected acute appendicitis confronts the surgeon with a dilemma. In the "open" era, the normal looking appendix found during exploration has been removed routinely because the presence of the typical scar in the right lower abdominal quadrant might cause confusion about the diagnosis in the future. Nowadays, diagnostic laparoscopy leaves us the opportunity for leaving the normal appearing appendix in place. Although, not removing an organ and just establishing a diagnosis is not a natural thing to do for a surgeon, this strategy might have advantages, considering the accompanied morbidity of removing a normal appendix, as mentioned before. During laparoscopy a normal appendix can be easily identified as a white, non-swollen, flexible appendix, whereas, the inflamed appendix is red, covered with fibrin, swollen and not flexible (Figs. 1 and 2). Also fluids or pus might be present in the abdominal cavity as signs of perforation. Other diagnoses as a Meckel's diverticulum, ovarian cysts, salpingitis, extra uterine gravidity or Crohn's disease are also easily established.

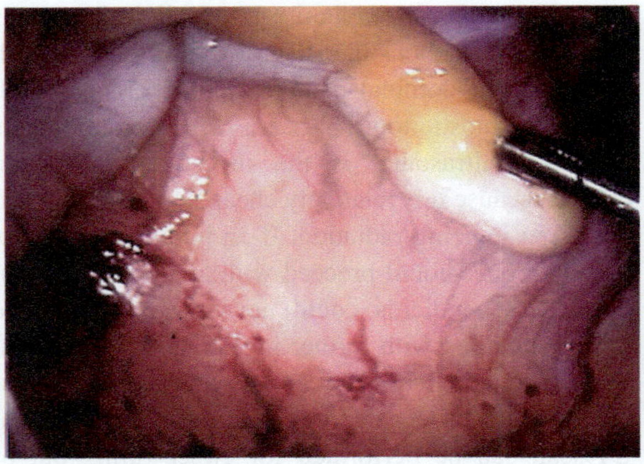

Fig. 1 A normal appendix seen by laparoscopy

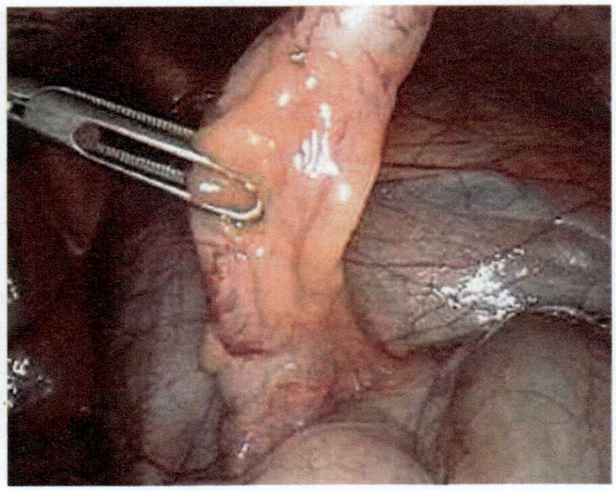

Fig. 2 An inflamed appendix seen by laparoscopy

As in daily life though, the definition of normal might not be that easy. Some surgeons advocate leaving the normal appearing appendix in place for the above mentioned benefits as others stress that the macroscopic normal appearing appendix should be removed because the surgeon's ability of diagnosing a normal appendix might not be adequate, the normal appendix might contain other diseases as neoplasms or the normal appendix might have neurogenic or other pathological conditions at histological examination that could have caused the patient's symptoms of right lower abdominal pain.

A review article, published in 2000, analyzed 54 studies in which a total of 4,281 laparoscopies were performed resulting in 2,683 (63%) appendectomies. In 1,598 (37%) cases the normal appearing appendix was left in place (Kraemer et al. 2000). There were only nine (0.2%) false negative diagnosis reported which resulted in two re-laparotomies. These re-laparotomies occurred in the period between 1975 and 1979 and it was concluded that it was caused by the relative lack of experience of laparoscopy where the top of the appendix was not clearly visualized. The other five false negative appendices were judged as normal during laparoscopy but despite these findings they were still removed. These appendices appeared to be macroscopically normal but showed histological signs of inflammation. Based on these findings it was concluded that it is safe to leave a normal appearing appendix in situ during laparoscopy for suspected acute appendicitis. In another study there were 109 normal appearing appendices left in place (Van den Broek et al. 2001). In 65 (60%) patients there was another diagnosis obtained during laparoscopy and in the remaining 44 (40%) patients no other diagnosis was found explaining the right lower quadrant abdominal pain. There were no false negative patients in the direct postoperative period but at a latter point in time eight patients underwent an appendectomy where in only one patient a histological inflamed appendix was removed. After a median follow up period of 4.4 years, nine patients still complained of recurrent pain in the right lower abdominal quadrant. There were no differences between patients in which another diagnosis was obtained and patients where no other diagnosis was found during laparoscopy. Also in this study it was concluded that is safe to leave a normal appendix in situ. These results are confirmed in another study where in 21 children the normal appendix was left in place (Dingemann et al. 2009). There were no false negative diagnosis and only one child had still recurrent abdominal pain during follow up but refused further diagnostic procedures or interventions.

On the other hand, others claim that a normal appearing appendix might not be normal at histological examination and should, therefore, not be left in place. In a retrospective study of 7,767 patients who underwent appendectomy for suspected acute appendicitis there were 37 (0.5%) carcinoid tumors found in normal appearing appendices during operation (Shapiro et al. 2010). When a strategy of leaving the normal appendix in place was performed there would be a delay in the diagnosis of a malignant disease. Also, a clinical entity as Neurogenic Appendicopathy has been suggested by others, based on the histological findings in 282 appendices where, based on hematoxylin-eosin staining, in 3,8% of the patients with acute appendicitis and in 47% of the patients with a normal appearing appendix the diagnosis neurogenic appendicopathy was established. The clinical importance of these findings was not reported (Franke et al. 2002). It is also shown that TNFα and IL-2 mRNA expression, as markers of inflammation of an appendix, are elevated in normally judged appendices (Wang et al. 1996). The clinical importance of these findings remains also unclear.

The reliability of the surgeon in establishing the correct diagnosis during operation has also been discussed. In a study of 1,225 appendices, which were removed, for suspected acute appendicitis there were 46 (3.8%) abnormal diagnosis revealed. In only two (two carcinoid tumors) these were recognized during operation (Jones et al. 2007). In 24 patients the abnormal diagnosis was clinically significant and consisted of adenocarcinoma's, carcinoid tumors, cystadenoma's, Crohn's disease and parasite infections. The authors concluded that intra-operative detection of abnormal appendices by the surgeon is unreliable and supports the sending of all appendectomy specimens for routine histopathological analysis. Others confirm these pathological findings where in a study of 876 patients 13 neoplastic lesions were not recognized by the surgeon (Roberts et al. 2008). This would imply that a normal appearing appendix judged by the surgeon might contain a clinically relevant diagnosis and should, therefore, not be left in situ.

Because in the large clinical studies false-negative laparoscopies are rare we may conclude that it is safe to leave a normal appendix in place to avoid added morbidity and costs as seen with removal of a normal appendix. Symptoms mimicking acute appendicitis are probably due to self-limiting diseases, such as gastro-enteritis. If an entity as endo-appendicitis or neurogenic appendicopathy exists the clinical importance remains unclear. The endo-appendicitis may be cured by a dose of 500 mg Metronidazole, usually given during the laparoscopy, or does not need further therapy at all.

One should realize though that in some pathological studies the correct diagnosis by the surgeon was not established. Therefore, care should be taken to not miss a diagnosis that needs further therapy such as carcinoid tumors which appear in 0,5% of the non-inflamed appendices. So, "when in doubt, during laparoscopy, take it out", should be the advice. During long-term follow the chance of developing appendicitis appears to be no higher than in a normal population. So there can be no rational reason for a "prophylactic appendectomy".

6 Changing Aspects in Treatment of Acute Appendicitis

In all the above we assume that we should lower the negative appendectomy rate to prevent an unnecessary operation. As acute appendicitis is a potential life-threatening disease we should perform an appendectomy when the diagnosis appendicitis is established. But nowadays, even this logical assumption is question of debate. In a recent study, 369 patients with appendicitis were randomized between appendectomy and treatment with antibiotics. Major complications were threefold higher in patients who had an appendectomy and it was concluded that antibiotic treatment is a safe first-line therapy in unselected patients with acute appendicitis (Hansson et al. 2009). If treatment with antibiotics will be the standard care for patients with acute appendicitis we don't have to worry about negative appendectomy rates anymore. The treatment of acute appendicitis including antibiotic treatment is further discussed in "Laparoscopy and Laparotomy" and "Treatment of Appendiceal Perforation ". The future, and more randomized trials, will provide us the data for optimizing the standard care for patients with suspected acute appendicitis. In the mean time we should lower the negative appendectomy rates by selectively applying our new diagnostic tools.

References

Addis DG, Shaffer N, Fowler BS, Tauxe RV (1990) The epidemiology of appendicitis and appendectomy in the United States. Am J Epidemiol 132:910–925

Anderson RE, Hugander A, Thulin AJ (1992) Diagnostic accuracy and perforation rate inappendicitis: association with age and sex of the patient and with appendectomy rate. Eur J Surg 158:37–41

Balthazar EJ, Megibow AJ, Gordon RB, Naidich DP, Birnbaum BA (1986) CT of appendicitis. Am J Roentgenol 147:705–710

Balthazar EJ, Megibow AJ, Siegel SE, Birnbaum BA (1991) Appendicitis: prospective evaluation with high-resolution CT. Radiology 180:21–24

Barrat C, Catheline J-M, Rizk N, Champault GG (1999) Does laparoscopy reduce the incidence of unnecessary appendectomies? Surg Laparosc Endosc 9:27–31

Bendeck SE, Nino-Murcia M, Berry GJ, Jeffrey RB Jr (2002) Imaging for suspected appendicitis: negative appendectomy and perforation rates. Radiology 225:131–136

Bijnen CL, van den Broek WT, Bijnen AB, de Ruiter P, Gouma DJ (2003) Implications of removing a normal appendix. Dig Surg 20:215–219 discussion 220-1.

Birnbaum BA, Wilson SR (2000) Appendicitis at the millennium. Radiology 215:337–348

Borgstein PJ, Gordijn RV, Eijsbouts QAJ, Cuesta MA (1997) Acute appendicitis: a clear-cut case in men, a guessing game in young women. Surg Endosc 11:923–927

Connor TJ, Garcha IS, Ramshaw BJ, Mitchell W, Wilson JP, Mason EM, Duncan TD, Dozier FA, Lucas GW (1995) Diagnostic laparoscopy for suspected appendicitis. Am Surg 61:187–189

Dingemann J, Metzelder M, Kuebler JF, Ure B (2009) Laparoscopy for suspected appendicitis in children: may a macroscopically normal appendix be left in situ? Eur J Pediatr Surg 19:153–156

Douglas T (2007) The vestigiality of the human vermiform appendix. A modern reappraisal. http://www.talkorigins.org

Franke C, Gerharz CD, Böhner H, Ohmann C, Heydrich G, Krämling HJ, Stock W, Rosen D, Kurpreugsch K, Röher HD (2002) Neurogenic appendicopathy: a clinical disease entity? Int J Colorectal Dis 17:185–191

Frei SP, Bond WF, Bazuro RK, Richardson DM, Sierzega GM, Reed JF (2008) Appendicitis outcomes with increasing computed tomographic scanning. Am J Emerg Med 26:39–44

Goodman M, Porter CA, Czelusniak J, Page SL, Schneider H, Shoshani J, Gunnell G, Groves CP (1998) Toward a phylogenetic classification of Primates based on DNA evidence complemented by fossil evidence. Mol Phylogenet Evol 9:585–598

Gough IR, Morris MI, Pertnikovs EI, Murray MR, Smith MB, Bestmann MS (1983) Consequences of removal of a "normal"appendix. Med J Aus 1:370–372

Hansson J, Körner U, Khorram-Manesh A, Solberg A, Lundholm K (2009) Randomized clinical trial of antibiotic therapy versus appendicectomy as primary treatment of acute appendicitis in unselected patients. Br J Surg 96: 473–481

Jadallah FA, Abdul-Ghani AA, Tibblin S (1994) Diagnostic laparoscopy reduces unnecessary appendicectomy in fertile women. Eur J Surg 160:41–45

John H, Neff U, Kelemen M (1993) Appendicitis diagnosis today: Clinical and ultrasonic deductions. World J Surg 17:243–249

Jones PF (2001) Ultrasonography in diagnosis of acute appendicitis. Active observation is often sufficient to make diagnosis. BMJ 322:615–616

Jones AE, Phillips AW, Jarvis JR, Sargen K (2007) The value of routine histopathological examination of appendicectomy specimens. BMC Surg 7:17

Kamel IR, Goldberg SN, Keogan MT, Rosen MP, Raptopoulos V (2000) Right lower quadrant pain and suspected appendicitis: Nonfocused appendiceal CT-review of 100 cases. Radiology 217:159–163

Kardong KV (2002) Vertebrates: Comparative anatomy, function, evolution, 3rd edn edn. McGraw-Hill, New York, pp 510–515

Kim K, Lee CC, Song KJ, Kim W, Suh G, Singer AJ (2008) The impact of helical computed tomography on the negative appendectomy rate: a multi-center comparison. J Emerg Med 34:3–6

Kraemer M, Ohmann C, Leppert R (2000) Yang Q Macroscopic assessment of the appendix at diagnostic laparoscopy is reliable. Surg Endosc 14:625–633 Review

Kum CK, Sim EKW, Goh PMY, Ngoi SS, Rauff A (1993) Diagnostic laparoscopy: reducing the number of normal appendectomies. Dis Colon Rectum 36:763–766

Lane MJ, Katz DS, Ross BA, Clautice-Engle TL, Mindelzun RE, Jeffrey RB (1996) Unenhanced helical CT for suspected acute appendicitis. Am J Roentgenol 168:405–409

Lessin MS, Chan M, Catallozzi M, Gilchrist BF, Richards C, Manera L, Wallach MT, Luks FI (1999) Selective use of ultrasonography for acute appendicitis in children. Am J Surg 177:193–196

Malone AJ, Wolf CR, Malmed AS, Melliere BF (1993) Diagnosis of acute appendicitis: value of unenhanced CT. Am J Roentgenol 160:763–766

Moberg AC, Montgomery A (2000) Introducing diagnostic laparoscopy for patients with suspected appendicitis. Surg Endosc 14:942–947

Moberg AC, Ahlberg G, Leijonmarck CE, Montgomery A, Reiertsen O, Rosseland AR, Stoerksson R (1998) Diagnostic laparoscopy in 1,043 patients with suspected acute appendicitis. Eur J Surg 164:833–840 discussion 841

Moore K (1982) The Developing Human. WB Saunders Company, 3rd edn, ISBN0-7216-6472-5, p 242

Mutter D, Vix M, Bui A, Evrard S, Tassetti V, Breton JF, Marescaux J (1996) Laparoscopy not recommended for routine appendectomy in men: Results of a prospective randomized study. Surgery 120:71–74

Mutter D, Navez B, Gury J-F, Guiot P, Russier Y, Vix M, Marescaux J (1998) Value of microlaparoscopy in the diagnosis of right iliac fossa pain. Am J Surg 176:370–372

Naganuma M, Iizuka B, Torii A, Ogihara T, Kawamura Y, Ichinose M, Kojima Y, Hibi T (2001) Tokyo G Club. Appendectomy protects against the development of ulcerative colitis and reduces its recurrence: results of a multicenter case-controlled study in Japan. Am J Gastroenterol 96:1123–1126

Olsen JB, Myren CJ, Haahr PE (1993) Randomized study of the value of laparoscopy before appendicectomy. Br J Surg 80:922–923

Pieper R, Kager L (1982) The incidence of acute appendicitis and appendectomy: an epidemiologic study of 971 cases. Acta Chirurgica Scandinavia 148:45–49

Puig S, Hörmann M, Rebhandl W, Felder-Puig R, Prokop M, Paya K (2003) US as a primary diagnostic tool in relation to negative appendectomy: six years experience. Radiology 226(1):101–104

Puylaert BCM, Rutgers PH, Lalisang RI, De Vries BC, Van der Werf SDJ, Dörr JPJ, Blok RAPR (1987) A prospective study of ultrasonography in the diagnosis of appendicitis. N Eng J Med 317:666–669

Ramachandran P, Sivit CJ, Newman KD, Schwartz MZ (1996) Ultrasonography as an adjunct in the diagnosis of acute appendicitis: a 4 year experience. J Pediatr Surg 31:164–167
Rao PM, Boland GW (1998) Imaging of acute right lower abdominal quadrant pain. Clin Radiol 53:639–649
Rao PM, Rhea JT, Novelline RA, McCabe CJ, Lawrason JN, Berger DL, Sackroff R (1997) Helical CT technique for the diagnosis of appendicitis: prospective evaluation of a focused appendix CT examination. Radiology 202:139–144
Rao PM, Rhea JT, Novelline RA, Mostafavi AA, McCabe CL (1998) Effect of computed tomography of the appendix on treatment of patients and use of hospital resources. N Eng J Med 338:141–146
Rhea JT, Halpern EF, Ptak T, Lawrason JN, Sacknoff R, Novelline RA (2005) The status of appendiceal CT in an urban medical center 5 years after its introduction: experience with 753 patients. Am J Roentgenol 184:1802–1808
Roberts JK, Behravesh M, Dmitrewski J (2008) Macroscopic findings at appendicectomy are unreliable: implications for laparoscopy and malignant conditions of the appendix. Int J Surg Pathol 16:386–390
Russel MG, Dorant E, Brummer RJ, van de Kruijs MA, Muris JW, Bergers JM, Goedhard J, Stockbrügger RW (1997) Appendectomy and the risk of developing ulcerative colitis or Crohn's disease: Results of a large case-control study. South limburg inflammatory bowel disease study group. Gastroenterology 113:377–382
Sandler RS (1998) Appendicectomy and ulcerative colitis. Lancet 352:1797–1798
Schuler JG, Shortsleeve MJ, Goldenson RS, Perez-Rossello JM, Perlmutter RA, Thorsen A (1998) Is there a role for abdominal computed tomographic scans in appendicitis? Arch Surg 133:373–377
Schwerk WB, Wichtrup B, Ruschoff J, Rothmund M (1990) Acute and perforated appendicitis: current experience with ultrasound-aided diagnosis. World J Surg 14:271–276
Semm K, Mettler L (1980) Progress in pelvic surgery via operative laparoscopy. Am J Obstet Gynecol 138:121–127
Shapiro R, Eldar S, Sadot E, Venturero M, Papa MZ, Zippel DB (2010) The significance of occult carcinoids in the era of laparoscopic appendectomies. Surg Endosc 24:2197–2199
Shoshani J, McKenna MC (1998) Higher taxonomic relationships among extant mammals based on morphology, with selected comparisons of results from molecular data. Mol Phylogenet Evol 9:572–584
Shoshani J, Groves CP, Simons EL, Gunnell GF (1996) Primate phylogeny: morphological versus molecular results. Mol Phylogenet Evol 5:102–154
Siegel MJ, Carel C, Surratt S (1991) Ultrasonography of acute abdominal pain in children. JAMA 266:1987–1989
Sivit CJ, Dudgeon DL, Applegate KE, Borisa VJ, Berlin SC, Morrison SC, Myers MT, Weinert DM, Stallion A, Grisoni ER (2000) Evaluation of suspected appendicitis in children and young adults: Helical CT. Radiology 216:430–433
Stroman DL, Bayouth CV, Kuhn JA, Westmoreland M, Jones RC, Fisher TL, McCarty TM (1999) The Role of computed tomography in the diagnosis of acute appendicitis. Am J Surg 178:485–489
Teh SH, O'Ceallaigh S, McKeon JGK, Tanner WA, Keane FBV (2000) Should an appendix that looks 'normal' be removed at diagnostic laparoscopy for acute right iliac fossa pain? Eur J Surg 166:388–389
Thorell A, Grondal S, Schedvins K, Wallin G (1999) Value of diagnostic laparoscopy in fertile women with suspected appendicitis. Eur J Surg 165:751–754
Tijtgat SHAJ, Bakker XR, Butzelaar RMJM (1998) Laparoscopic evaluation of patients with suspected appendicitis. Surg Endosc 12:918–920
Ure BM, Bax NMA, Van der Zee DC (2000) Laparoscopy in infants and children: a prospective study on feasibility and the impact on routine surgery. J Pediatr Surg 35:1170–1173
Van den Broek WT, Bijnen AB, Van Eerten PV, De Ruiter P, Gouma DJ (2000) Selective use of diagnostic laparoscopy in patients with suspected appendicitis. Surg Endosc 14: 938–941
Van den Broek WT, Bijnen AB, De Ruiter P, Gouma DJ (2001) A normal appendix found during diagnostic laparoscopy should not be removed. Br J Surg 88:251–255
van den Broek WT, Bijnen BB, Rijbroek B, Gouma DJ (2002) Scoring and diagnostic laparoscopy for suspected appendicitis. Eur J Surg 168:349–354
Verroken R, Penninckx F, Van Hoe L, Geboes K, Kerremans R (1996) Diagnostic accuracy of ultrasonography and surgical decision-making in patients referred for suspicion of appendicitis. Acta Chir Belg 96:158–160
Wade DS, Morrow SE, Balsara ZN, Burkhard TK, Goff WB (1993) Accuracy of Ultrasound in the diagnosis of acute appendicitis compared with the surgeon's clinical impression. Arch Surg 128:1039–1046
Wang Y, Reen DJ, Puri P (1996) A histologically normal appendix following emergency appendicectomy alway normal? Lancet 347:1076–1079
Zielke A, Hasse C, Sitter H, Rothmund M (1998) Influence of ultrasound on clinical decision making in acute appendicitis: a prospective study. Eur J Surg 164:201–209

Laparoscopy and Laparotomy

Ravikrishna Mamidanna and Omar Faiz

Contents

Abstract

The mainstay for management of acute appendicitis is appendicectomy. Apart from clinical judgement, radiological modalities such as ultrasound, computerized tomography (CT) and magnetic resonance imaging (MRI) may aid in the diagnosis of appendicitis. Prior optimization of the patient with analgesia, fluid resuscitation and antibiotics are adjuncts for a smooth recovery. Pre-operative antibiotic prophylaxis is generally considered for all cases and a post-operative course of intravenous/oral antibiotics for cases of complicated appendicitis including those presenting with gangrene or perforation. Peri-operative antibiotic guidelines have been set for paediatric patients. Antibiotic treatment alone may be considered in special circumstances where surgery is either contraindicated or not feasible. Traditional open surgery and minimal invasive surgery such as laparoscopic appendicectomy are currently the procedures of choice. Evidence from randomized trials and meta-analyses suggest some benefits of the laparoscopic approach such as decreased length of stay, earlier recovery and return to work and lower incidence of superficial wound infections. Newer treatment modalities such as Single Incision Laparoscopic Surgery (SILS) and Natural orifice transluminal endoscopic surgery (NOTES) are currently being developed.

R. Mamidanna · O. Faiz (✉)
Department of Surgery and Cancer,
Imperial College, St. Mary's Hospital,
10th floor QEQM building, South Wharf Road,
Paddington, London, W2 1NY, UK
e-mail: o.faiz@imperial.ac.uk

C. Keyzer and P. A. Gevenois (eds.), *Imaging of Acute Appendicitis in Adults and Children*, Medical Radiology. Diagnostic Imaging, DOI: 10.1007/174_2011_214,

1 Introduction

Reginald Fitz first described appendicitis in 1886 (Fitz 1886). Acute appendicitis still remains the most common intra-abdominal surgical emergency. The definitive treatment of acute appendicitis is appendicectomy. The first published report of an appendicectomy was in 1887 by Thomas Morton who diagnosed appendicitis, drained the abscess and removed the appendix (O'Connell 2004). Since, then appendicectomy has come a long way with surgeons describing variations in the type of incision, excision of the appendix from its attachment to the caecum and recently minimally invasive approach to appendicectomy. However, despite numerous randomized trials, prospective studies and case series, there seems to be no universal consensus on the best approach to appendicectomy. Ironically, this is still the most commonly performed emergency surgical procedure.

2 Treatment

2.1 General Treatment

Supportive management is the first step in the management of any acute abdominal condition. If and when the diagnosis of appendicitis has been established efforts should be made to undertake appendicectomy promptly. In the interim, supportive management should be established as follows:

1. Admit the patient and establish intravenous (IV) access
2. Administer intravenous fluid resuscitation, antiemetic therapy and analgesia
3. Monitor observations such as pulse, blood pressure, temperature and urine output as indicated
4. Observe for signs or symptoms of differential diagnoses
5. Inform the anaesthetic team and theatre co-ordinator to prepare for surgery
6. Commence antibiotics once the diagnosis is established
7. Re-assess the clinical situation frequently in order to be able to change priorities at any stage during management.

2.2 Specific Treatment

2.2.1 Appendicectomy

The mainstay of treatment of acute appendicitis is appendicectomy (O'Connell 2004). This is to prevent the morbidity associated with peritonitis where the appendix becomes gangrenous or is perforated. Although appendicectomy is undertaken as an emergency, prior resuscitation of the patient is of vital importance.

2.2.1.1 Open Appendicectomy

Appendicectomy is performed in an operating theatre under general anaesthesia. The patient is consented prior to the anaesthetic. Open appendicectomy remained the gold standard treatment for almost a century (O'Connell 2004). Different incisions have been described (Fig. 1). The McBurney's point is identified, named after Charles McBurney who described the symptoms of appendicitis and demonstrated the point of maximal tenderness (McBurney 1894). This is a point lying on an imaginary line drawn from the umbilicus to the anterior superior iliac spine and divides the line into medial two-thirds and lateral one-thirds. The classical or 'gridiron' incision in centered over the McBurney's point right at angles to the imaginary line mentioned above. This is so called due to its resemblance to a framework of cross beams or 'grid iron'. Following skin and subcutaneous fat incision, the external oblique sheath is incised in line of its fibers and the muscles (internal oblique and transversus abdominis) are split. If required, these muscles are cut along the line of the incision to give better retraction and access to the peritoneal cavity. This is called the Rutherford Morison modification. The most popular incision however is a cosmetic transverse incision described by Otto Lanz (O'Connell 2004). The 'Lanz' incision is a skin crease incision. This is centered on a line joining the mid-point of the right clavicle and the mid-inguinal point on the right side, about 2 cm below the level of the umbilicus. In cases where doubt exists in relation to the diagnosis of appendicitis a lower midline incision can be beneficial providing access to the pelvis with ease of extension if required. A right paramedian incision has been used historically but is now rarely employed. This is due to the fact that a paramedian incision tends to weaken the muscles resulting in atrophy as well as exposing the inferior epigastric vessels to potential injury. Each of the above mentioned incisions has its own benefits and

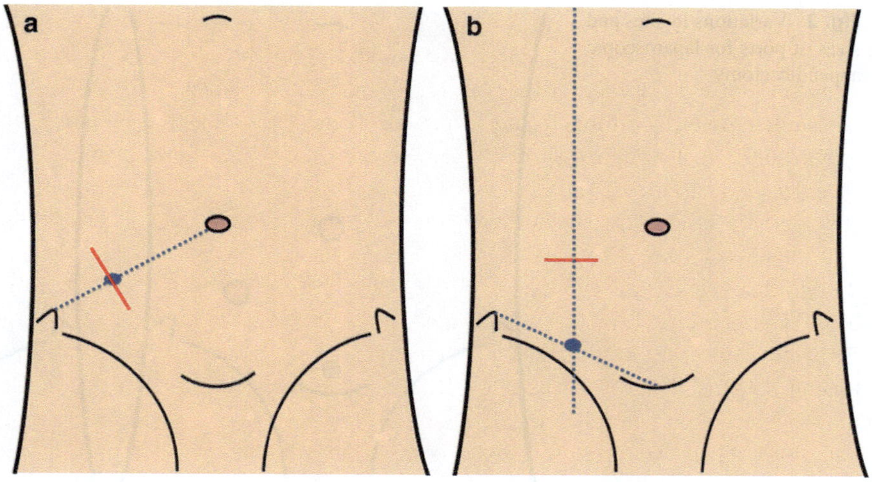

Fig. 1 Incisions described for open approach to appendicectomy **a** Gridiron incision centered on McBurney's point **b** Lanz incision centred on a line from mid-inguinal point to the center of the clavicle, placed about 2 cm below the umbilicus

disadvantages. The gridiron incision provides good access but results in an unsightly scar. The Lanz incision is more cosmetic, however difficulty arises in case of a superiorly lying appendicular base.

Once the peritoneum is opened, the appendix is identified by locating the caecum as the lateral most structure and following the Taenia Coli to the base of the appendix. Although different positions of the appendix have been described such as pelvic, pre-ileal and post-ileal, the appendix can lie in any position as it is fixed only by its base with its free end mobile along the arc. From a surgical point of view, a retro-caecal appendix poses a challenge as it is difficult to approach and dissect the appendix. Once the appendix is identified and freed, the next step is to deliver it through the wound and gain control over the blood supply. The appendicular artery is an end-artery arising from the ileo-colic vessel. The vessel lies in the mesoappendix and is clipped, cut and tied in a stepwise manner through the mesoappendix to the appendix base. It is important to note that the mesoappendix may be thickened in case of severe, or long standing, infection making it friable. The base of the appendix is then crushed and then clamped distal to the crushed area. A ligature is secured at the crushed area and the appendix is separated distally with a sharp knife. Some surgeons prefer to bury the appendicular stump in a purse string suture applied around the junction of the appendix with the caecum (Figs. 3 and 4).

2.2.2 Variations

Caution should be exercised in case of edema of the caecal wall as a purse string suture may cut-through. In case of gangrenous appendicitis the base should not be crushed, but ligated. In case of a perforation at the base of the appendix, sutures should be used to close the caecal defect which should be applied prior to disconnection of the appendix. In presence of severe inflammation with a thickened mesoappendix or if the appendix is retrocaecal, one may undertake a retrograde appendicectomy. Here, a window is created in the mesoappendix at the base of the appendix and the appendix is amputated from the caecum. Then the rest of the appendix is carefully dissected and delivered. In extreme cases, partial caecectomy or even ileocaecal resection may be required.

Once the appendicectomy is completed, the specimen is sent for histological examination. Hemostasis is achieved using diathermy or ligatures. In the presence of pus or contamination of the peritoneal cavity, a peritoneal toilet or wash-out should be undertaken. The peritoneum is closed using a continuous suture, although some surgeons choose not to close it. The muscles are approximated and the external oblique is closed. This is the most important layer for closure. The skin may be closed using interrupted stitches or continuous subcuticular sutures for cosmesis. In the presence of severe infection, one may choose to allow healing by secondary intention and only approximate the skin with interrupted sutures with a gauze wick soaked in antiseptic solution placed between sutures.

2.2.3 Laparoscopic Appendicectomy

Laparoscopic appendicectomy was first described and performed by Semm (1983), a gynaecologist. Since

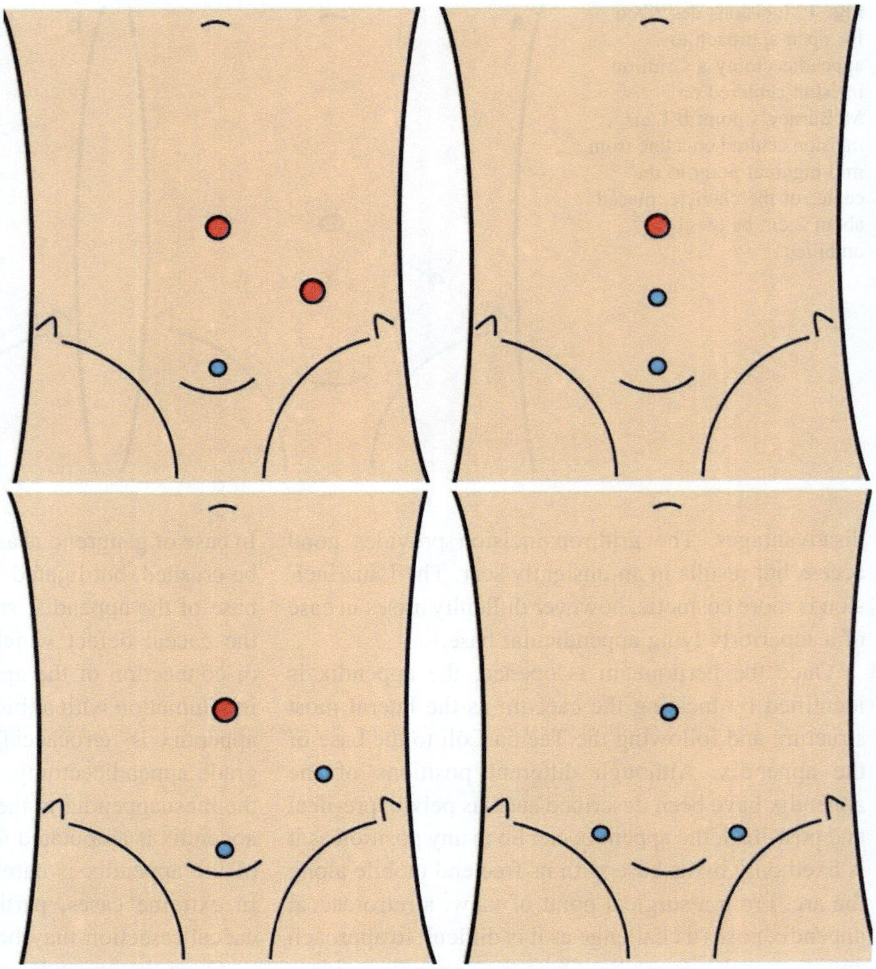

Fig. 2 Variations in sites and sizes of ports for laparoscopic appendicectomy

then, laparoscopic appendicectomy (LA) has been extensively studied and evaluated against the traditional open approach. With the rapid uptake of minimally invasive surgery (MIS) for cholecystectomy and colorectal surgery, there have been significant improvements in the techniques, instruments and expertise of surgeons all over the world. This has made laparoscopic appendicectomy a safe procedure even in the paediatric patient (Faiz et al. 2008a). Laparoscopy is also invaluable as a diagnostic tool, especially in women of reproductive age-group as it enables direct visualization of the uterus, ovaries and fallopian tubes.

The patient is consented for LA with the risk of conversion to open surgery clearly documented and explained to the patient. The procedure is performed under a general anaesthetic with the legs either together or in Lloyd-Davies position. Although different variations in position of ports are described, the surgeon is generally standing to the left of the patient with the assistant to the surgeon's right hand side. The creation of pneumoperitoneum is undertaken either blindly using a Verres needle or by the open Hasson technique. Different combinations of the sizes and locations of ports are shown in Fig. 2. Moderate Trendenlenburg position (head down) with a tilt to the left promotes easy shift of small bowel from the surgical field. A thorough diagnostic laparoscopy is undertaken and diagnosis of appendicitis is established. The appendix is located as in open approach by following the taenia coli. A window is created in the mesoappendix and the appendicular vessels are either coagulated or clipped and cut. Once the appendix is free from the mesentery, the base is ligated using a loop suture or a linear stapling device. The specimen is delivered in a bag and sent for histology.

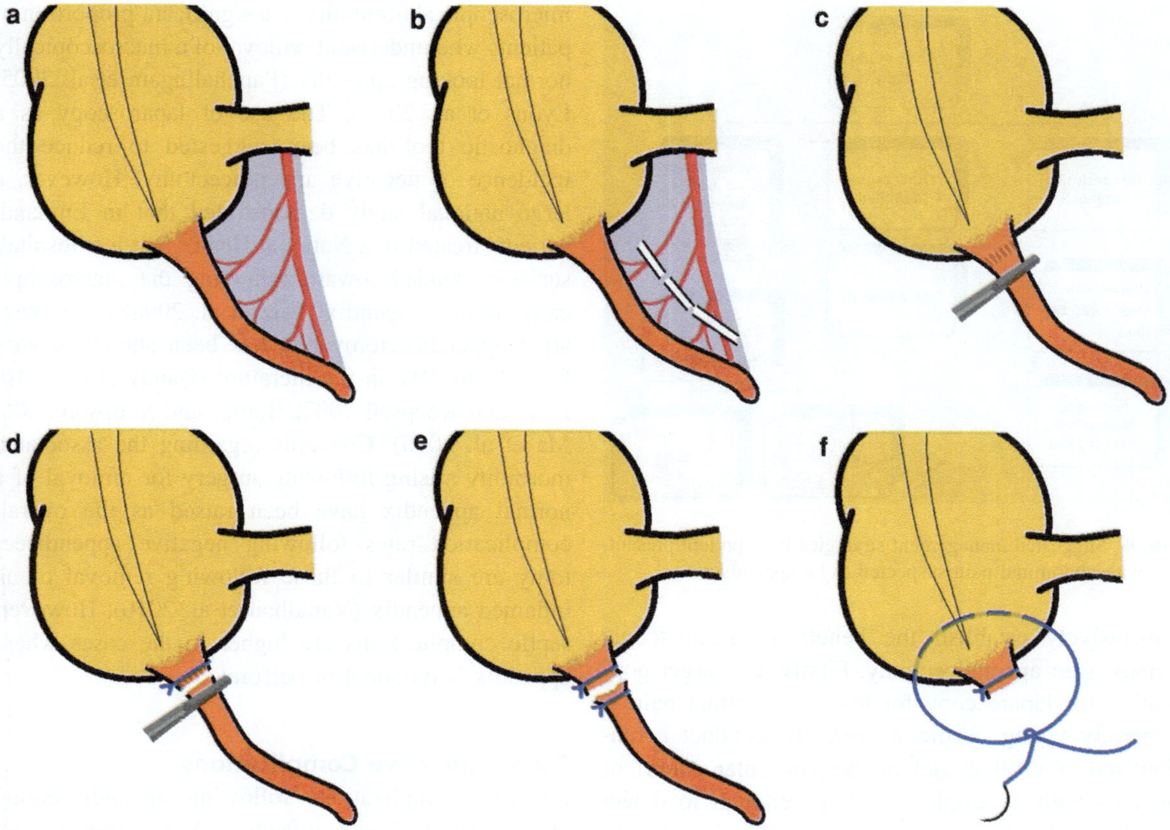

Fig. 3 Important steps in appendicectomy **a** Identification and dissection of appendix and mesoappendix **b** Ligation of appendicular artery and branches in the mesopappendix **c** Crushing the base of the appendix and reapplying clamp distally **d** Ligature across the base of appendix and excision of specimen **e** Excision by cutting between two ligatures (usually laparoscopically) **f** Burying the appendicular stump with a purse string suture

The abdominal cavity is inspected for hemostasis and peritoneal irrigation is carried out if necessary. In women, if not performed earlier, an inspection of the reproductive organs is done. Each port is withdrawn carefully inspecting for bleeding and closed in layers. Large port sites need closure of the sheath to prevent herniation in future.

2.2.4 Laparoscopic Versus Open Appendicectomy

During first half of the 20th century almost 16% of the population in Europe, America and Autralasia underwent appendicectomy for suspected acute appendicitis (O'Connell 2004). However, the incidence has fallen dramatically; especially in the developed nations and currently 6–8% of the population undergo an appendicectomy in their lifetime (Sauerland et al. 2010; Faiz et al. 2008b). The diagnosis and management of appendicitis has been improved with the introduction of newer and better imaging modalities and minimally invasive surgery. Laparoscopic appendicectomy, although popular, has not yet gained widespread acceptance as the gold standard. Although initial studies demonstrated equivocal results from the two surgical approaches, recent large studies have suggested potential advantages of laparoscopic appendicectomy with regard to length of stay and early return to work (Sauerland et al. 2010; Page et al. 2010; Kouhia et al. 2010). The benefits of the laparoscopic approach with regard to post-operative pain, time to recovery and earlier discharge have also been clearly demonstrated in cholecystectomy and colorectal resection (Ballal et al. 2009; Faiz et al. 2009; Jayne et al. 2007; Braga et al. 2002; Uchiyama et al. 2004). There are various issues surrounding the inability of studies to

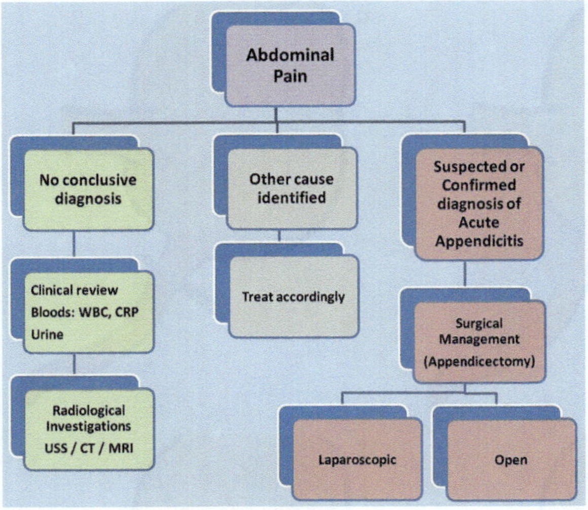

Fig. 4 Suggested management strategies for a patient presenting with abdominal pain suspected to be appendicitis

conclusively establish the benefit of laparoscopic versus open appendicectomy. Firstly, the target population for laparoscopy for lower abdominal pain is generally young, fertile women. To conduct a randomized controlled trial in this particular cohort of patients with a sample size large enough to detect small differences in complication rates is difficult. Secondly, emergency appendicectomy is often undertaken by trainees and there may be reluctance among senior surgeons to permit trainees to perform unsupervised laparoscopic procedures. A systematic review by Kapischke et al. (2006) demonstrated that in many studies, the more experienced surgeon performed laparoscopic appendicectomy when compared to those that performed open surgery during the course of the study. The same study also showed variation in the number of surgeons in a trial performing laparoscopic surgery. This leads to variation in the operative time and other outcomes for laparoscopic appendicectomy depending on the expertise and level of the surgeon.

2.2.5 Diagnostic Laparoscopy

The extent of exposure achievable by laparoscopy offers an ability to undertake a complete peritoneal survey. Laparoscopy is certainly gaining popularity in the diagnostic investigation of chronic right iliac fossa pain (Siriwardana et al. 2010; Onders 2003). Although the merits of excision of a normal looking appendix are debatable, studies have demonstrated microscopic abnormality in a significant proportion of patients who underwent removal of a macroscopically normal looking appendix (Panchalingam et al. 2005; Lyons et al. 2001). The use of laparoscopy as a diagnostic tool has been suggested to reduce the incidence of negative appendicectomy. However, a large national study demonstrated that in England, patients treated in a National Health Service hospital, surgeons tended toward removing the macroscopically normal appendix (Faiz et al. 2008b). The negative appendicectomy rate has been shown to vary from 15 to 25% in the literature (Gandy et al. 2010; Flum and Koepsell 2002; Humes and Simpson 2006; Ma et al. 2010). Concerns regarding the associated morbidity arising following surgery for removal of a normal appendix have been raised as the overall complication rates following negative appendicectomy are similar to those following removal of an inflamed appendix (Varadhan et al. 2010). However, septic complications are higher in the cases where appendix is inflamed or perforated.

2.2.6 Infective Complications

Infective complications following appendicectomy include surgical site infection (SSI), deep wound infection and deep or organ space infection (OSI) such as an intra-abdominal abscess. The incidence of these complications is higher in cases of complicated appendicitis such as perforation or gangrene. A Cochrane review and other large studies have demonstrated that wound infections were half as likely after laparoscopic appendicectomy as compared to open surgery; however, laparoscopic surgery was associated with higher incidence of intra-abdominal abscess (Sauerland et al. 2010; Page et al. 2010; Ingraham et al. 2010). Randomized trials have also supported this finding and described lower rates of wound infection and better cosmesis with laparoscopic appendicectomy (Pedersen et al. 2001). It has been postulated that inability to visualize or clearly identify the base of the appendix in a case of perforated appendicitis may contribute toward higher OSI in the laparoscopic group (Bennett et al. 2007). Also, dissemination of the infection due to pneumoperitoneum may be a contributing factor. A very large American study suggested the increased risk of OSI with laparoscopic appendicectomy depends on patient characteristics and there may be a specific cohort of patients in whom this higher risk is overshadowed by other potential benefits of laparoscopy (Fleming et al. 2010).

2.2.7 Length of Stay

Length of stay (LOS) is an outcome of relevance to both surgeons and managers alike. A frequently cited benefit of minimal access surgery is an associated reduction in LOS. In appendicectomy, however, studies have not demonstrated an unequivocal reduction in LOS following utilization of the laparoscopic approach. Although large studies have shown a significant shorter LOS after laparoscopic appendicectomy (Faiz et al. 2008), the number of re-admissions following surgery is higher in this cohort. In hospitals with a longer than average LOS after open appendicectomy, a significant reduction in LOS is seen with a laparoscopic approach. However, centres that already have a short LOS after open surgery, demonstrate no difference (Sauerland et al. 2010; Pedersen et al. 2001). Laparoscopic appendicectomy is a higher cost operative procedure than the open approach (McCahill et al. 1996; Ali et al. 2010). This combined with increase in re-admissions has serious economic implications. However, with increasing surgeon experience, operative time and costs have been shown to be lower as compared to a few years ago. This combined with shorter LOS and early return to work, may offset the higher cost of equipment in the longer run (Korndorffer et al. 2010).

2.2.8 Morbidity

Laparoscopic appendicectomy has been found to be associated with an overall lower risk of morbidity when compared with the open approach (Ingraham et al. 2010). This may be explained in part by the fact that minimal access surgery is generally associated with reduced surgical trauma and a diminished stress response (Madbouly et al. 2010; Saenz et al. 2007). The majority of studies in the past have reported longer operating times associated with the laparoscopic approach. However, with changing surgical practice and training laparoscopic expertise is increasing and operative times for open and laparoscopic appendicectomy are reaching comparable levels (Page et al. 2010). However, the fact cannot be discounted that the more difficult and complicated appendicectomies are performed using the open approach (Page et al. 2010).

In centres with the facilities and expertise for laparoscopic surgery, this may be considered as the option of choice in the absence of contraindications to laparoscopy. Its validity is most recogonizable in cases where diagnostic uncertainty exists. Laparoscopic appendicectomy is yet to be established as the gold standard for management of acute appendicitis. In selected patient groups such as young females or obese patients, there may be an added advantage of using the laparoscopic approach.

2.2.9 Rare Presentations of Appendicitis

A left-sided appendix occurs in about 0.2% of adult population (Bedoui et al. 2009). Patients with intestinal malrotation or situs invertus may present with left-sided abdominal pain and appendicitis. Radiological modalities such as Computerised Tomography (CT) Scan are beneficial in such cases as is a diagnostic laparoscopy. Retroperitoneal abscess formation may occur with a perforated appendicitis, however, Diana et al. (2010) have reported a case of rectal perforation and hepatic portal venous gas associated with necrotizing appendicitis. Another important yet rare complication after an appendicectomy is stump appendicitis which is re-inflammation of the residual tissue. It is postulated that a stump that is left too long is the most common aetiology for this pathology. Various case reports have been published, however, due to its rarity there has been no quantification of its incidence. Currently just under forty cases have been identified in English literature (O'Leary et al. 2010). Appendicitis may also present as small bowel obstruction and this may be due to a paralytic ileus or even a mechanical obstruction. A radiologist may achieve this diagnosis on the basis of a CT scan, however, the diagnosis may not be apparent until the patient undergoes a laparotomy. De Garengeot first described a case of acute appendicitis in a femoral hernia (Sharma et al. 2007). Fortunately the appendix is found in an abdominal wall hernia in less than 1% of cases (See Fig. 2 in "Historical Background, Anatomy and Function, Etiology and Epidemiology" of this volume).

2.2.10 Antibiotics in Appendicitis

Conservative treatment of acute appendicitis with antibiotic therapy has been suggested in the past. Various studies have attempted to compare the outcome among patients with appendicitis treated only with antibiotic therapy with those undergoing

Table 1 Summary of guidelines based on a systematic review by the American Pediatric Surgical Association Outcomes and Clinical Trials Committee

Pathology	Evidence[a]	Antibiotics	Timing/Duration
Non-perforated Appendicitis	Grade A	Broad-spectrum antibiotics	Pre-operative
Perforated Appendicitis	Grade B	Broad spectrum, single or double agent	5 day IV antibiotics OR 7 day IV + Oral antibiotics
Non-surgical Management	Grade D	Broad-spectrum IV antibiotics	Based on clinical criteria, such as fever, pain, return of bowel function, and WBC count

[a] Evidence—Grade A (>=two large prospective randomized controlled trials or meta-analysis)
Grade B (1 = one large prospective randomized controlled trials or meta-analysis)
Grade C (Small randomized trials with uncertain results)
Grade D (>=one non-randomized trial with controls)
Grade E (Expert opinion, case reports, uncontrolled studies) (Howdieshell et al. 2006; Mazuski et al. 2002)

appendicectomy (Eriksson and Granstrom 1995; Hansson et al. 2009; Styrud et al. 2006). Evidence suggests that antibiotics may be safely used as an alternative to surgery in selected patients with appendicitis where perforation or peritonitis has been carefully excluded. A meta-analysis of randomized controlled trials has shown that only 68% of patients randomized to the antibiotic group were successfully treated with antibiotics alone with a 15% re-admission rate (Varadhan et al. 2010). The remaining 32% of patients initially treated with antibiotics required surgery either during same admission or at a later date. Thus currently there is no strong evidence suggesting that antibiotics offer a safe and definite alternative to surgery. Appendicectomy, therefore, remains the gold standard treatment for simple and complicated appendicitis. The role of antibiotic therapy alone is restricted to special circumstances where surgery is either too risky or otherwise contraindicated.

Antibiotic prophylaxis is one of many measures considered to reduce post-operative morbidity such as infective complications. Whether the operation is clean, contaminated or clean-contaminated there are currently no definitive guidelines as to prescription of antibiotics in adult population. Antibiotic therapy in the pre, intra or post-operative management of acute appendicitis has been shown to reduce the risk of post-operative wound infection and intra-abdominal septic complications (Andersen et al. 2005; Winslow et al. 1983; Lee et al. 2010). Although debate is ongoing whether antibiotics are beneficial in only complicated appendicitis such as perforation or gangrene of the appendix, some surgeons choose to prescribe antibiotics in cases of simple appendicitis. In case of appendicitis in paediatric patients, the American Pediatric Surgical Association Outcomes and Clinical Trials Committee published guidelines based on a systematic review (Lee et al. 2010). This report suggested that children with non-perforated appendicitis should receive preoperative, broad-spectrum antibiotics. They also recommended that in patients with perforated appendicitis, the duration of broad-spectrum, intravenous antibiotics should be based on clinical symptoms. The summary of these recommendations are shown in Table 1.

2.2.11 Newer Advances in Minimal Access Appendicectomy

Since first being described, laparoscopic or minimal access surgery has seen significant advances in the techniques and instrumentation. Improvements in the ergonomic properties of instruments, higher definition cameras and hemostatic and stapling devices have made minimal access surgery faster and less challenging than a decade ago. The two principal advances in minimally invasive appendicectomy have been Single Incision Laparoscopic Surgery (SILS) and Natural Orifice Transluminal Endoscopic Surgery (NOTES). Although there is still a long way to go before these procedures are widely performed, there is an increasing popularity for incision-less surgery among patients and surgeons.

2.2.12 Single Incision Laparoscopic Surgery

Advances in surgery are often driven by an attempt to reduce post-operative LOS, pain and improve cosmesis. Single Incision Laparoscopic Surgery (SILS) is an innovation that allows minimal access surgery to be performed through a single umbilical incision (Chow et al. 2010). SILS has been shown to be effective and safe for operations, such as tubal ligation, hysterectomy, appendicectomy, cholecystectomy, sleeve gastrectomy, colectomy and nephrectomy (Chow et al. 2010). To date, however, evidence is available from small trials and case series. Results from large prospective randomized controlled trials are yet to establish the benefits of this procedure. The potential advantages over other approaches for SILS are proposed as reduced port site complications, diminished post-operative pain and reduction in post-operative length of stay (Ahmed et al. 2011). The unique selling point to this approach is, however, that SILS offers virtual "scarless surgery", thereby proving popular with some patients.

In this procedure, the anaesthesia and patient position are similar to conventional laparoscopic surgery. The umbilicus is everted and incised between stay sutures taking care to not damage the umbilical ring. Once the fascia is incised, the peritoneum is entered under direct vision. A special SILS port with multiple entry sites is used or conventional ports are inserted using the same skin incision but different entry sites in the fascia. Conventional instruments may be used by experienced surgeons, specially designed ergonomic instruments that can roticulate and/or flex may be used for ease. Retraction in SILS is usually a strong suture on a straight needle that is used to hitch the required tissue up against the abdominal wall. The actual process of dissection and removal of the appendix varies among surgeons. Loops, linear staples or sutures may be used as per availability and preference. Closure of the fascia needs careful attention as multiple port sites may be present. The skin is closed in a manner in which the incision is hidden inside the umbilicus giving the 'scarless' appearance. SILS is not a naturally ergonomic technique (Chow et al. 2010). The surgeon has to adapt to operate in a mirror image because his right-hand instrument may control the left-sided instrument on screen and vice versa. The traditional laparoscopic principals of triangulation are also lost due to the shared access points of the camera and instruments. This can, however, be offset by the use of angled laparoscopes or flexible endoscopes.

SILS- appendicectomy has been shown to be safe even in the paediatric population (Chandler and Danielson 2010; Tam et al. 2010). Outcomes have been shown to be comparable with conventional laparoscopic surgery with the added advantage of cosmesis. Using the conventional instruments and reducing the number of ports may seem a cost-effective strategy. However, specifically designed instruments and ports for use in SILS are currently more expensive and this may ultimately determine its uptake. This is a developing technique and well designed prospective trials are needed to demonstrate the superiority of this technique over conventional methods.

2.2.13 Natural Orifice Transluminal Endoscopic Surgery

Natural orifice transluminal endoscopic surgery is a technique that utilizes the body's natural orifices (mouth, anus, vagina and urethra) to access the abdominal cavity. The concept is based upon avoidance of the complications associated with abdominal incisions such as wound infection, pain, hernias and also to minimize adhesion formation (Sodergren et al. 2009). The majority of the evidence currently available is from studies on porcine models; however, various series have been published recently from different centres from across the world. Natural orifice transluminal endoscopic surgery (NOTES) is currently at a very early stage of development, but the literature published about this approach has exponentially increased over the last few years. Currently the procedures that have been performed via this approach are cholecystectomy, nephrectomy, appendicectomy, colectomy and distal pancreatectomy. It is too early to quantify the morbidity associated with this procedure as the number of cases performed on human subjects is currently small. The transvaginal approach is probably the most developed in human series, but the transgastrically approach also holds future promise. Appendicectomy via the NOTES approach has been described both transgastric and transvaginally (Palanivelu et al. 2008; Rao et al. 2008). Some surgeons choose a hybrid variety where a trans-abdominal or umbilical port is inserted for further ease of dissection or retraction. NOTES is currently under review and it may be a few years before this procedure becomes a common surgical practice.

2.2.14 Appendicits in Pregnancy

It is estimated that about 1 in 500–1 in 635 women undergo non-obstetrical abdominal surgery during their pregnancy (Yumi 2008). Acute appendicitis is the most common indication for surgery in this group with a reported incidence of about 1 in 1,440 pregnancies (Walsh et al. 2008). This condition poses a diagnostic challenge due to the changes in the physiology as well as intra-abdominal anatomy as the gravid uterus increases in size. Patients often present with atypical symptoms. There is also an attempt to minimize ionising radiation, leading to limited imaging modalities being available at smaller centers. Fetal loss and early or preterm delivery are important and well-known risks of appendicectomy in pregnancy. Previously published literature has reported fetal loss rates of 3–15% following appendicectomy (McGee 1989; Maslovitz et al. 2003; Ghazanfar et al. 2002; Andersen and Nielsen 1999). However, a recent population based study by McGory et al. (2007) demonstrated a fetal loss rate of 4%, but this was higher in cases of complicated appendicitis (6%). Early delivery occurred in 7% of patients following appendicectomy in this study although older literature from the 1980s report rates ranging between 13 and 45%. Society of American Gastrointestinal and Endoscopic Surgeons (SAGES) published guidelines in 2008 which suggested that laparoscopy was safe in any trimester during pregnancy and that laparoscopic appendicectomy (LA) could be performed safely in a pregnant woman with appendicitis (Yumi 2008).

Laparoscopy has been shown to be beneficial in pregnancy by reducing narcotic requirements, shortening length of stay and decreasing risk of thromboembolic complications. LA is also noted be associated with lower intra-operative and wound complications. It has been suggested that the reduced need for uterine manipulation leads to decreased irritability and lower rates of spontaneous abortion or preterm delivery (Yumi 2008; Curet 2000). However, two large studies have found a fetal loss rate of 5.6–7% following LA and around 3% following open surgery (Walsh et al. 2008; McGory et al. 2007). Overall spontaneous abortion is higher is cases of complicated appendicitis such as perforation, abscess formation or generalized peritonitits. Importantly, negative appendicectomy is also associated with a 4% fetal loss rate, highlighting the fact that pre-operative diagnosis is of utmost importance. Newer radiological modalities such as MRI may contribute toward lower negative appendicectomy rates in pregnant women. Imaging of pregnant women suspected of acute appendicitis is extensively discussed in chapter "Imaging of Acute Appendicitis in Adults: MRI" (by C Schmid-Tannwald and A Oto) and "Current Practice in Pregnant Women" (by T Jaffe) of this volume.

The use of open Hasson's technique against Verres needle, subcostal rather than umbilical entry for the first port and lower insufflation pressure are some variations depending on surgeon or center. In the absence of level 1 evidence from large randomized controlled trials, currently there seems to be no clear procedure of choice for approach to appendicectomy in pregnancy. LA, if undertaken, should be performed by a skilled and experienced surgeon only. Risks and benefits of laparoscopy and open surgery to both mother and fetus should be thoroughly considered. In every pregnant woman with non-obstetric abdominal pain, a surgical consult should be sought at the earliest.

3 Summary

This chapter attempts to provide an insight into the available treatment modalities and surgical options for treatment of appendicitis. The current evidence available for choosing the surgical approach and important steps in performing an appendicectomy has been discussed. Benefits of minimally invasive surgery such as laparoscopy and its role in special circumstances are mentioned. Concepts of newer techniques in minimally invasive surgery such as SILS and NOTES have been introduced.

References

Ahmed K, Wang TT, Patel VM, Nagpal K, Clark J, Ali M, Deeba S, Ashrafian H, Darzi A, Athanasiou T, Paraskeva P (2011) The role of single-incision laparoscopic surgery in abdominal and pelvic surgery: a systematic review. Surg Endosc 25(2):378–396

Ali R, Khan MR, Pishori T, Tayeb M (2010) Laparoscopic appendectomy for acute appendicitis: is this a feasible option for developing countries? Saudi J Gastroenterol 16:25–29

Andersen BR, Kallehave FL, Andersen HK (2005) Antibiotics versus placebo for prevention of postoperative infection after appendicectomy. Cochrane Database Syst Rev 3:CD001439

Andersen B, Nielsen TF (1999) Appendicitis in pregnancy: Diagnosis, management and complications. Acta Obstet Gynecol Scand 78:758–762

Ballal M, David G, Willmott S, Corless DJ, Deakin M, Slavin JP (2009) Conversion after laparoscopic cholecystectomy in England. Surg Endosc 23:2338–2344

Bedoui R, Ali Ouaer M, Nouira R, Dziri C (2009) Acute left-sided appendicitis. Tunis Med 87:873–874

Bennett J, Boddy A, Rhodes M (2007) Choice of approach for appendicectomy: a meta-analysis of open versus laparoscopic appendicectomy. Surg Laparosc Endosc Percutan Tech 17:245–255

Braga M, Vignali A, Gianotti L, Zuliani W, Radaelli G, Gruarin P et al (2002) Laparoscopic versus open colorectal surgery a randomized trial on short-term outcome. Ann Surg 236:759–766 discussion 767

Chandler NM, Danielson PD (2010) Single-incision laparoscopic appendectomy versus multiport laparoscopic appendectomy in children: a retrospective comparison. J Pediatr Surg 45:2186–2190

Chow A, Purkayastha S, Nehme J, Darzi LA, Paraskeva P (2010) Single incision laparoscopic surgery for appendicectomy a retrospective comparative analysis. Surg Endosc 24:2567–2574

Curet MJ (2000) Special problems in laparoscopic surgery. Previous abdominal surgery, obesity, and pregnancy. Surg Clin North Am 80:1093–1110

Diana M, Paroz A, Demartines N, Schafer M (2010) Retroperitoneal abscess with concomitant hepatic portal venous gas and rectal perforation a rare triad of complications of acute appendicitis. A case report. World J Emerg Surg 5:3

Eriksson S, Granstrom L (1995) Randomized controlled trial of appendicectomy versus antibiotic therapy for acute appendicitis. Br J Surg 82:166–169

Faiz O, Blackburn SC, Clark J, Bottle A, Curry JI, Farrands P et al (2008a) Laparoscopic and conventional appendicectomy in children outcomes in English hospitals between 1996 and 2006. Pediatr Surg Int 24:1223–1227

Faiz O, Clark J, Brown T, Bottle A, Antoniou A, Farrands P et al (2008b) Traditional and laparoscopic appendectomy in adults outcomes in English NHS hospitals between 1996 and 2006. Ann Surg 248:800–806

Faiz O, Warusavitarne J, Bottle A, Tekkis PP, Darzi AW, Kennedy RH (2009) Laparoscopically assisted versus open elective colonic and rectal resection a comparison of outcomes in English National Health Service Trusts between 1996 and 2006. Dis Colon Rectum 52:1695–1704

Fitz R (1886) Perforating inflammation of the vermiform appendix with special reference to its early diagnosis and treatment. Am J Med Sci 92:321–346

Fleming FJ, Kim MJ, Messing S, Gunzler D, Salloum R, Monson JR (2010) Balancing the risk of postoperative surgical infections: a multivariate analysis of factors associated with laparoscopic appendectomy from the NSQIP database. Ann Surg 252:895–900

Flum DR, Koepsell T (2002) The clinical and economic correlates of misdiagnosed appendicitis: Nationwide analysis. Arch Surg 137:799–804 discussion

Gandy RC, Truskett PG, Wong SW, Smith S, Bennett MH, Parasyn AD (2010) Outcomes of appendicectomy in an acute care surgery model. Med J Aust 193:281–284

Ghazanfar A, Nasir SM, Choudary ZA, Ahmad W (2002) Acute appendicitis complicating pregnancy; experience with the management of 50 patients. J Ayub Med Coll Abbottabad 14:19–21

Hansson J, Korner U, Khorram-Manesh A, Solberg A, Lundholm K (2009) Randomized clinical trial of antibiotic therapy versus appendicectomy as primary treatment of acute appendicitis in unselected patients. Br J Surg 96:473–481

Howdieshell TR, Heffernan D, Dipiro JT (2006) Surgical infection society guidelines for vaccination after traumatic injury. Surg Infect (Larchmt) 7:275–303

Humes DJ, Simpson J (2006) Acute appendicitis. BMJ 333:530–534

Ingraham AM, Cohen ME, Bilimoria KY, Pritts TA, Ko CY, Esposito TJ (2010) Comparison of outcomes after laparoscopic versus open appendectomy for acute appendicitis at 222 ACS NSQIP hospitals. Surgery 148:625–635 discussion 635–637

Jayne DG, Guillou PJ, Thorpe H, Quirke P, Copeland J, Smith AM et al (2007) Randomized trial of laparoscopic-assisted resection of colorectal carcinoma 3 year results of the UK MRC CLASICC Trial Group. J Clin Oncol 25:3061–3068

Kapischke M, Caliebe A, Tepel J, Schulz T, Hedderich J (2006) Open versus laparoscopic appendicectomy a critical review. Surg Endosc 20:1060–1068

Korndorffer JR Jr, Fellinger E, Reed W (2010) SAGES guideline for laparoscopic appendectomy. Surg Endosc 24:757–761

Kouhia ST, Heiskanen JT, Huttunen R, Ahtola HI, Kiviniemi VV, Hakala T (2010) Long-term follow-up of a randomized clinical trial of open versus laparoscopic appendicectomy. Br J Surg 97:1395–1400

Lee SL, Islam S, Cassidy LD, Abdullah F, Arca MJ (2010) Antibiotics and appendicitis in the pediatric population an American Pediatric Surgical Association Outcomes and Clinical Trials Committee systematic review. J Pediatr Surg 45:2181–2185

Lyons TL, Winer WK, Woo A (2001) Appendectomy in patients undergoing laparoscopic surgery for pelvic pain. J Am Assoc Gynecol Laparosc 8:542–544

Ma KW, Chia NH, Yeung HW, Cheung MT (2010) If not appendicitis, then what else can it be? A retrospective review of 1492 appendectomies. Hong Kong Med J 16:12–17

Madbouly KM, Senagore AJ, Delaney CP (2010) Endogenous morphine levels after laparoscopic versus open colectomy. Br J Surg 97:759–764

Maslovitz S, Gutman G, Lessing JB, Kupferminc MJ, Gamzu R (2003) The significance of clinical signs and blood indices for the diagnosis of appendicitis during pregnancy. Gynecol Obstet Invest 56:188–191

Mazuski JE, Sawyer RG, Nathens AB, DiPiro JT, Schein M, Kudsk KA et al (2002) The surgical infection society guidelines on antimicrobial therapy for intra-abdominal infections: an executive summary. Surg Infect (Larchmt) 3:161–173

McBurney C IV (1894) The incision made in the abdominal wall in cases of appendicitis with a description of a new method of operating. Ann Surg 20:38–43

McCahill LE, Pellegrini CA, Wiggins T, Helton WS (1996) A clinical outcome and cost analysis of laparoscopic versus open appendectomy. Am J Surg 171:533–537

McGee TM (1989) Acute appendicitis in pregnancy. Aust N Z J Obstet Gynaecol 29:378–385

McGory ML, Zingmond DS, Tillou A, Hiatt JR, Ko CY, Cryer HM (2007) Negative appendectomy in pregnant women is associated with a substantial risk of fetal loss. J Am Coll Surg 205:534–540

O'Connell PR (2004) The vermiform appendix. In: Russel RCG, Christopher NsW, Bulstrode JK (eds) Bailey and Love's short practice of surgery. Arnold Publishers, London, pp 1203–1218
O'Leary DP, Myers E, Coyle J, Wilson I (2010) Case report of recurrent acute appendicitis in a residual tip. Cases J 3:14
Onders RP (2003) Mittendorf EA Utility of laparoscopy in chronic abdominal pain. Surgery 134:549–552 discussion 552–554
Page AJ, Pollock JD, Perez S, Davis SS, Lin E, Sweeney JF (2010) Laparoscopic versus open appendectomy an analysis of outcomes in 17, 199 patients using ACS/NSQIP. J Gastrointest Surg 14:1955–1962
Palanivelu C, Rajan PS, Rangarajan M, Parthasarathi R, Senthilnathan P, Prasad M (2008) Transvaginal endoscopic appendectomy in humans: a unique approach to NOTES—world's first report. Surg Endosc 22:1343–1347
Panchalingam L, Driver C, Mahomed AA (2005) Elective laparoscopic appendicectomy for chronic right iliac fossa pain in children. J Laparoendosc Adv Surg Tech A 15:186–189
Pedersen AG, Petersen OB, Wara P, Ronning H, Qvist N, Laurberg S (2001) Randomized clinical trial of laparoscopic versus open appendicectomy. Br J Surg 88:200–205
Rao GV, Reddy DN, Banerjee R (2008) NOTES: Human experience. Gastrointest Endosc Clin N Am 18:361–370
Saenz J, Asuero MS, Villafruela J, Correa C, Galindo J, Cuevas B et al (2007) Immunohumoral response during laparoscopic and open living donor nephrectomy an experimental model. Transplant Proc 39:2102–2104
Sauerland S, Jaschinski T, Neugebauer EA (2010) Laparoscopic versus open surgery for suspected appendicitis. Cochrane Database Syst Rev 10:CD001546
Semm K (1983) Endoscopic appendectomy. Endoscopy 15:59–64
Sharma H, Jha PK, Shekhawat NS, Memon B, Memon MA (2007) De Garengeot hernia an analysis of our experience. Hernia 11:235–238
Siriwardana RC, Renuka S, Kumarage S (2010) Laparoscopy as a diagnostic and therapeutic option in evaluating chronic unexplained right iliac fossa pain. Surg Endosc 24:2793–2795
Sodergren MH, Clark J, Athanasiou T, Teare J, Yang GZ, Darzi A (2009) Natural orifice translumenal endoscopic surgery: Critical appraisal of applications in clinical practice. Surg Endosc 23:680–687
Styrud J, Eriksson S, Nilsson I, Ahlberg G, Haapaniemi S, Neovius G et al (2006) Appendectomy versus antibiotic treatment in acute appendicitis a prospective multicenter randomized controlled trial. World J Surg 30:1033–1037
Tam YH, Lee KH, Sihoe JD, Chan KW, Cheung ST, Pang KK (2010) Initial experience in children using conventional laparoscopic instruments in single-incision laparoscopic surgery. J Pediatr Surg 45:2381–2385
Uchiyama K, Onishi H, Tani M, Kinoshita H, Ueno M, Yamaue H (2004) Timing of laparoscopic cholecystectomy for acute cholecystitis with cholecystolithiasis. Hepatogastroenterology 51:346–348
Varadhan KK, Humes DJ, Neal KR, Lobo DN (2010) Antibiotic therapy versus appendectomy for acute appendicitis a meta-analysis. World J Surg 34:199–209
Walsh CA, Tang T, Walsh SR (2008) Laparoscopic versus open appendicectomy in pregnancy: a systematic review. Int J Surg 6:339–344
Winslow RE, Dean RE, Harley JW (1983) Acute nonperforating appendicitis. Efficacy of brief antibiotic prophylaxis. Arch Surg 118:651–655
Yumi H (2008) Guidelines for diagnosis, treatment, and use of laparoscopy for surgical problems during pregnancy: This statement was reviewed and approved by the Board of Governors of the Society of American Gastrointestinal and Endoscopic Surgeons (SAGES), September 2007. It was prepared by the SAGES Guidelines Committee. Surg Endosc 22:849–861

Treatment of Appendiceal Perforation

Alex M. Almoudaris and Omar Faiz

Contents

Abstract

The treatment of appendiceal perforation is subject to considerable debate in current surgical literature. In perforated appendicitis radiologists have an important role both as diagnosticians and in offering interventional treatment options. As a result, knowledge and understanding of the current debate surrounding the treatment of appendiceal perforation is vital for radiologists and surgeons alike. The focus of this chapter is to discuss the treatment of appendiceal perforation with reference to contemporary evidence. General and specific management of the patient with an appendiceal perforation is offered including important pre-operative considerations for both radiologists and surgeons. Timing of surgery, use of laparoscopy and the current debate with respect to interval appendectomy is discussed in an evidence based manner.

1 Introduction

Appendicitis with obstruction of the appendiceal lumen by faecoliths can lead to increased intraluminal pressure and reduced venous return. In turn, appendiceal artery thrombosis may follow leading to gangrene and subsequent appendiceal perforation. Perforation of the appendix occurs most commonly in young children. Perforation rates as high as 82% have been reported in children with appendicitis less than 5 years (Newman et al. 2003). Delayed diagnosis has been cited as a factor contributing to perforation. This in turn has been attributed to other causes including socio-economic factors, ethnicity, insurance status

A. M. Almoudaris · O. Faiz (✉)
Department of Surgery and Cancer, Imperial College, St. Mary's Hospital, 10th floor QEQM building, South Wharf Road, Paddington, London, W2 1NY, UK
e-mail: o.faiz@imperial.ac.uk

C. Keyzer and P. A. Gevenois (eds.), *Imaging of Acute Appendicitis in Adults and Children*, Medical Radiology. Diagnostic Imaging, DOI: 10.1007/174_2011_215, © Springer-Verlag Berlin Heidelberg 2011

and which hospital service patients are originally referred to (Morrow and Newman 2007). Perforation rate and time interval between the onset of the symptoms and surgery is further discussed in "Appendicitis Perforation Rates and Time Interval between Symptom Onset and Surgery". In comparison to 'simple' or 'uncomplicated' appendicitis once perforation occurs, the subsequent risk of morbidity and mortality is significantly increased. Studies report complication rates of 18 (Styrud et al. 1998)–58% (David et al. 1982) in cases with perforation in comparison with approximately 10% (Styrud et al. 1998) in uncomplicated cases. Pre-operative radiology may provide further evidence of suspected perforation of the appendix although the type of imaging modality initially utilized may be influenced by patient factors such as age and concurrent pregnancy as well as local resource availability.

Unlike in 'uncomplicated' appendicitis where prompt surgical excision is favored to prevent the development of complications, the treatment of the perforated appendix often demands a pragmatic approach. The principal aim of treating a patient with a perforated appendix is to mitigate the risks of subsequent complications. Viewpoints on best practice of managing perforated appendicitis vary and this makes development of a prescriptive management strategy difficult. However, what is intended is to present sensible approaches supported by the surgical literature for the different strategies, while explaining the reasons underlying these decisions. This should inform readers as to the conceptual framework that underpins management strategies in appendiceal perforation.

1.1 Causes of Appendiceal Perforation

By far the commonest cause of perforation of the appendix is as an evolution of appendicitis. However, it is important to note that other causes of appendiceal perforations do exist. The causes of appendiceal perforation are listed in Table 1.

Table 1 Commonest causes of appendiceal perforation

Causes of Appendiceal Perforation
Appendicitis
Foreign body
Perforated malignancy (including carcinoid)

2 Treatment Strategy

The treatment of any patient with suspected intra-abdominal sepsis demands that they undergo:

1. Physiological optimization, plus
2. Definitive timely treatment of the underlying cause.

It must be noted that in any patient with suspected appendiceal perforation physical optimization should commence without delay and ideally should run alongside preparations for definitive treatment. Early senior surgical involvement is essential, especially in patients at the extremes of age where less physiological reserve often exists and consequently these patients may deteriorate rapidly. Older children have a greater capacity to withstand considerable physiological insult, however, they can decompensate rapidly and the clinician must be aware of this.

2.1 General Treatment of the Unwell Patient with Perforated Appendicitis

Patients with perforated appendicitis are usually in pain, febrile, dehydrated and septic. The key primary treatment aims are thus to initially address the above-

Therefore, the essential initial aims of treatment should include (Fig. 1)

1. Fluid Resuscitation
2. Analgesia
3. Antibiotics
4. Surgical Consult
5. Thromboprophylaxis
6. Monitoring
7. Decompression-gastric (optional discretionary consideration).

Firstly, every patient should have venous access with appropriate crystalloid fluid administration in order to replace daily requirements and to offset insensible losses. This is because any patient suspected of harboring a perforated appendix should be restricted orally (i.e., placed: 'nil-by-mouth') until a senior surgeon responsible for care has clinically reviewed them. Therefore, all further medications should be administered parenterally.

No surgical patient should be denied suitable and adequate analgesia for fear of masking clinical signs.

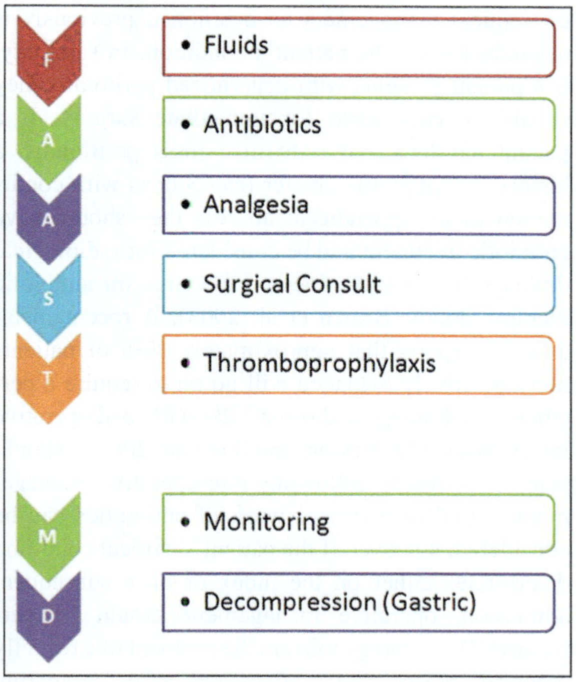

Fig. 1 Schematic memory aid for treatment strategy (FAAST MD)

The view of withholding analgesia is outdated and it is now accepted that analgesia is safe and does not affect diagnostic accuracy (Gallagher et al. 2006; Amoli et al. 2008). Appropriate dosing of opiate analgesia should therefore, not be restricted and should be accompanied by anti-emetic medication also. Acetaminophen (Paracetamol) should be given intravenously for its antipyretic and analgesic properties followed by titrated additional analgesia where necessary.

Intravenous antibiotics should be administered promptly and ideally within 1 h (Dellinger et al. 2008). Antibiotic therapy should follow local guidelines, however, broad cover against the aerobic and anaerobic pathogens that constitute the bacterial flora of the colon is mandatory. In the case of perforated appendicitis specific protection against gram negative bacteria is essential. Where allergies conflict with normal prescribing methods, specialist local advice should be sought. Antibiotic courses for perforated appendicitis should be continued for 5–7 days beyond the operation in the first instance (i.e., a full treatment dose). A didactic approach to antimicrobial therapy is difficult in patients with perforated appendicitis who do not undergo early surgery. A recent systematic review by the American Pediatric Surgical Association outcomes and clinical trials committee concluded that the duration of antibiotic use in children with perforated appendicitis who are undergoing an appendectomy should continue based on clinical criteria (Lee et al. 2010). Furthermore, they concluded that broad-spectrum, single, or double agent therapy is as effective as triple agent therapy for the treatment of perforated appendicitis (Lee et al. 2010). Antibiotics should be converted from the intravenous route to oral when the patients are able to tolerate oral intake and gut absorption has resumed.

Patients with perforated appendicitis (especially at the extremes of age) and signs of generalized peritonitis or general systemic sepsis must be observed closely pre- and post-operatively. These patients are liable to rapid decompensation and indicative trends should be realized as early as possible to allow for timely intervention. The High Dependency Unit (HDU) setting is appropriate for this patient group—especially older patients with multiple co-morbidities. Furthermore, it is essential that adequate fluid balance is maintained and the use of urinary catheters, nasogastric decompression tubes may be required. Gastric decompression with a nasogastric (NG) tube is not essential but may be indicated in patients with concurrent reactive small bowel ileus and vomiting. Evidence in a non-randomized retrospective record review of 159 patients with perforated appendicitis demonstrated a significantly longer time to eating and length of stay in post-operative children after using NG tubes as compared to those without (St Peter et al. 2007). Therefore, judicious use of gastric decompression is advised.

Given the lack of patient mobility, coupled with a hyper dynamic and pro-thrombotic state all adult patients with perforated appendicitis should receive thromboprophylaxis unless contraindicated. Aside from the pre-operative phase, some patients, especially those who proceed to laparotomy may be immobile for some time post-operatively thus warranting ongoing prophylaxis.

2.2 Overview of Specific Treatment Options

There are essentially two interventional treatment options for perforated appendicitis—surgery or radiological drainage. Conservative management solely with antibiotics and expectant management is the only non-interventional treatment. The chosen option depends upon two further factors. Firstly, the clinical condition of the patient (i.e., the presence of localized versus generalized clinical signs) and the radiological intra-abdominal findings. Duration of symptoms may also guide a clinician as to what treatment pathway is most appropriate—with a shorter course favoring surgery. There is debate in the literature about whether patients with confirmed localized perforated appendicitis should be treated operatively or considered for conservative management with antibiotics ± percutaneous drainage of any appendicular abscess (Weber et al. 2003; Henry et al. 2007; Roach et al. 2007). Several studies have demonstrated either lower or acceptable complication rates in patients with confirmed perforated appendicitis who have undergone conservative management and usually followed by interval appendectomy (Kogut et al. 2001; Weber et al. 2003; Simillis et al. 2010). There have also been studies that have demonstrated no worse outcomes when immediate surgery was undertaken citing reduction in diagnostic uncertainty and subsequent hospital visits as benefits to this approach (Goh et al. 2005). Initial pilot results from a prospective randomized trial of patients with a perforated appendix with an intra-abdominal abscess who were randomized to laparoscopic appendectomy or intravenous antibiotics with percutaneous drainage of the abscess followed by interval laparoscopic appendectomy 10 weeks later have showed no significant differences in length of stay, recurrent abscess rate and costs between the groups (St Peter et al. 2010). The overall shift is seemingly toward avoiding surgery at the time of the index admission favoring antibiotic therapy with radiological drainage if required followed by a planned interval appendectomy several weeks later.

3 Management Options in Pre-Operatively Suspected Perforated Appendicitis

In patients in whom a perforated appendix is suspected pre-operatively either due to radiological suggestion or on identifying a mass in the right lower quadrant (where malignancy is not suspected), consequent management as mentioned previously is dependent upon the patient's condition. In summary, if a patient presents with generalized peritonitis they should be considered for immediate surgery. If a patient has localized right iliac fossa peritionitis, a history of symptoms greater than 3 days with confirmation of an appendiceal abscess they should have antibiotic treatment and be considered for radiological drainage (if the septic focus is too large for antibiotic therapy alone) (Brown et al. 2003). A recent meta-analysis reports that approximately 20% of patients non-operatively managed will go on to require a percutaneous drainage and some 7.2% will need operative intervention (Andersson and Petzold 2007). Should symptoms return following non-operative management, a trial of a further week of antibiotics can be considered, however, if the patient's clinical condition deteriorates either on the index or on a subsequent admission, operative management should be performed. This strategy mirrors the protocol of a recently reported prospective randomized trial comparing immediate surgery versus immediate drainage with delayed surgery (St Peter et al. 2010). A final consideration is whether or not a patient who has successfully undergone non-operative management need to go onto have a planned interval appendectomy and this is discussed in the Sect. 3.3 of this chapter. Figure 2 is a flow diagram summarizing the treatment options.

3.1 Surgery

The indications for surgery in a patient with perforated appendicitis are numerous. At presentation if a patient is septic and displays signs of generalized peritonitis immediate surgery following a short period of optimization is warranted. Similarly patients with complex loculated abdominal or pelvic abscesses who are not amenable to percutaneous drainage should proceed to surgery also. Patients with a localized mass or abscess in whom conservative measures fail resulting in ongoing sepsis should also be considered candidates for surgery. The surgical approach is dependent upon the surgeon's experience with laparoscopy (see discussion on laparotomy and laparoscopy in "Laparoscopy and Laparotomy" of this book and in Sect. 5 of this Chapter). Some surgeons who are proficient with laparoscopy may decide to perform minimal access examination and proceed if feasible.

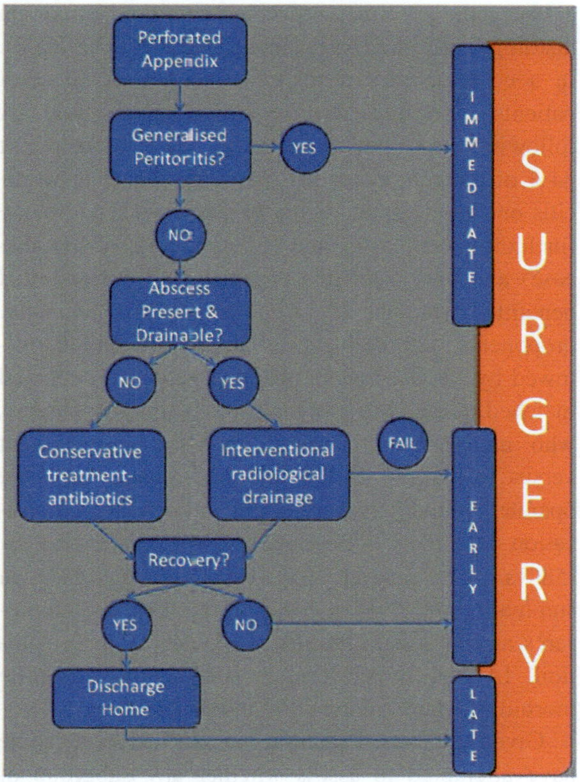

Fig. 2 A proposed overview schematic for the management of perforated appendicitis

The principles of surgery apply irrespective of the technical approach. Securing safe appendectomy while ensuring no collateral damage to surrounding structures and thorough lavage represent the essential components of intervention in these circumstances (see Laparoscopy versus laparotomy chapter).

3.2 Radiologically Guided Percutaneous Drainage

In patients who are clinically stable and have evidence of a radiologically confirmed abscess, consideration should be made to manage these patients radiologically in the first instance alongside the general measures highlighted above (Hogan 2003). The feasibility of this depends upon the anatomical location of the abscess, its size, the presence of additional or disparate septic foci and the presence or absence of loculations within its cavity. The ultimate aim of radiological percutaneous drainage is to achieve adequate drainage of localized sepsis with the avoidance of general anesthesia and surgery. This treatment strategy has been shown to safe and effective and is associated with a low recurrence rate of further abscess formation (Zerem et al. 2007). From a radiological perspective several considerations must be made. Firstly the patient must consent to the procedure and the plan as well as be made aware of possible complications including placement failure. Secondly the patient should be clinically suitable for drainage- this includes ensuring the patients clotting status is suitable and ensuring any coagulopathy is corrected or within acceptable limits. Anatomical considerations must also be taken into account to include whether the abscess is multiloculated, accessible or likely to contain necrotic tissue that will not benefit from radiological intervention and that will require surgical debridement (Wallace et al. 2010).

3.3 Interval Appendectomy

Considerable debate surrounds the need to perform an interval appendectomy (IA) following initial non-operative management. Those who do not support IA cite that if a patient has not needed surgery on an index admission for appendicitis 'routine' IA should not be performed due to low risk of future problems (Tekin et al. 2008). Furthermore, if recurrence does occur it tends to be less severe (Dixon et al. 2003). One of the stated reasons for avoiding IA is the reported low recurrence rates (Deakin and Ahmed 2007). Contemporary studies cite recurrence rates of approximately 5 (Kaminski et al. 2005)–14% (Dixon et al. 2003; Tekin et al. 2008) inferring that >85% of patients will thus not have another episode after the index presentation (wider variation is observed in older literature), however, this is obviously dependent upon the follow-up period. A pooled recurrence rate from a contemporary meta-analysis of seven studies reported a recurrence rate of 8.9% with a variable follow-up period (Andersson and Petzold 2007). This questions the value of 'routine' IA in these cases as IA in itself carries operative risk and additional hospital stay. Other authors have suggested that the benefit of preventing recurrence is small when undertaking routine IA and has been quantified at preventing recurrence in <16% of patients if performed within 6 weeks of discharge and preventing recurrence in <10% of patients if performed at 12 weeks or later (Lai et al. 2006) suggesting that recurrence tends to occur sooner. This viewpoint is also reflected in the conclusions of a recent review, however, this was in patients without recurrent symptoms (Deakin and Ahmed 2007). A further study with a mean follow-up of 7.5 years in children who had been non-operatively managed for perforated appendicitis found all recurrences occurred within 3 years and 80% of these occurred within 6 months yielding an overall recurrence rate of 8% (Puapong et al. 2007). Similar findings have been demonstrated in adult patients with recurrence rates of 5% at 4 years and furthermore among those who recurred one-third did not need an operation (Kaminski et al. 2005). Finally, it should be acknowledged that IA also carries an associated operative risk and hospital stay. Median length of hospital stay has been shown to be longer in patients treated with IA than in the few patients who have recurrent disease (Kaminski et al. 2005) and the morbidity associated with IA has been cited at 18% including superficial and deep infections, small bowel obstruction and wound problems (Willemsen et al. 2002). In summary, the low likelihood of recurrent appendicitis, the associated morbidity and hospital stay associated with IA and associated costs are cited as reasons for re-considering 'routine' IA after conservative management of a perforated appendix.

Proponents of IA cite the benefits or IA are not only those of preventing recurrent appendicitis but also that of obtaining histological diagnosis. Interestingly, in a paper that examined the histological diagnoses of IA specimens, all were found to have patent appendiceal lumens (as opposed to obliterated lumens) indicating a risk of a recurrent episode and furthermore in 5 out of 17 specimens unsuspected histological finding were discovered (Mazziotti et al. 1997). It has also been shown in a prospective, non-randomized study of IA in children, up to 45.8% of specimens demonstrated chronic active inflammation and 2.1% a serious unpredicted histology (in these cases—carcinoid tumor) (Samuel et al. 2002). A further study of 103 children that were initially non-operatively managed with 97 going on to undergo IA as planned some 4–6 weeks later has shown that the mean length of stay for the IA was 2.5 days (range 1–5 days) and only 3.1% of the children developed a complication, all of which were minor. Furthermore 2.1% of the specimens revealed carcinoid tumor on histology from the IA specimens (Gillick et al. 2008). In a contemporary retrospective series of 46 adult patients who underwent elective laparoscopic IA following perforated appendicitis the authors report 84% of patients either had persistent acute appendicitis or chronic appendicitis or some other pathology (including neoplastic and inflammatory bowel disease) and thus state this proportion of patients had benefitted from the IA (Lugo et al. 2010). Finally, proponents of initial conservative management followed by IA cite that in matched patient groups and matched presentation signs and symptoms patients who underwent immediate operative management versus primary drainage and IA, those who were operated initially had a significantly higher complication rate than those patients who underwent IA (58 vs. 15%, respectively) (Brown et al. 2003). In summary, obtaining a histological diagnosis represents an important argument in favor of IA. In addition, IA can be performed safely and with little morbidity when compared with early surgery.

Given the varied opinions in the literature, some have attempted to assess whether any subgroup of patients would likely benefit from an IA. Evidence exists that those with an appreciable appendicolith on CT or those with a past history of appendicitis would benefit from IA within 6 weeks of the original presentation, otherwise watchful waiting is acceptable (Tsai et al. 2006). Furthermore in adult patients in whom an IA is not performed following a period of conservative management for presumed perforated appendicitis, further imaging of the bowel is also recommended as these are the patients most likely to have some form of unexpected histology. It has been suggested that in patients non-operatively managed over the age of 40 years, they should undergo some form of further imaging of the bowel to include colonoscopy, barium study of the colon or a virtual CT colonoscopy (Andersson and Petzold 2007). The authors are more in favor of a non-operative approach in the first instance utilizing percutaneous drainage and antibiotics where possible. In terms of IA, the authors feel that patients should be fully involved in the decision-making process with knowledge of the risks and benefits for both IA and leaving the appendix in situ. This said, all patients over the age of 40 years or those patients who decline IA with recurrent symptoms should undergo full colonic imaging and surgical follow-up.

4 Management Options in Intra-Operatively Discovered Perforated Appendicitis

In the presence of appendicitis the discovery of a faecolith/faeces within the abdominal cavity, or an abscess cavity with or without inter-loop abscesses or the presence of a foreign body (e.g., fish bone) all reflect that the appendix has perforated. Under such circumstances the anesthetist should be informed as significant bacteraemia often occurs when handling grossly infected tissues. Surgically, the appendix should be removed in the usual fashion, noting that burying the appendix stump may be difficult due to an edematous and fragile caecum that may not withhold a purse-string suture. In rare circumstances, where there is heavy local contamination and the risk of stump breakdown is considered high ileo-caecal resection may be necessary. The decision to anastomose following ileo-caecal resection is made upon the degree of local contamination and the current stability of the patient alongside their pre-morbid health status. Gross peritoneal contamination in an unstable patient with significant cardio-respiratory disease may render ileostomy a safer option than restoring intestinal continuity. Abdominal drainage in this instance is highly recommended.

In cases where an appendix mass is identified pre-operatively and no generalized intra-abdominal sepsis exists placement of an abdominal drain and wound closure may be preferable over attempted appendectomy. Such a decision should involve an experienced surgeon as inappropriate dissection of a fragile appendix may incur iatrogenic damage to adherent bowel loops rendering fistulisation likely. With increasing access to ultrasound and CT scanning fewer such cases should arise.

With respect to closure of the wound there are several considerations. Firstly, the traditional view has been that in cases where a perforation has been encountered skin closure should not be performed due to the increased risk of subsequent wound infection (Bower et al. 1981; Lemieur et al. 1999) with rates as high as 58% being reported (David et al. 1982). In patients with perforated appendicitis managed by either primary closure (PC) or open wound management (OWM), patients were significantly more likely to develop wound infections in the PC group in a series of 65 patients (Chiang et al. 2006). Patients managed with PC had a wound infections rate of 43.9% compared to the OWM rate of 4.2%. The primarily closed group also had a significantly longer length of stay and were re-admitted more often (Chiang et al. 2006). The figures are higher than other contemporary Western series with numbers >10 patients who report much lower rates of wound infection after perforated appendicitis and PC of the wound ranging from 7.7 (McGreal et al. 2002) to 9% (Chatwiriyacharoen 2002). There are practical problems with OWM that includes the pain and distress especially young children may suffer with this form of wound management which must be considered. In contrast a recent systematic review and meta-analysis has suggested that PC is the preferred method of wound closure in perforated appendicitis incorporating a search from all published data from 1980–2003 (Henry and Moss 2005). This meta-analysis was, however, limited to non-laparoscopic cases and the method of closure was not controlled for (Henry and Moss 2005). In another observational study of 400 patients equally split between those with simple and those with perforated appendicitis, all patients had the wounds primarily closed. There was no statistical difference in the wound infection rates between the two groups with an overall wound infection rate of 3.7% (Mehrabi Bahar et al. 2010).

5 Open Versus Laparoscopic Surgery for Perforated Appendicitis

Only a surgeon proficient in minimally invasive surgery (MIS) should consider performing laparoscopic appendectomy in situations where perforation is suspected. The benefits of laparoscopy over the conventional technique are less clear in cases of perforation. A recent Cochrane review concluded that the benefits of laparoscopy included shorter hospital stay, reduced pain and earlier return to work and normal activity when compared to open appendectomy. A reduction in the negative appendectomy rate was also cited as a benefit of laparoscopy especially in fertile young women. The final recommendations were, however, restricted to patients without perforation as the authors' state in such cases the likelihood of postoperative intra-abdominal abscess formation is greater (Sauerland et al. 2010). The literature is divided on whether laparoscopic appendectomy in itself is likely to confer a greater risk of subsequent postoperative infective complications in patients with suspected perforated appendicitis. Several authors report that in complicated appendectomies patients who have undergone laparoscopic excisions are more likely to suffer from intra-abdominal abscess formation (Horwitz et al. 1997; Krisher et al. 2001). However, these findings are not reproduced in a large contemporary series (of 1,747 patients) which observed no outcome differences between LA and OA (Park et al. 2009). In a national study of LA versus OA rates of 89,497 children in England, no differences were observed in re-admission rates or mortality between the operative methods used (Faiz et al. 2008a). In a further study of 259,735 adult patients from England, LA conferred benefit in terms of reduced mortality and length of stay, but patients undergoing LA were re-admitted more often within 28 days of their original procedure (Faiz et al. 2008b). It must be noted, however, that in neither aforementioned studies, subgroup analysis was performed to determine any difference in outcome between simple and perforated appendicitis and the operative method utilized.

Some surgeons prefer commencing directly with OA in small children. Firstly, the OA wound in children is small and procedure times are generally shorter when this approach is employed. Furthermore no special equipment is required. Lastly, laparoscopy can be difficult when the size of the abdominal cavity is small and, as mentioned above, recovery appears similar irrespective of the surgical approach utilized.

In adults, the authors own preference is to commence with laparoscopic examination using an infra-umbilical incision. This allows for a diagnostic laparoscopy, attempted LA if this is deemed appropriate or alternatively conversion to open using an appropriately placed incision. The latter wound may represent a conventional McBurneys or Grid Iron incision or in rare cases a midline laparotomy depending on the clinical circumstances.

6 Treatment of Rarer Causes of Appendiceal Perforation

Causes of appendiceal perforation other than appendicitis is highlighted in Table 1. The former sections have dealt with treatment that relates to appendicitis. This section will consider the management of the less common causes of appendiceal perforation, namely perforation secondary to foreign bodies and malignancies.

6.1 Foreign Body Perforations

Perforations of the appendix due to foreign bodies have been reported in the literature ranging from ingestion of needles (Renner et al. 2000), pins (Bingham and King 1999) and fish bones (Ball 1967). In most cases of foreign body appendiceal perforation a standard appendectomy with removal of the foreign body is sufficient as treatment. This is obviously dependent on finding the foreign body in the first place, but most foreign bodies that go on to perforation are reported to be radio-opaque in the literature, thus there is likely to be a pre-operative clue (Klingler et al. 1998). If the foreign body is suspected pre-operatively, this should be sought at operation and removed. Similarly, if a foreign body is discovered at the time of operation it is important to search for any other areas of the bowel that may have been damaged either as the foreign body was traveling intra-luminally or post perforation. Fluoroscopy intra-operatively can also be used to help localize a pre-operatively suspected foreign body (Klingler et al. 1998).

6.2 Perforated Malignancies

Malignancies of the appendix are rare, however, treatment strategies in certain circumstances differ from that of a histologically benign appendiceal perforation. In order of incidence (most common first) mucinous adenocarcinoma, adenocarcinoma, carcinoid, goblet and signet-ring cell tumors are considered (McGory et al. 2005). It is rare to pre-operatively suspect an appendiceal perforation due to malignancy. Similarly it can also be difficult to distinguish a malignancy from an inflammatory process intra-operatively (Roberts et al. 2008). Some features which may lead to suspicion are enlarged mesenteric lymph nodes or the presence of a cystic lesion originating from the appendix itself. If an appendicular mucocele is discovered intra-operatively this should be handled with extreme caution so as to resect the cyst completely and without rupture. This is to reduce the possibility of disseminating cells that may lead to pseudomyxoma peritonei (Haritopoulos et al. 2001; Roberge and

Park 2006). In the case of obvious peritoneal disease, the primary resection should be undertaken with biopsies of the deposits as well and subsequent referral to specialist centers. However, more often than not, the diagnosis is made once the original histology is returned and thus the subsequent treatment should be tailored accordingly with consultation of an appropriate oncological multi-disciplinary team. Current guidelines specify that an appendectomy be performed for carcinoid tumors <1 cm if there are no features present that would dictate a more extensive resection. More extensive resections are indicated if there is lymphatic invasion or if there is lymph node involvement, spread to the mesoappendix or positive resection margins. Currently, right hemicolectomy (rather than an appendectomy) is indicated for carcinoid tumors >2 cm (McGory et al. 2005; Fornaro et al. 2007; Pinchot et al. 2008; Deschamps and Couvelard 2010). There is some debate, however, as to whether a more extensive resection such as a right hemi-colectomy confers actual survival benefit (Fornaro et al. 2007).

7 Conclusion

In this chapter the general and specific management strategies for the treatment of the perforated appendix are discussed. Rapid commencement of resuscitation in patients with a suspected perforated appendix is necessary. The initial condition of the patient will dictate the timing of surgical intervention, as will preoperative detection of an appendiceal abscess- which may favor radiological intervention with possible delayed surgery for those with recurrent symptoms or signs. Surgical follow-up with colonic imaging should be performed on every patient >40 years old that is initially conservatively managed for perforated appendicitis. Despite advancements in both medical and surgical care, deaths still occur as a result of a perforated appendix. Prompt surgical consultation and senior review is essential in managing these patients and thus mitigating this risk.

References

Amoli HA, Golozar A et al (2008) Morphine analgesia in patients with acute appendicitis: a randomised double-blind clinical trial. Emerg Med J 25:586–589

Andersson RE, Petzold MG (2007) Nonsurgical treatment of appendiceal abscess or phlegmon: a systematic review and meta-analysis. Ann Surg 246:741–748

Ball JR (1967) Complete perforation of appendix by a fish bone. Br J Clin Pract 21(2):99

Bingham S, King PA (1999) Sewing-pin perforation of the appendix into the bladder. Pediatr Surg Int 15(1):66–67

Bower RJ, Bell MJ et al (1981) Controversial aspects of appendicitis management in children. Arch Surg 116(7): 885–887

Brown CV, Abrishami M et al (2003) Appendiceal abscess: Immediate operation or percutaneous drainage? Am Surg 69(10):829–832

Chatwiriyacharoen W (2002) Surgical wound infection post surgery in perforated appendicitis in children. J Med Assoc Thai 85(5):572–576

Chiang RA, Chen SL et al (2006) Comparison of primary wound closure versus open wound management in perforated appendicitis. J Formos Med Assoc 105(10):791–795

David IB, Buck JR et al (1982) Rational use of antibiotics for perforated appendicitis in childhood. J Pediatr Surg 17(5): 494–500

Deakin DE, Ahmed I (2007) Interval appendicectomy after resolution of adult inflammatory appendix mass–is it necessary? Surgeon 5(1):45–50

Dellinger RP, Levy MM et al (2008) Surviving Sepsis Campaign: International guidelines for management of severe sepsis and septic shock. Crit Care Med 36(1): 296–327

Deschamps L, Couvelard A (2010) Endocrine tumors of the appendix: a pathologic review. Arch Pathol Lab Med 134(6): 871–875

Dixon MR, Haukoos JS et al (2003) An assessment of the severity of recurrent appendicitis. Am J Surg 186(6): 718–722; discussion 722

Faiz O, Blackburn SC et al (2008a) Laparoscopic, conventional appendicectomy in children: outcomes in English hospitals between 1996 and 2006. Pediatr Surg Int 24(11):1223–1227

Faiz O, Clark J et al (2008b) Laparoscopic, conventional appendicectomy in children: Outcomes in English hospitals between 1996 and 2006. Ann Surg 248(5):800–806

Fornaro R, Frascio M et al (2007) Appendectomy or right hemicolectomy in the treatment of appendiceal carcinoid tumors? Tumori 93(6):587–590

Gallagher EJ, Esses D et al (2006) Randomized clinical trial of morphine in acute abdominal pain. Ann Emerg Med 48(2): 150–160, 160 e151–154

Gillick J, Mohanan N et al (2008) Laparoscopic appendectomy after conservative management of appendix mass. Pediatr Surg Int 24(3):299–301

Goh BK, Chui CH et al (2005) Is early laparoscopic appendectomy feasible in children with acute appendicitis presenting with an appendiceal mass? A prospective study. J Pediatr Surg 40(7):1134–1137

Haritopoulos KN, Brown DC et al (2001) Appendiceal mucocoele: a case report and review of the literature. Int Surg 86(4):259–262

Henry MC, Gollin G et al (2007) Matched analysis of nonoperative management versus immediate appendectomy for perforated appendicitis. J Pediatr Surg 42(1):19–23; discussion 23–14

Henry MC, Moss RL (2005) Primary versus delayed wound closure in complicated appendicitis: an international systematic review and meta-analysis. Pediatr Surg Int 21(8):625–630
Hogan MJ (2003) Appendiceal abscess drainage. Tech Vasc Interv Radiol 6(4):205–214
Horwitz JR, Custer MD et al (1997) Should laparoscopic appendectomy be avoided for complicated appendicitis in children? J Pediatr Surg 32(11):1601–1603
Kaminski A, Liu IL et al (2005) Routine interval appendectomy is not justified after initial nonoperative treatment of acute appendicitis. Arch Surg 140(9):897–901
Klingler PJ, Seelig MH et al (1998) Ingested foreign bodies within the appendix: a 100 year review of the literature. Dig Dis 16(5):308–314
Kogut KA, Blakely ML et al (2001) The association of elevated percent bands on admission with failure and complications of interval appendectomy. J Pediatr Surg 36(1):165–168
Krisher SL, Browne A et al (2001) Intra-abdominal abscess after laparoscopic appendectomy for perforated appendicitis. Arch Surg 136(4):438–441
Lai HW, Loong CC et al (2006) Interval appendectomy after conservative treatment of an appendiceal mass. World J Surg 30(3):352–357
Lee SL, Islam S et al (2010) Antibiotics and appendicitis in the pediatric population: an American Pediatric Surgical Association Outcomes and Clinical Trials Committee Systematic Review. J Pediatr Surg 45(11):2181–2185
Lemieur TP, Rodriguez JL et al (1999) Wound management in perforated appendicitis. Am Surg 65(5):439–443
Lugo JZ, Avgerinos DV et al (2010) Can interval appendectomy be justified following conservative treatment of perforated acute appendicitis? J Surg Res 164(1):91–94
Mazziotti MV, Marley EF et al (1997) Histopathologic analysis of interval appendectomy specimens: Support for the role of interval appendectomy. J Pediatr Surg 32(6):806–809
McGory ML, Maggard MA et al (2005) Malignancies of the appendix: Beyond case series reports. Dis Colon Rectum 48(12):2264–2271
McGreal GT, Joy A et al (2002) Antiseptic wick: Does it reduce the incidence of wound infection following appendectomy? World J Surg 26(5):631–634
Mehrabi Bahar M, Jangjoo A et al (2010) Wound infection incidence in patients with simple and gangrenous or perforated appendicitis. Arch Iran Med 13(1):13–16
Morrow SE, Newman KD (2007) Current management of appendicitis. Semin Pediatr Surg 16(1):34–40
Newman K, Ponsky T et al (2003) Appendicitis 2000: variability in practice, outcomes, and resource utilization at thirty pediatric hospitals. J Pediatr Surg 38(3):372–379; discussion 372–379
Park HC, Yang DH et al (2009) The laparoscopic approach for perforated appendicitis, including cases complicated by abscess formation. J Laparoendosc Adv Surg Tech A 19(6):727–730
Pinchot SN, Holen K et al (2008) Carcinoid tumors. Oncologist 13(12):1255–1269
Puapong D, Lee SL et al (2007) Routine interval appendectomy in children is not indicated. J Pediatr Surg 42(9):1500–1503
Renner K, Holzer B et al (2000) Needle perforation of the appendix. Dig Surg 17(4):413–414
Roach JP, Partrick DA et al (2007) Complicated appendicitis in children: a clear role for drainage and delayed appendectomy. Am J Surg 194(6):769–772; discussion 772–763
Roberge RJ, Park AJ (2006) Mucocele of the appendix: an important clinical rarity. J Emerg Med 30(3):303–306
Roberts JK, Behravesh M et al (2008) Macroscopic findings at appendicectomy are unreliable: Implications for laparoscopy and malignant conditions of the appendix. Int J Surg Pathol 16(4):386–390
Samuel M, Hosie G et al (2002) Prospective evaluation of nonsurgical versus surgical management of appendiceal mass. J Pediatr Surg 37(6):882–886
Sauerland S, Jaschinski T et al (2010) Laparoscopic versus open surgery for suspected appendicitis. Cochrane Database Syst Rev 10: CD001546
Simillis C, Symeonides P et al (2010) A meta-analysis comparing conservative treatment versus acute appendectomy for complicated appendicitis (abscess or phlegmon). Surgery 147(6):818–829
St Peter SD, Valusek PA et al (2007) Does routine nasogastric tube placement after an operation for perforated appendicitis make a difference? J Surg Res 143(1):66–69
St Peter SD, Aguayo P et al (2010) Initial laparoscopic appendectomy versus initial nonoperative management and interval appendectomy for perforated appendicitis with abscess: a prospective, randomized trial. J Pediatr Surg 45(1):236–240
Styrud J, Eriksson S et al (1998) Treatment of perforated appendicitis: an analysis of 362 patients treated during 8 years. Dig Surg 15(6):683–686
Tekin A, Kurtoglu HC et al (2008) Routine interval appendectomy is unnecessary after conservative treatment of appendiceal mass. Colorectal Dis 10(5):465–468
Tsai HM, Shan YS et al (2006) Clinical analysis of the predictive factors for recurrent appendicitis after initial nonoperative treatment of perforated appendicitis. Am J Surg 192(3):311–316
Wallace MJ, Chin KW et al (2010) Quality improvement guidelines for percutaneous drainage/aspiration of abscess and fluid collections. J Vasc Interv Radiol 21(4):431–435
Weber TR, Keller MA et al (2003) Is delayed operative treatment worth the trouble with perforated appendicitis is children? Am J Surg 186(6):685–688; discussion 688–689
Willemsen PJ, Hoorntje LE et al (2002) The need for interval appendectomy after resolution of an appendiceal mass questioned. Dig Surg 19(3):216–220; discussion 221
Zerem E, Salkic N et al (2007) Comparison of therapeutic effectiveness of percutaneous drainage with antibiotics versus antibiotics alone in the treatment of periappendiceal abscess: is appendectomy always necessary after perforation of appendix? Surg Endosc 21(3):461–466

Part III

Imaging of Acute Appendicitis in Adults

Imaging of Acute Appendicitis in Adults: Radiography

Ronald L. Eisenberg

Contents

Abstract

The clinical symptoms of acute appendicitis can be so characteristic that there is no difficulty in making the correct diagnosis. In some patients, however, the clinical findings may be obscure or minimal. In these patients, imaging studies may be required to make a correct diagnosis and permit prompt surgical intervention before perforation occurs. Today, this is accomplished rapidly and accurately by ultrasound and computed tomography. In the past, abdominal radiography has traditionally been considered an essential part of the workup of patients presenting with acute abdominal pain. Although it has a low diagnostic yield, this procedure is still frequently performed in patients with abdominal pain suggestive of acute appendicitis to detect abnormal bowel gas patterns or an appendicolith. There is no current indication for barium enema examination for acute appendicitis, but a short presentation of this technique provides younger readers an idea of how appendicitis was diagnosed before the age of cross-sectional imaging.

1 Introduction

The clinical symptoms of acute appendicitis can be so characteristic that there is no difficulty in making the correct diagnosis. In some patients, however, the clinical findings may be obscure or minimal. In these patients, imaging studies may be required to make a correct diagnosis and permit prompt surgical intervention before perforation occurs. Today, this is

R. L. Eisenberg (✉)
Department of Radiology,
Beth Israel Deaconess Medical Center—
Harvard Medical School,
330 Brookline Avenue, Boston, MA 02215, USA
e-mail: rleisenb@bidmc.harvard.edu

C. Keyzer and P. A. Gevenois (eds.), *Imaging of Acute Appendicitis in Adults and Children*,
Medical Radiology. Diagnostic Imaging, DOI: 10.1007/174_2011_212,

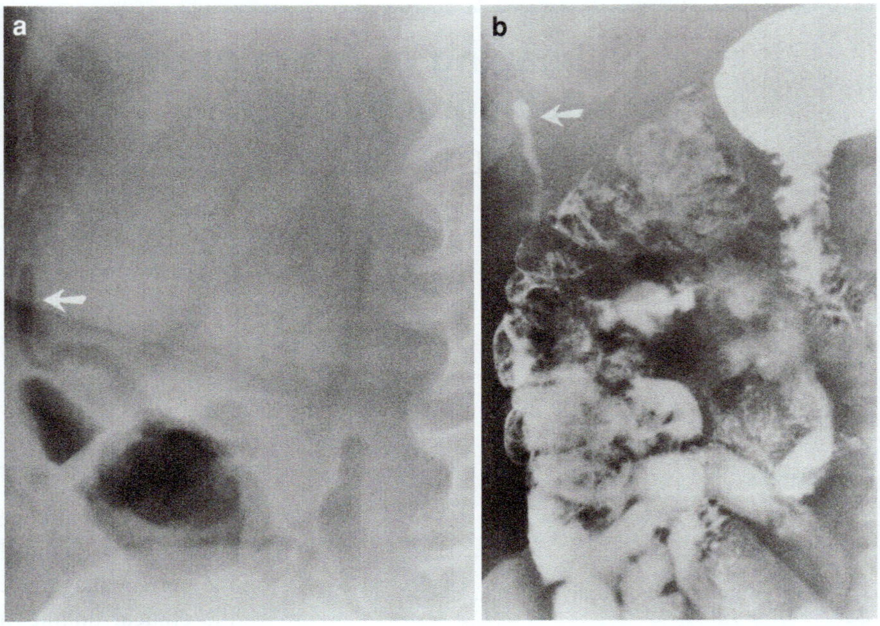

Fig. 1 Gas in a normal retrocecal appendix (*arrow*). **a** Plain abdominal radiograph and **b** barium enema examination

accomplished rapidly and accurately by ultrasound (US) and computed tomography (CT). In the past, however, conventional radiographs and barium enema examination were the only imaging tools available for making this diagnosis.

2 Conventional Radiography

Abdominal radiography has traditionally been considered an essential part of the workup of patients presenting with acute abdominal pain. However, the diagnostic yield of abdominal radiography is very poor, due to the inherent low soft-tissue contrast of the modality and the fact that many abdominal diseases do not have specific radiographic features. Indeed, one study reported a 0% sensitivity for acute appendicitis (as well as for pyelonephritis, pancreatitis, and diverticulitis) (Ahn et al. 2002). These authors conclude that abdominal radiography is not indicated in patients with a high clinical suspicion of intra-abdominal disease and that abdominal CT should be the initial imaging procedure. A more recent study reports a high incidence of positive CT and US imaging findings in patients with non-traumatic abdominal pain, even in more than 80% whose initial abdominal radiographs were interpreted as normal or nonspecific (Kellow et al. 2008). The authors argue that "when imaging is needed, the emergency physician should be encouraged to immediately request more definitive imaging abnormalities (e.g., US and/or CT)".

Although the empirical evidence so overwhelmingly favors eliminating abdominal radiography, this procedure is still frequently performed in patients with abdominal pain. It is unclear whether the emergency physician ordering this procedure actually expects to discover an abnormality on the abdominal radiograph, or whether the study was ordered merely to placate the patient, to assure someone with a low probability of disease that there was no acute abnormality (Eisenberg 2008).

In most patients with acute appendicitis, the bowel gas pattern is normal or "non-specific", with scattered loops of gas-containing bowel that are often mildly dilated but show no recognizable pattern indicating the underlying disease. Nevertheless, at times an abnormal gas collection or calcification may be a sign suggestive of acute appendicitis on conventional abdominal radiographs.

Air in the appendix is a normal finding, especially when the organ is located in a retrocecal location (Fig. 1). Extra luminal bubbles of air in the right lower quadrant, when associated with an ill-defined soft-tissue mass, suggest an appendiceal abscess (Jacobs and Balthazar 2008).

An isolated distended loop of small or large bowel, reflecting a localized adynamic ileus (so-called the sentinel loop), is often associated with an adjacent

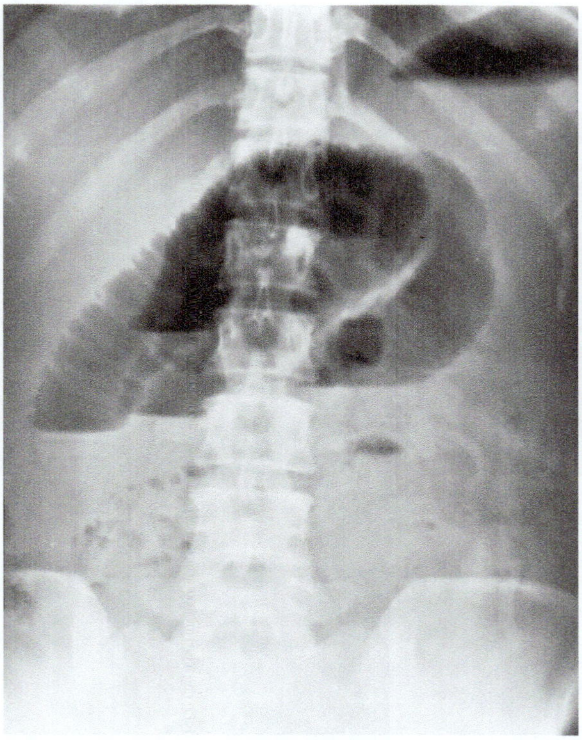

Fig. 2 Adynamic ileus in acute appendicitis. Although mechanical obstruction was suggested by the dilated small bowel loops with a paucity of distal gas, no evidence of obstruction was found at surgery

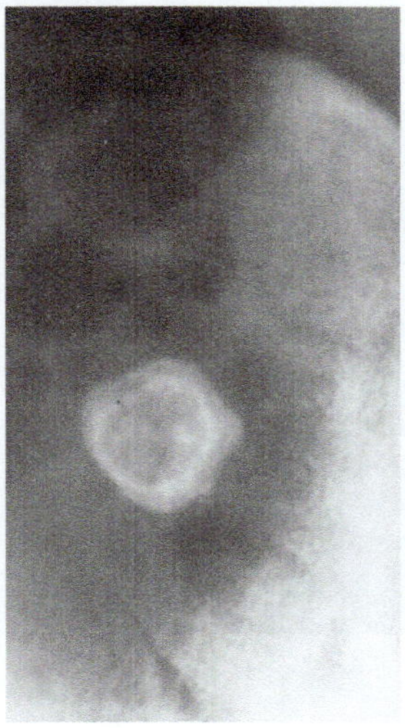

Fig. 3 Appendicolith. Laminated pattern of calcification in a stone overlying the right iliac bone

acute inflammatory process. The portion of the bowel involved may offer a clue to the underlying disease. Dilatation of the terminal ileum raises the possibility of acute appendicitis.

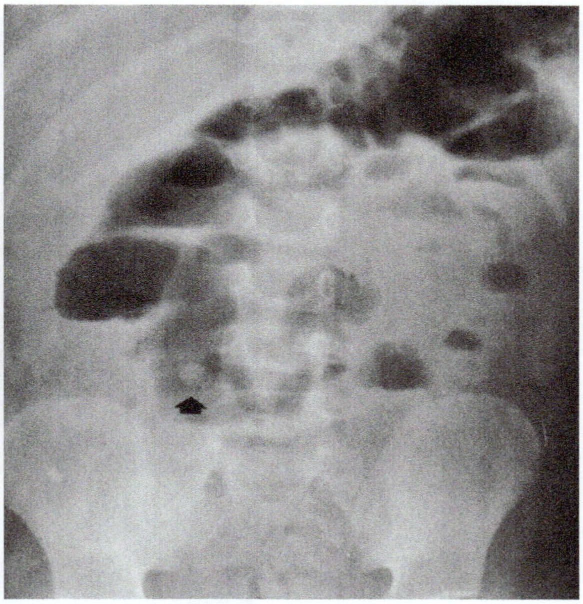

Fig. 4 Appendicolith (*arrow*) in acute appendicitis

Some inflammatory intra-abdominal processes can cause both a mechanical block and adynamic ileus. Both conditions may be present at the same time and produce a confusing appearance. For example, an acute periappendiceal abscess can cause true mechanical obstruction, with gas-fluid levels at different heights in the same loop, in addition to the characteristic adynamic ileus seen in patients with appendicitis (Fig. 2).

Whenever the diagnosis of acute appendicitis is being considered, it is essential that the right lower quadrant be examined for evidence of an appendicolith. These are round or oval, laminated stones of varying size (0.5–2 cm) that are found in about 10% of cases of acute appendicitis (Fig. 3). In the past, the radiographic demonstration of an appendicolith in a patient with fever, leukocytosis, and right lower quadrant pain was considered as highly suggestive of acute appendicitis (Fig. 4). Moreover, surgical experience suggested that the presence of an appendicolith in combination with symptoms of acute appendicitis usually implied that the appendix was gangrenous and likely to perforate. However, CT imaging has shown that small appendicoliths can be detected in patients without acute appendicitis, so that the presence of an appendicolith is now considered as only a secondary finding on this modality (Lane et al. 1999; Daly et al. 2005; Pereira et al. 2004; Benjaminov et al. 2002).

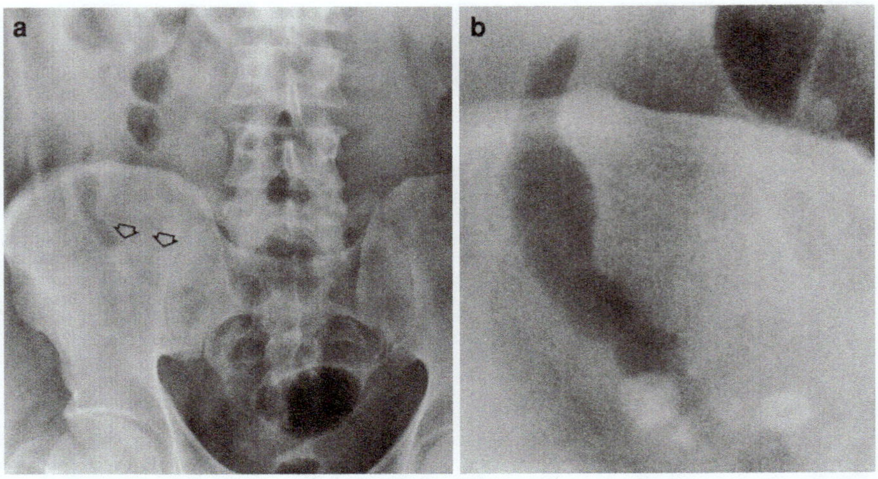

Fig. 5 Appendicoliths in a periappendiceal abscess. **a** Full and **b** coned views show that the appendicoliths (*arrows*) lie in an abscess outside of the gas-filled appendix

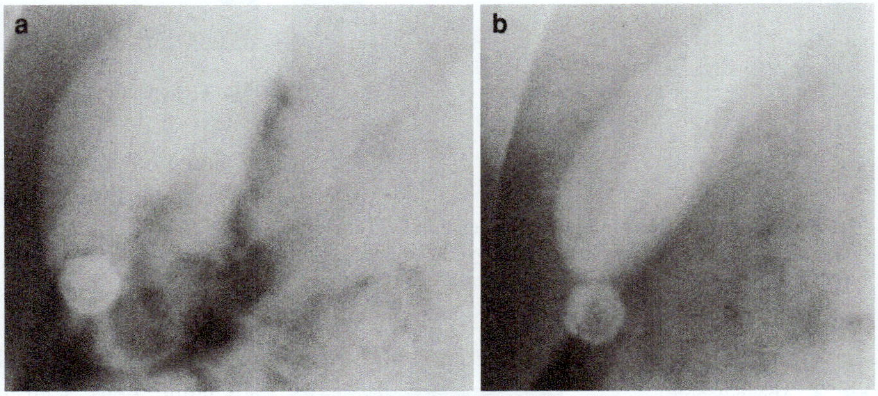

Fig. 6 Appendicolith in a retrocecal appendix mimicking a gallstone. **a** On a cholecystogram, the calcified appendicolith appears to lie in the opacified gallbladder. **b** After a fatty meal, the appendicolith is clearly seen to lie outside the confines of the shrunken gallbladder

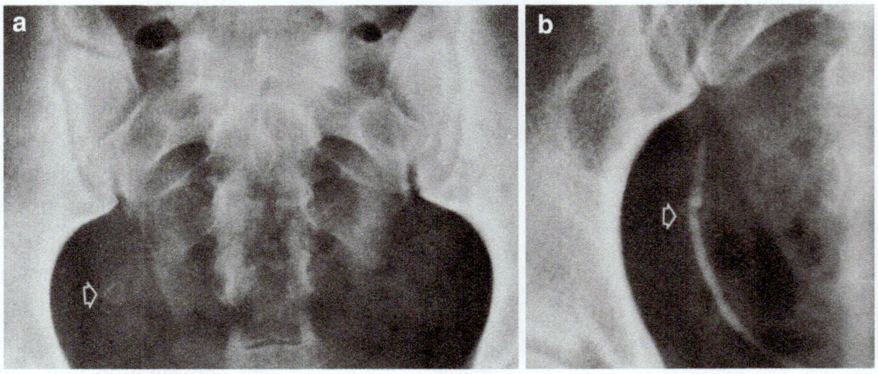

Fig. 7 Appendicolith mimicking a ureteral stone in a patient with hematuria. **a** Plain abdominal radiograph demonstrates a calcification in the region of the lower right ureter (*arrow*). **b** Excretory urogram shows the appendicolith (*arrow*) as separate from the nonobstructed right ureter

Appendicoliths are generally situated within the lumen of the appendix but in rare instances may penetrate through the wall and lie free in the peritoneal cavity or in a periappendiceal abscess (Fig. 5). Most appendicoliths are located in the right lower quadrant. Depending on the length and position of the appendix, an appendicolith can also be seen in the pelvis or in the right upper quadrant (in the case of a retrocecal appendix), where it can simulate a gallstone (Fig. 6). An appendicolith located near the midline can mimic a ureteral stone (Fig. 7); this is of great clinical significance because an inflamed

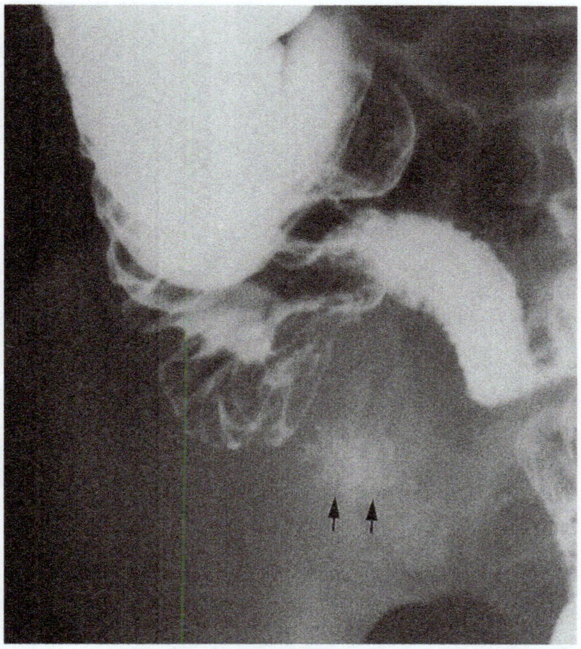

Fig. 8 Appendicitis. Barium enema shows a mass effect on the base of the cecum with no visualization of the appendix. Note the ill-defined calcification (*arrows*) representing an appendicolith within the inflammatory mass

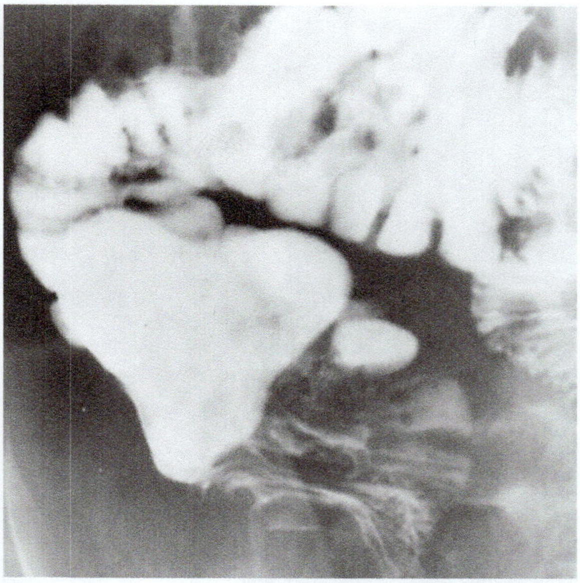

Fig. 9 Periappendiceal abscess. Fixation and a mass effect are seen at the base of the cecum, with no filling of the appendix

appendix in this region can cause hematuria and lead the physician to mistakenly suspect renal colic rather than appendicitis.

3 Barium Enema

There is no current indication for barium enema examination for acute appendicitis and this section is included purely for historical value. Nevertheless, it will give younger readers an idea of how appendicitis was diagnosed before the age of cross-sectional imaging.

When performing an emergency or semi-emergency barium enema in a patient suspected of having appendicitis, it is not necessary to prepare the colon with cleansing enemas or laxatives. Indeed, laxatives may actually be contraindicated. Once the barium reaches the cecum, it is important to evaluate the cecum in various degrees of obliquity to determine whether an extrinsic mass is present. Sequentially, lowering and raising the enema bag and using intravenous glucagon and post evacuation films are techniques that may help to obtain maximal filling of the appendix. It is impossible to be certain that the appendix is entirely filled unless a globular tip is seen.

Acute appendicitis and appendiceal abscesses can produce characteristic appearances on barium enema examinations. An irregular impression at the base of the cecum due to inflammatory edema, in association with failure of barium to enter to appendix, has been considered to be virtually pathognomonic of acute appendicitis (Fig. 8) or appendiceal abscess (Fig. 9). Nevertheless, failure of barium to fill the appendix alone is not a reliable sign of appendicitis because the appendix does not fill in about 20% of normal patients. Sometimes there is partial filling of the appendix with distortion in its shape or caliber. This appearance strongly suggests acute appendicitis, especially when there is a cecal impression. In contrast, a patent appendiceal lumen effectively excludes the diagnosis of acute appendicitis, especially when barium extends to fill the rounded appendiceal tip.

Although highly suggestive of acute appendicitis, especially when there are appropriate clinical symptoms, a mass impression on the cecum with nonfilling of the appendix can be caused by other pathologic entities. Endometriosis, ovarian cyst, and tube-ovarian abscess can produce an identical radiographic appearance. *Yersinia enterocolitis* is notorious for mimicking appendicitis clinically and occasionally may be associated with an

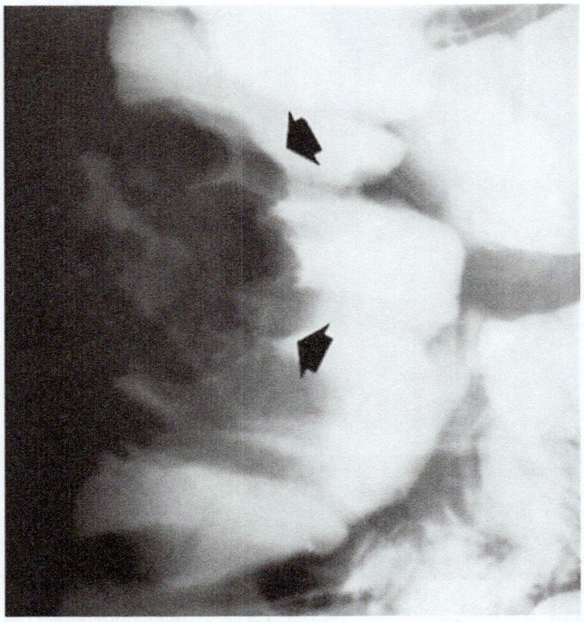

Fig. 10 Periappendiceal abscess. Severe inflammatory mucosal changes and a mass of the lateral aspect of the ascending colon (*arrows*) in a patient with a ruptured retrocecal appendix

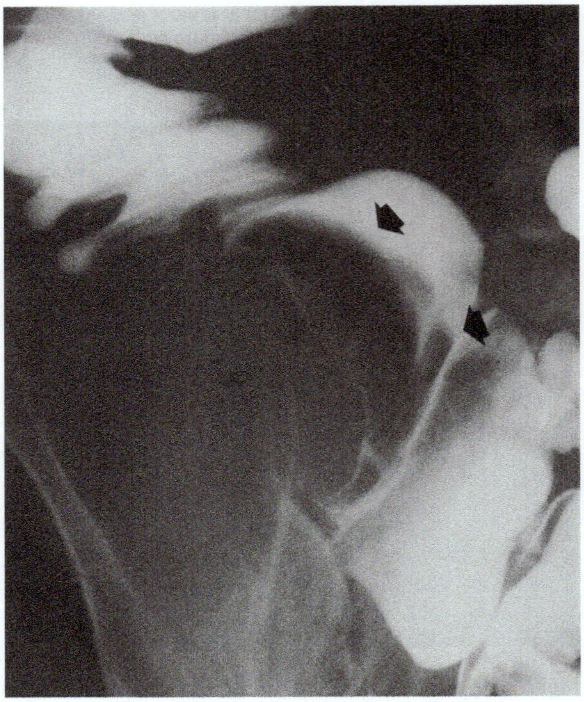

Fig. 11 Periappendiceal abscess. This large extrinsic mass involving the lateral aspect of the ascending colon (*arrows*) was seen in a patient with a ruptured retrocecal appendix

inflammatory process suggesting an appendiceal abscess. Crohn's disease is a well-known cause of right lower quadrant inflammatory processes and occasionally may produce a pattern indistinguishable from appendicitis. Patients with distal small bowel obstruction may have dilated fluid-filled loops of ileum causing extrinsic compression of the cecum that may mimic a pericecal inflammatory mass.

In the proper clinical context, most patients with nonfilling of the appendix and a large extrinsic compression of the base of the cecum have an appendiceal abscess. The contour defect in the cecum adjacent to an appendiceal abscess is accompanied by increased irritability and inflammatory edema of the mucosa, with local obliteration of cecal haustration (Fig. 10). Depending on the size and extent of the inflammatory process, the contour deformity may involve the cecum, ascending colon, bladder, ileum, ureter, adnexa, uterus, or sigmoid. In rare instances, barium enters the abscess cavity itself, implying that the appendiceal lumen has remained partially patent. Supine plain abdominal radiographs occasionally demonstrate a mottled gas pattern in an appendiceal abscess, and a gas-fluid level can sometimes be noted on upright or decubitus views.

In some patients, a large appendiceal inflammatory process may not involve the tip of the cecum. When the appendix is in a retrocecal position and the inflammatory process is limited to the tip of the appendix, there may be a more proximal mass on the posterolateral aspect of the cecum but sparring of the cecal tip (Fig. 11). In some patients, an appendiceal abscess may be entirely pelvic in location, with an extrinsic process involving the rectum or sigmoid but with no detectable pericecal component. In such cases, it may be impossible radiographically to exclude the possibility of an abscess arising from diverticulitis, pelvic inflammatory disease, or some other source. Appendiceal abscesses may be in locations remote from the right lower quadrant because of positional anomalies of the cecum and appendix or as a result of spread of the inflammatory process. Extension of the inflammatory process superiorly from the pelvis into the right or left paracolic gutter may result in a subdiaphragmatic or subhepatic abscess.

An oval, round, or finger-like filling defect resembling a coiled-spring in the medial wall of the cecum, when associated with non-filling of the appendix, may

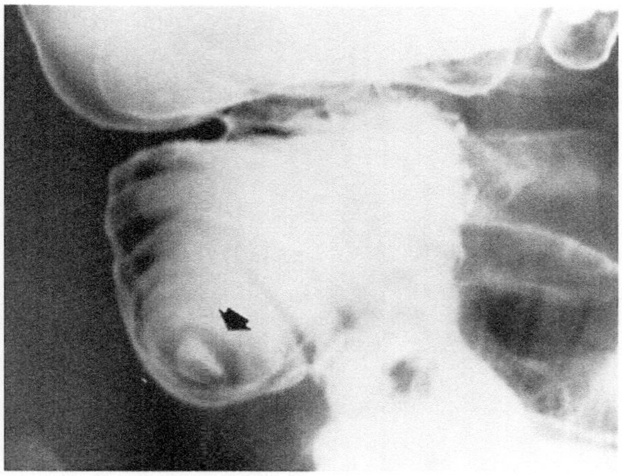

Fig. 12 Primary appendiceal intussception (*arrow*). After reduction, the cecum and appendix appeared normal on a subsequent barium enema examination

be an indication of acute appendicitis. However, this appearance also may represent an uncommon primary appendiceal intussusception (Fig. 12), in which the appendix invaginates into the cecum and simulates a cecal tumor, or even a mucocele, carcinoma, or endometriosis of the appendix.

Acknowledgments The author expresses thanks to Wolters Kluwer Publishers for permitting him to use illustrations from their book, Gastrointestinal Radiology: A Pattern Approach (4th edition). Philadelphia: Lippincott, 2002.

References

Ahn SH, Mayo-Smith WW, Murphy BL et al (2002) Acute nontraumatic abdominal pain in adult patients: abdominal radiography compared with CT evaluation. Radiology 225:159–164

Benjaminov O, Atri M, Hamilton P, Rappaport D (2002) Frequency of visualization and thickness of normal appendix at nonenhanced helical CT. Radiology 225:400–406

Daly CP, Cohan RH, Francis IR, Caoili EM, Ellis JH, Nan B (2005) Incidence of acute appendicitis in patients with equivocal CT findings. AJR 184:1813–1820

Eisenberg RL (2008) The role of abdominal radiography in the evaluation of the nontrauma emergency patient: new thoughts on an old problem. Radiology 248:715–716

Jacobs JE, Balthazar EJ (2008) Diseases of the appendix. In: Gore RM, Levine MS (eds). Textbook of gastrointestinal radiology, 3rd edn. Saunders, Philadelphia

Kellow Z, Macinnes M, Kurzebcwyg D et al (2008) The role of abdominal radiography in the evaluation of the nontrauma emergency patient. Radiology 248:887–893

Lane MJ, Liu DM, Huynh MD, Jeffrey RB Jr, Mindelzun RE, Katz DS (1999) Suspected acute appendicitis: nonenhanced helical CT in 300 consecutive patients. Radiology 213: 341–346

Pereira JM, Sirlin CB, Pinto PS, Jeffrey RB, Stella DL, Casola G (2004) Disproportionate fat stranding: a helpful CT sign in patients with acute abdominal pain. Radiographics 24:703–715

Imaging of Acute Appendicitis in Adults: Ultrasonography

R. Brooke Jeffrey

Contents

R. Brooke Jeffrey (✉)
Department of Radiology,
Stanford University School of Medicine,
300 Pasteur Drive, H1307, Stanford,
CA 94305-5105, USA
e-mail: bjeffrey@stanford.edu

Abstract
Although ultrasound has been used diagnostically in patients with right lower quadrant pain and possible appendicitis since the 1980s, there has recently been renewed interest in this technique due to increasing concerns over radiation exposure with abdominal CT. Although overall slightly less accurate than CT for the diagnosis of appendicitis, ultrasonography has several distinct advantages, such as lack of ionizing radiation or intravenous contrast and low cost. Keys to success for this technique include a thorough understanding of the graded-compression technique using both gray-scale and color-Doppler sonography. In addition, the concept of "staging of appendicitis" is presented, since different treatment options may be selected for patients who have gangrenous or perforated appendicitis, rather than the standard laparoscopic appendectomy for early uncomplicated appendicitis. Finally, alternative diagnoses of the gastrointestinal and genitourinary tract that clinically mimic appendicitis are discussed.

1 Clinical Overview

Appendicitis was first described as a distinct pathologic entity in 1886 by Reginald Fitz, who recognized that the appendix, rather than the cecum, was the primary source of inflammation (Fitz 1886). To the present day, appendicitis remains an important clinical problem, and is the most common cause of the acute abdomen requiring surgical intervention in the

C. Keyzer and P. A. Gevenois (eds.), *Imaging of Acute Appendicitis in Adults and Children*,
Medical Radiology. Diagnostic Imaging, DOI: 10.1007/174_2011_223,

Western world (de Dombal 1994). Each year in the United States there are over 250,000 appendectomies performed, and the lifetime risk for developing appendicitis is estimated at 7% in females and 9% in males (Wagner et al. 1996). Despite our familiarity with this disease and its ongoing clinical importance, the challenge of clinical diagnosis of appendicitis in a substantial number of patients is formidable. The classic symptom complex of periumbilical pain followed by nausea and vomiting with pain migrating to the right lower quadrant may be absent in up to one-third of patients (Addiss et al. 1990). In addition, the clinical difficulty in distinguishing acute appendicitis from acute gynecologic disorders has been well documented by many observers due to the broad overlap of clinical symptomatology (Bendeck et al. 2002). If surgery is performed on the clinical findings alone, the negative appendectomy rate in women of reproductive age is approximately 28% (Bendeck et al. 2002).

Depending on the pathologic stage of appendicitis and the degree of inflammatory response, a wide variety of treatment options exist. In the vast majority of patients with early, uncomplicated appendicitis, prompt surgery, most often via laparoscopic appendectomy, is the therapy of choice (Garbutt et al. 1999; Hansen et al. 1996). However, once perforation develops it is important to clinically differentiate patients with liquefied abscesses versus those patients with merely indurated periappendiceal inflammatory masses (periappendiceal phlegmon) (Jeffrey et al. 1988). A small periappendiceal abscess may be treated surgically; however, there is some evidence to suggest that laparoscopic appendectomy via insufflation of a large amount of gas into the peritoneal cavity may in fact increase the incidence of postoperative abscess and wound infection (Pokala et al. 2007; Yau et al. 2007) In these patients, an open surgical approach with either a midline or McBurney incision may be preferred. In other patients with larger periappendiceal abscesses, percutaneous drainage guided by imaging is a safe and effective treatment method. Conversely, patients with periappendiceal phlegmons without liquefied abscesses are often best managed alone by primary antibiotic therapy (Jeffrey et al. 1988). In selected instances, interval appendectomy can be performed at a later date once the inflammatory process has resolved, but a number of studies have shown that this is not mandatory or cost effective (Raval et al. 2010; Keckler et al. 2008). Because of the wide variety of treatment options, not only is it important for the radiologist to establish the diagnosis of appendicitis, but also to determine whether perforation is likely and if there is a liquefied abscess or phlegmon. Treatment of acute appendicitis and appendiceal perforation is further discussed in "Laparoscopy and Laparotomy" and "Treatment of Appendiceal Perforation" by Mamidanna, Almoudaris and Faiz.

2 Role of Sonography and CT

For the past two decades, sonography and CT have been widely utilized in the preoperative diagnosis and management of patients with suspected acute appendicitis (Birnbaum and Wilson 2000; Strouse 2010; Puylaert 1986, 1988; Puylaert et al. 1987; Raja et al. 2010; Coursey et al. 2010; McDonald et al. 2001). In male patients with a classic symptom complex and physical findings indicating appendicitis, there is little evidence to support routine preoperative CT or sonography (Bendeck et al. 2002). Male patients with atypical signs and symptoms, however, may benefit from preoperative imaging (Bendeck et al. 2002). In pediatric patients it is often difficult to obtain an accurate history and perform a reliable physical examination, and routine preoperative imaging with sonography should strongly be considered.

Much has been made in the imaging literature of the "operator dependency" in the performance of sonography (Strouse 2010). This is undoubtedly true, and there is a clear learning curve to becoming proficient in the graded-compression technique. Nevertheless, it is also important to point out that although the creation of images is standardized and automated with the performance of CT, interpretation can be quite difficult, particularly in thin patients with little intra-abdominal fat. Therefore, interpretation of CT often requires considerable experience in order to achieve optimal results. Intravenous or oral contrast, or both, is also required for accurate diagnosis in these patients. It is, therefore, important for radiologists to work with their clinical colleagues to optimize referrals for the appropriate imaging modalities.

Sonography is most accurate in patients who are either thin or of normal body habitus. Computed tomography often relies on identification of periappendiceal fat stranding for the diagnosis of appendicitis, and this is often difficult to assess in very thin patients. Conversely, obese patients are often a challenge with sonography, as it is often difficult to obtain adequate penetration in order to adequately visualize the iliac fossa. In patients with appendiceal perforation, pain from peritoneal signs often precludes adequate graded compression. These patients often present with prolonged symptom duration (>48 h), high fever and leukocytosis (Jeffrey et al. 1988; Borushok and Jeffrey 1990). The pregnant female patient presents another distinct challenge, and graded compression may be quite difficult past the first trimester. There has been a trend toward the utilization of MR in pregnant patients with suspected appendicitis due to the concern for ionizing radiation from CT (Oto et al. 2009; Singh et al. 2007). Current imaging practice in pregnant women suspected of acute appendicitis is further discussed in "Imaging of Acute Appendicitis in Adults: Current Practices in Pregnant Women" by Jaffe.

When comparing the overall accuracy of sonography and CT, most studies have consistently demonstrated CT to have a higher sensitivity and specificity (see "Ultrasonography Versus Computed Tomography: Evidence-Based Imaging" by Keyzer) (Hermanz-Schulman 2010; Doria AS 2009; Poortman et al. 2009; Wan et al. 2009; Gaitini et al. 2008; Rybkin and Thoeni 2007; Johansson et al. 2007; Doria et al. 2006; Kaiser et al. 2002). Nevertheless, the lower cost and lack of ionizing radiation are compelling arguments for sonography. Over the past decade there has been an increased concern about the potential harmful effects of radiation exposure with CT (Brody et al. 2007). Due to the lifetime accumulated risk of radiation exposure, this is of particular relevance to patients with suspected appendicitis because the majority of patients are pediatric patients or young adult (Addiss et al. 1990). It has been estimated that, with the assumption of a radiation dose of 5 mSv for a single-phase abdominal CT, the lifetime risk of radiation-induced cancer for a 5-year-old girl is 26.1 per 100,000, and 20.4 per 100,000 for a 5-year-old boy (Addiss et al. 1990; Hall and Brenner 2008). Radiation issues and dose optimization for abdominal CT in children and adults is further discussed in "Imaging of Acute Appendicitis in Children: Computed Tomography Including Radiation Issues" by Spencer and in "Radiation Dose from MDCT Examinations for Suspected Acute Appendicitis" by Tack. The cost of contrast-enhanced CT is many fold greater than sonography, and therefore, in children, it appears more cost effective to initially screen patients with ultrasound, then perform CT if sonography is negative (see "US Versus CT: Evidence-Based Medicine and Cost-Effectiveness in Imaging Acute Appendicitis in Children" by Kamat, Garcia-Pena, Blackmore and Medina) (Wan et al. 2009).

In summary, sonography performs best in thin patients with suspected early appendicitis, pediatric patients and female patients of reproductive age. Computed tomography is often the imaging method of choice in patients who are obese or are suspected of having possible appendiceal perforation.

3 Sonographic Technique

The graded-compression sonographic technique for imaging the right lower quadrant for appendicitis was first described by Puylaert (1986) using linear-array transducers (Puylaert 1988). Over the ensuing two decades this technique has largely been refined with the use of higher-resolution linear probes, the introduction of color- and power-Doppler imaging, and higher-frequency curved-array transducers (Birnbaum and Wilson 2000). The graded-compression technique relies on the principle that normal bowel loops are readily compressible with mild to moderate application of pressure; however, the inflamed and obstructed appendix will not compress. Compression is particularly valuable to express bowel gas and fluid from the cecum and terminal ileum, in order to visualize the inflamed appendix that will not compress. Achieving excellent results with graded-compression sonography requires not only state-of-the-art equipment, but also dedication and experience.

Prior to scanning the adult patient, a brief history is obtained. The patient should always be asked to point with a single finger to his/her site of maximal pain. This maneuver of "self localization" of the pain is often very helpful for the sonographer (Chesbrough et al. 1993). It may provide an important clue to an aberrantly positioned appendix or a site of other pathology. In addition, in patients who are unable to localize their pain and do not have a focal point of maximal tenderness, the suspicion for appendicitis is often much lower. Chesbrough et al. (1993) demonstrated in a series of

236 patients referred to sonography for possible appendicitis that 85% (121 of 142) patients, when handed the transducer and asked to localize their pain, were able to localize it to a specific site. Conversely, in patient without significant disease in the right lower quadrant, only 15% were able to localize their pain (Chesbrough et al. 1993).

Following self-localization of maximal pain, the examination begins with a linear-array transducer, often 8–12 MHz; in very thin patients, 12–14 MHz may be adequate for penetration. The scan is performed initially in the transverse plane using light pressure from the edge of the liver tip, slowly migrating caudally to the iliac fossa. An attempt is made to identify the hepatic flexure, ascending colon, and ultimately the cecum. Light pressure is used initially in order not to elicit peritoneal signs and make the patient uncomfortable. The right colon is the largest structure having the sonographic signature of the gut layers (specifically the echogenic submucosal layer and the hypoechoic muscular layer), and should be readily compressed in the normal patient. The initial scanning sweeps are performed with very light pressure in order not to make the patient more uncomfortable. As the transducer is slowly migrated into the iliac fossa, application of pressure by the transducer is gently increased in order to express bowel gas and fluid from the cecum. An attempt is then made to identify the point of insertion of the peristalsing terminal ileum into the cecum, which denotes the region of the ileocecal valve. The cecal tip is then visualized with moderate pressure at this point.

Although the tip of the appendix may be in an ectopic or aberrant location, the base of the appendix invariably arises from the cecal caput, and therefore visualizing the termination of the cecum is essential for appreciating the origin of the base of the appendix. If the appendix is not visualized, more successive medial sweeps are then identified in succession until the anatomic landmarks have been fully elucidated. Important anatomic landmarks in the iliac fossa include the iliopsoas muscle and the external iliac artery and vein. Unless there is sufficient penetration with the scanning transducer to visualize these landmarks, a lower-frequency linear-array transducer or a curved-array transducer should be utilized. In moderate to severely obese patients, however, a linear-array transducer may not be adequate for penetration, and therefore, a curved-array transducer has the advantage of depth of penetration and wider field of view; 5–7 MHz curved-array transducers are often employed in these patients.

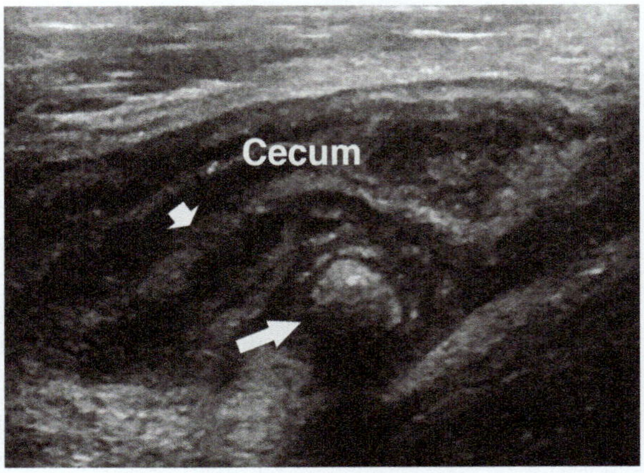

Fig. 1 Coronal view of cecum to visualize retrocecal appendicitis. By turning patient into steep left posterior oblique position and scanning in parasagittal plane, near-coronal acquisition can be obtained to visualize retrocecal space. Note mural thickening of cecum, with prominence of echogenic submucosal layer indicating edema (*short white arrow*). Note appendicolith within enlarged appendix, consistent with retrocecal appendicitis (*long white arrow*)

The original graded-compression technique described by Puylaert used only the pressure on the anterior abdominal wall from the handheld transducer (Puylaert 1986, 1988; Puylaert et al. 1987). Lee et al. (2002) has, since modified this technique to include simultaneous posterior manual compression as an adjunct in patients in whom the appendix is not visualized by the standard anterior approach. We have found this particularly useful in patients with retrocecal pathology, including retrocecal appendicitis or retrocecal perforation of cecal diverticulitis. If the appendix is not visualized in the transverse plane, it may be very useful to perform a dedicated maneuver to directly visualize the retrocecal appendix by having the patient turn in a left posterior oblique position, and scanning in a parasagittal plane to reproduce a coronal view of the retroperitoneal space behind the cecum (Fig. 1). Retrocecal appendices are often very challenging to visualize from a transverse anterior approach, and therefore, this dedicated maneuver in addition to posterior manual compression is often valuable for the laterally positioned appendix in the retrocecal position.

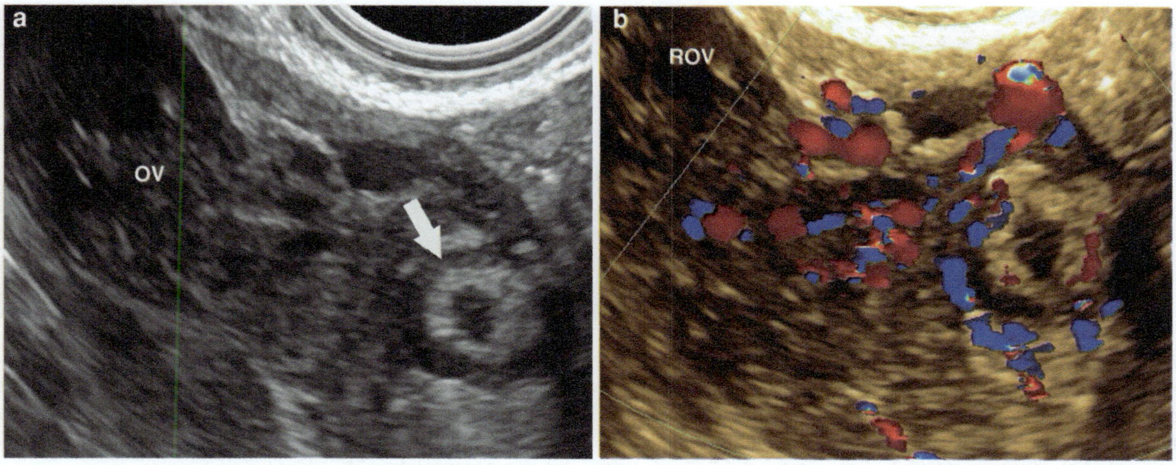

Fig. 2 **a, b** Value of endovaginal probe for detection of pelvic appendicitis. Note identification of inflamed appendix in short axis (*white arrow*) adjacent to right ovary ("OV") on grayscale endovaginal sonogram. In **b**, color Doppler endovaginal sonogram, note marked hyperemia around inflamed appendix. Appendix could not be visualized via anterior transabdominal approach

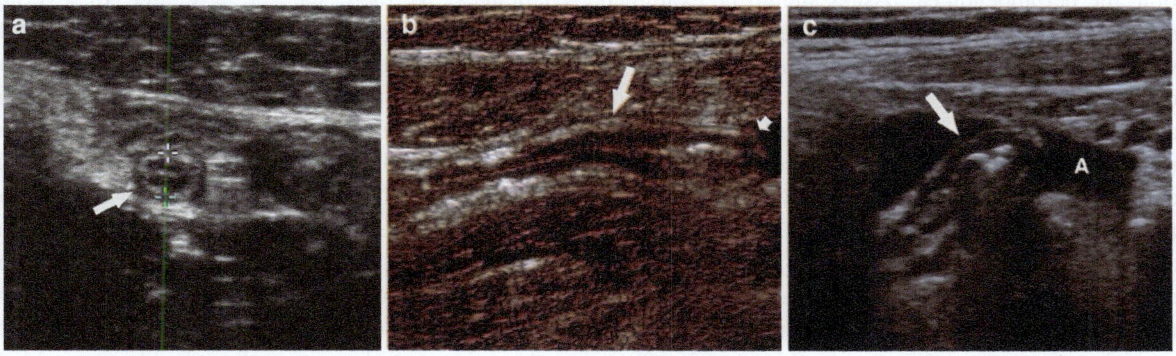

Fig. 3 **a, b, c** Normal appendices in three different patients. In **a**, note ovoid-appearing appendix scanned in short axis (*arrow*). In **b**, note normal appendix seen in long axis (*long arrow*) with bulbous, slightly enlarged tip of normal appendix, ending in blind pouch (*short white arrow*). In **c**, normal appendix is noted in right lower quadrant, containing gas in distal lumen (*white arrow*). Note adjacent ascites ("A")

In adult female patients, it is essential to always perform scans with an endovaginal probe to assess ovaries and fallopian tubes. Pelvic appendicitis in many patients can only be visualized with an endovaginal probe, and therefore, relying solely on linear-array transducers from an anterior abdominal approach will often be inadequate (Fig. 2). Similarly, the endovaginal probe may be used to visualize the ureteral insertion into the bladder and may be helpful to diagnose distal ureteral calculi (Laing et al. 1994).

Once a normal or abnormal appendix is identified, it is important to scan both longitudinally and transversely throughout its entire course to confirm that one is actually visualizing the appendix, due to its blind-ending pouch. It is a common pitfall to misconstrue the terminal ileum for the appendix; however, by rigidly adhering to the principle that the appendix must originate from the cecal tip and end in a blind pouch, this pitfall can be avoided. It is also important to recognize that early appendicitis may only be confined to the tip of the appendix, and therefore visualization of the blind-ending pouch is essential to avoid missing tip appendicitis (Nghiem and Jeffrey 1992; Lim et al. 1996). Once the appendix has been identified, specific observation should be made in real time on the degree of compressibility,

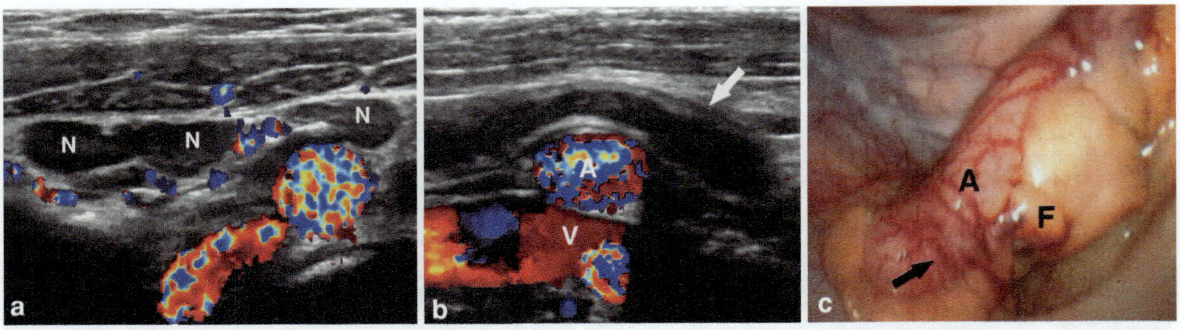

Fig. 4 **a, b, c** Appendicitis associated with enlarged mesenteric lymph nodes in young adult. In **a**, color Doppler sonogram demonstrates multiple enlarged mesenteric nodes ("N"). In **b**, note enlarged appendix with distended fluid-filled lumen (*arrow*) draped over external iliac artery ("A") and vein ("V"). Note that echogenic submucosal layer of appendix is visible throughout length of appendix, and at surgery early appendicitis was noted without evidence of gangrenous change. Figure **c** is laparoscopic view of inflamed appendix ("A"); note engorged blood vessels at appendiceal tip (*arrow*) and inflamed fat in mesoappendix ("F")

and its maximal anteroposterior (AP) diameter should be measured at the site of largest diameter. In addition, the periappendiceal tissues should be examined specifically for edema within the mesoappendix, which produces an echogenic mass often triangular or ovoid in appearance immediately adjacent to the appendix. The use of color Doppler has become routine, particularly in patients who have borderline appendicitis by size criteria (Lim et al. 1996). Normal flow of the vasa recta in the bowel wall is not visualized with the ultrasound technology currently available, and therefore any appreciable flow confirmed by spectral Doppler should immediately raise suspicion for acute appendicitis (Lim et al. 1996). Edema within the mesoappendix increases acoustic interfaces, and therefore, inflamed fat is characteristically hyperechoic on sonography (Borushok and Jeffrey 1990). Color-Doppler imaging may also be valuable to identify areas of infarction within the appendix. Often there is focal loss of visualization of the echogenic submucosal layer in conjunction with absent flow in this portion of the appendix. This should prompt consideration for gangrenous appendicitis (Jeffrey 1989; Yacoe 1994).

4 Sonographic Criteria for the Diagnosis of Appendicitis

The most widely utilized criterion for the sonographic diagnosis of appendicitis has reliance on the identification of a non-compressible appendix with a maximal AP diameter 6 mm or greater. However, reliance on a single measurement does pose some challenges, as there can be a degree of overlap between the size of the normal appendix (usually felt to be 5 mm or less) and early appendicitis. Use of 6 mm or greater as the threshold for diagnosing appendicitis results in nearly 100% sensitivity, but specificity is only 68% (Rettenbacher et al. 2001). However, by utilizing a 7 mm or greater criteria for acute appendicitis, Rettenbacher et al. (2001) noted a sensitivity of 94% and a specificity of 88%. In patients with "borderline" appendices that range in maximal AP diameters from 5 to 6 mm, other secondary signs can be extremely valuable to establish the diagnosis. The identification of intramural flow in the appendix should always be considered suspicious for appendicitis, and therefore, may be a very useful clue in borderline cases (Lim et al. 1996). Similarly, the identification of inflamed echogenic fat within the mesoappendix is also a very helpful secondary sign (Noguchi 2005).

The normal appendix is compressible, often resulting in an ovoid configuration, and has a maximal AP diameter of 5 mm or less (Rettenbacher et al. 2003; Lee 2003) (Fig. 3). There is generally no visible color-Doppler flow within the wall of the normal appendix (Jeffrey et al. 1994). Linear high-amplitude echoes casting reverberation artifacts ("dirty distal acoustic shadowing") indicate gas within the appendix (Fig. 3). Reliance on the presence of intraluminal gas, however, should not be utilized exclusively as a criterion for the normal appendix, as in some patients

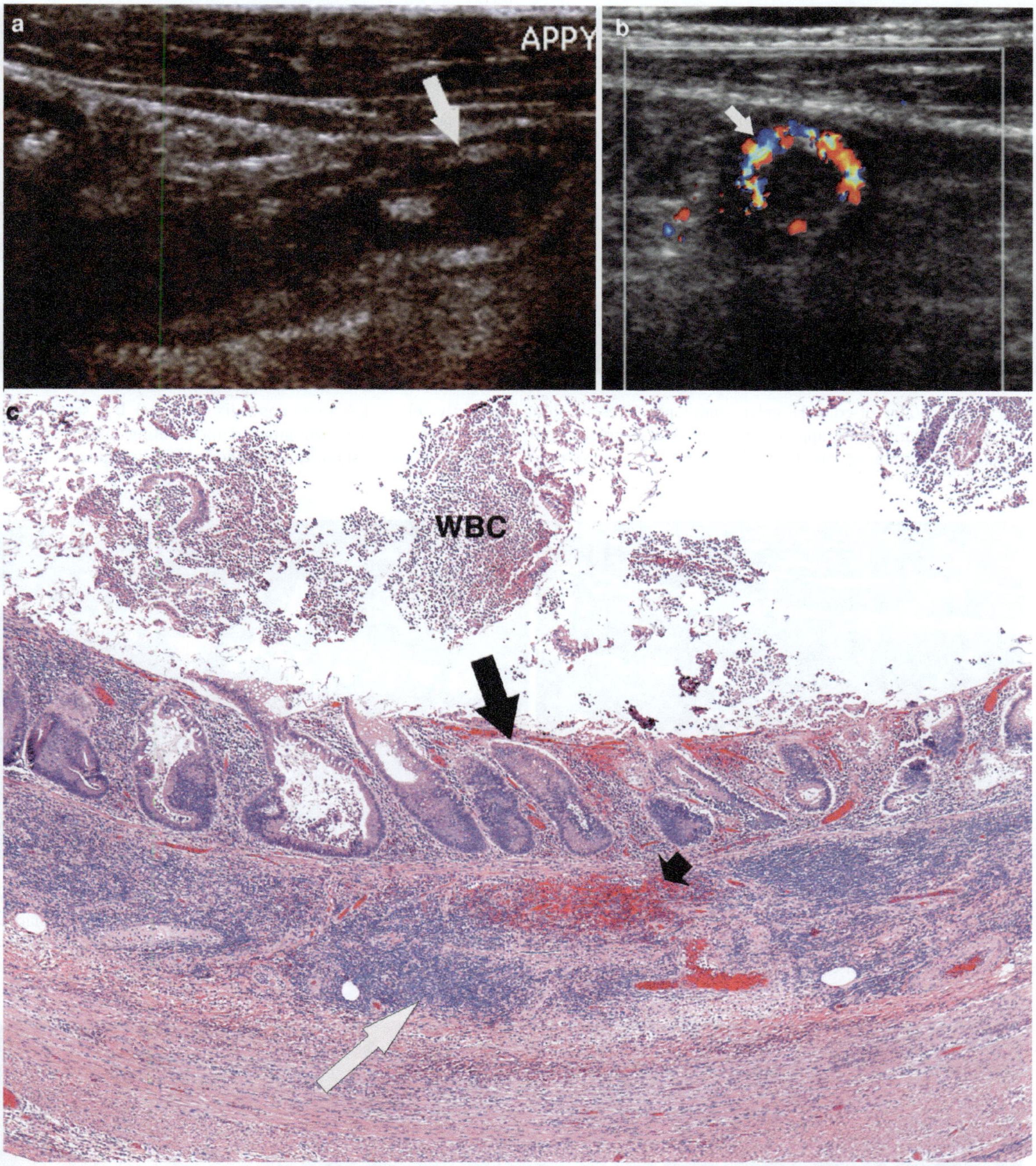

Fig. 5 **a, b, c** Early uncomplicated acute appendicitis. In **a**, grayscale sonogram of long axis of distended appendix, note preserved echogenic submucosal layer at distal end of appendix (*arrow*). In **b**, transverse color Doppler sonogram of short axis of appendix demonstrates mural hyperemia (*arrow*). Figure **c** is histologic section of appendiceal wall in same patient demonstrating white cell debris within appendiceal lumen ("WBC"). Columnar epithelium of appendiceal mucosa is preserved (*long black arrow*), and there is intramural hemorrhage (*short black arrow*) and inflammatory infiltrate in wall (*long white arrow*), indicating acute appendicitis. No evidence of mural necrosis or perforation

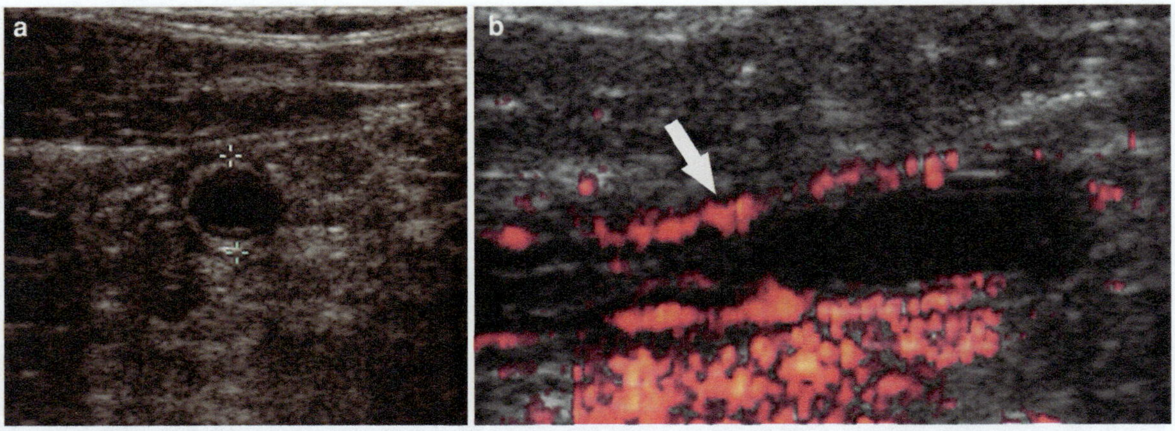

Fig. 6 **a, b** Value of color Doppler sonography in establishing diagnosis of early acute appendicitis. Transverse graded-compression sonogram of short axis of appendix demonstrates slightly enlarged, 6.5 mm appendix (calipers). **b** in same patient is power Doppler sonogram demonstrating hyperemia and intramural flow, establishing diagnosis of early acute appendicitis

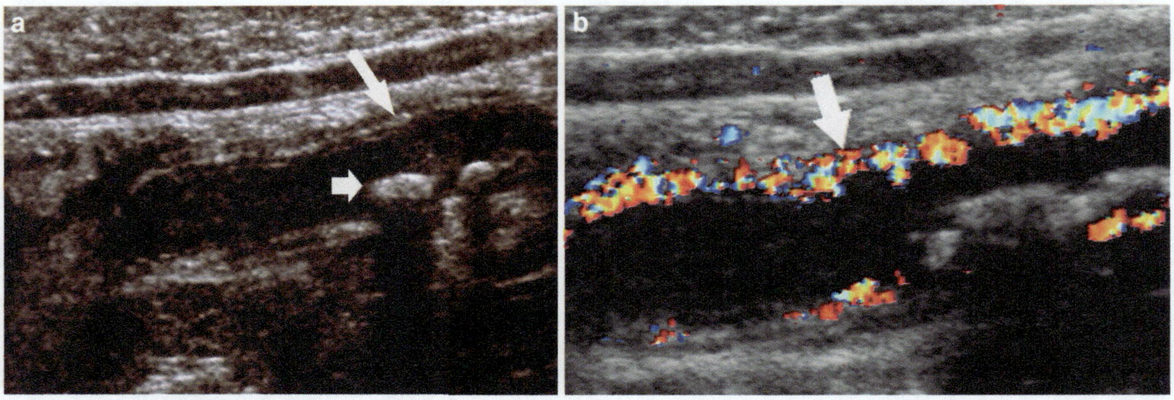

Fig. 7 **a, b** Value of color Doppler in establishing diagnosis of early, uncomplicated acute appendicitis. **a** is graded-compression grayscale long-axis sonogram of appendix demonstrating preservation of normal echogenic submucosal line (*long white arrow*); note appendicoliths within distal appendix (*short arrow*). **b** is color Doppler sonogram demonstrating marked mural hyperemia (*white arrow*), establishing diagnosis of early acute appendicitis

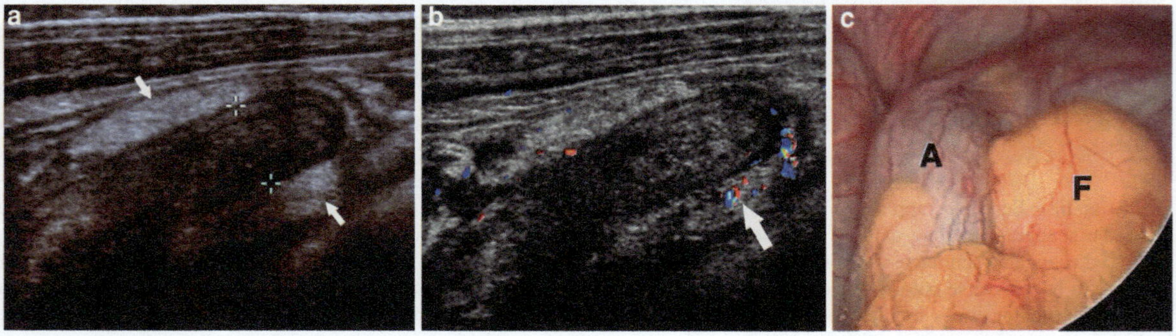

Fig. 8 **a, b, c** Early acute appendicitis with echogenic periappendiceal fat within mesoappendix. In **a**, grayscale graded-compression sonogram of long axis of appendix, notice dilated appendix (calipers). In addition, there is echogenic fat within mesoappendix (*white arrows*). In **b**, color Doppler sonogram demonstrates slight hyperemia with visible vessels within inflamed periappendiceal fat (*arrow*). **c** is laparoscopic image of inflamed appendix ("A") with adjacent hyperemic mesoappendiceal fat ("F")

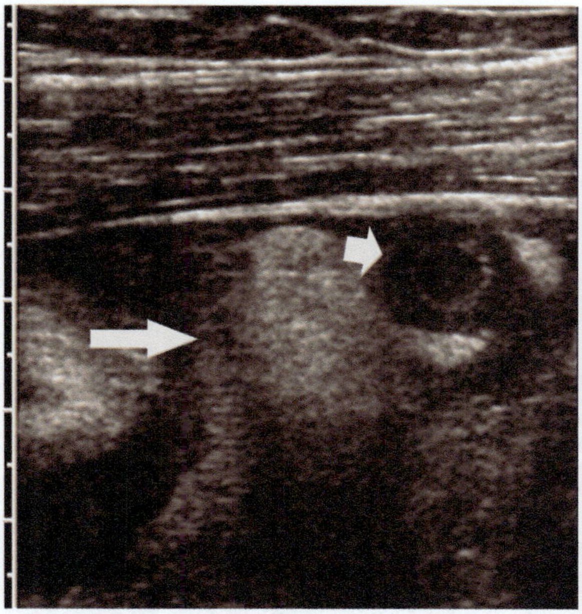

Fig. 9 Inflamed periappendiceal fat as secondary sign of appendicitis. Grayscale sonogram through short axis of appendix (*short arrow*) demonstrates mural thickening of wall of appendix. Note prominent echogenic fat adjacent to inflamed appendix (*long arrow*)

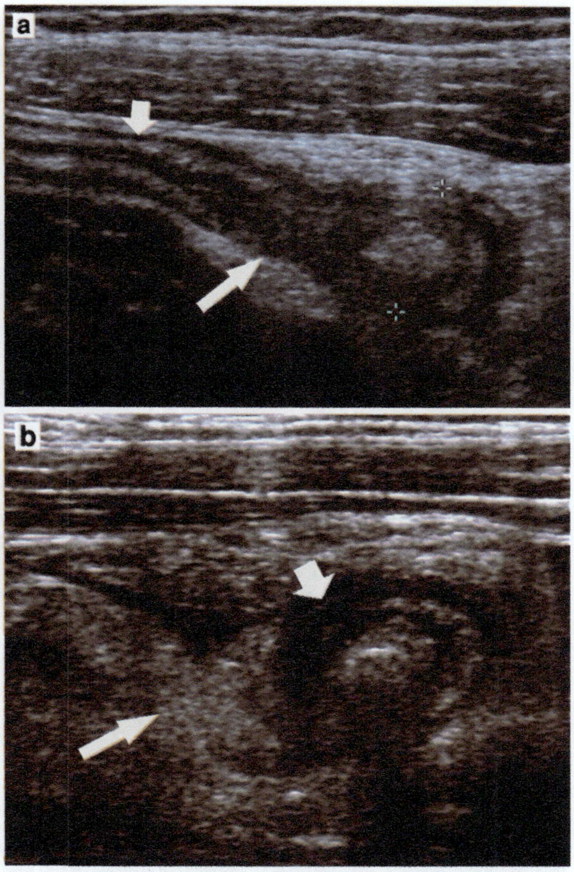

Fig. 10 **a, b** Tip appendicitis with early gangrenous change. **a** is grayscale long-axis sonogram of appendix demonstrating normal proximal appendix with preserved echogenic submucosal layer (*short arrow*). Distal tip of appendix is enlarged (calipers); note focal loss of echogenic submucosal layer in distal third of appendix (*long arrow*). In **b**, transverse scan through short axis of appendix, note prominent echogenic inflamed periappendiceal fat (*long arrow*). Note focal loss of echogenic submucosal layer adjacent to this fat (*short arrow*). At surgery, tip appendicitis with early gangrenous change was noted

gas-forming appendiceal intraluminal abscesses may produce a similar finding (Jeffrey et al. 1994; Poljak et al. 1991).

Having identified the normal appendix, an attempt should be made to establish alternative diagnosis by carefully scanning again where the patient points to a site of maximal tenderness (van Breda Vriesman and Puylaert 2006; Jain et al. 1996; Townsend et al. 1989; Gaensler et al. 1989; Loh et al. 2005; Tarantino et al. 2003; Birnbaum 1998). It should be noted that, especially in young adults, prominent ileocecal lymph nodes are often present, both in patients with and without appendicitis. Therefore, in the absence of visualization of a normal appendix, the mere identification of these nodes should not be a criterion to establish the diagnosis of mesenteric adenitis, as this is a difficult diagnosis to establish on imaging grounds alone (Fig. 4). The right kidney, ileocecal areas, pelvis, and mid-abdomen should then be carefully scrutinized with a combination of linear- and curved-array transducers to establish an alternative diagnosis to appendicitis. Identification of hydronephrosis from ureteral calculus, inflammation of the right colon or terminal ileum, and/or gynecologic or adnexal pathology is often an invaluable contribution that can be established by sonography.

5 Staging Appendicitis

Determining the stage of appendicitis is critical to directing appropriate patient management. In patients with early acute uncomplicated appendicitis, there is primarily luminal distension, with or without mild

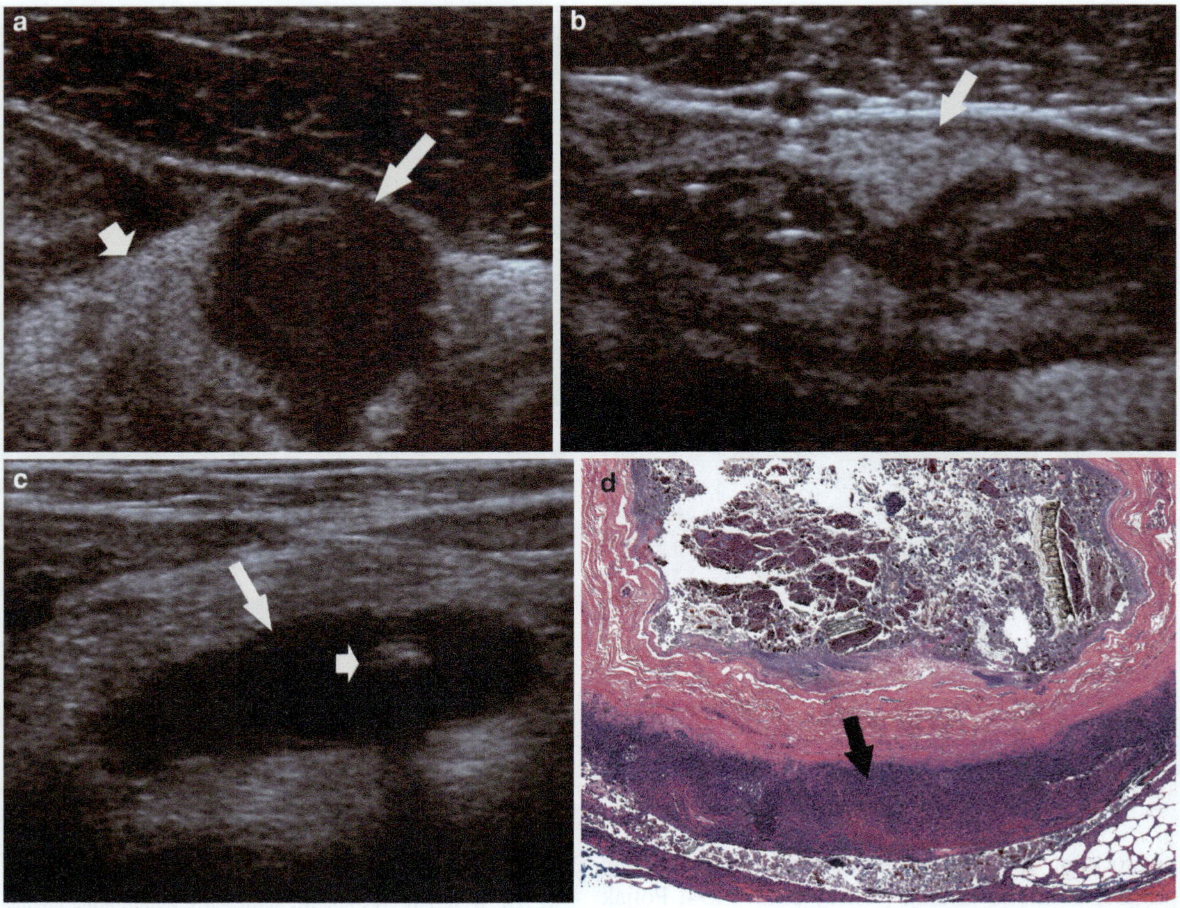

Fig. 11 **a, b, c, d** Gangrenous appendicitis with focal loss of echogenic submucosal layer and cecal edema in two different patients. **a** is transverse sonogram of short axis of appendix demonstrating marked mural thickening and loss of echogenic submucosal layer (*long arrow*); note inflamed periappendiceal fat with increased echogenicity (*short arrow*). In **b**, transverse grayscale sonogram of cecum in same patient, note marked mural thickening with prominence of echogenic submucosal layer related to edema and inflammation from adjacent gangrenous appendix. In different patient with gangrenous appendicitis (Fig. **c**), note complete loss of echogenic submucosal layer on long-axis view of appendix (*long arrow*), as well as appendicolith near tip (*short arrow*). **d** is histologic section through gangrenous appendix in same patient, demonstrating complete loss of mucosal and submucosal layer with transmural inflammation (*arrow*)

mural thickening (Figs. 4, 5, 6 and 7). The maximal AP diameter of the appendix is greater than 6 mm and in some, but not all, patients there is demonstrable flow within the wall of the appendix. There may be associated edema in the mesoappendix with inflamed echogenic fat. Increased vasculature within this inflamed fat may be demonstrated with color of power Doppler (Figs. 8 and 9). Of note is the fact that the echogenic submucosal layer is intact and the entire wall of the appendix can be visualized. While there may in some instances be pericecal free fluid that is often triangular in configuration and conforming to the confines of the peritoneal cavity, there should be no loculated complex fluid indicating an abscess. Most abscesses demonstrate mass effect on adjacent organs and are often walled-off by inflamed echogenic mesenteric and omental fat. With color Doppler, this inflamed fat is often hyperemic.

Unless treated promptly, acute appendicitis may evolve to gangrene, necrosis, and ultimately result in perforation. Increasing intraluminal pressure and increasing intramural inflammation often lead to vascular compromise in the appendix and gangrenous appendicitis (Quillin et al. 1992; Hayden et al. 1992; Bixby et al. 2006). This may be evident by loss of the sonoreflectivity of the echogenic submucosal layer

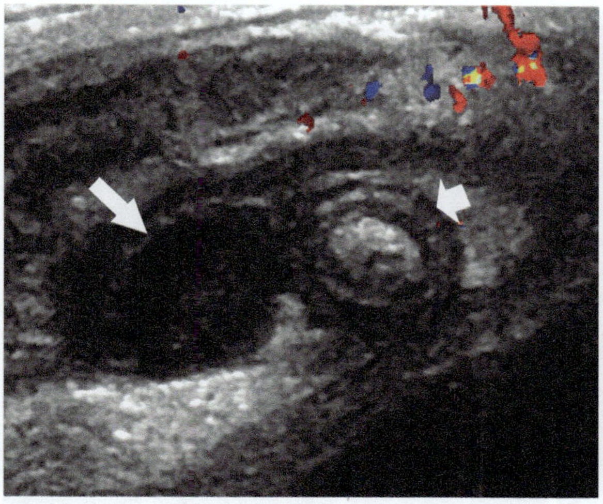

Fig. 12 Small periappendiceal abscess adjacent to appendiceal tip. Note hypoechoic mass with minimal enhanced through-sound transmission (*long white arrow*) adjacent to enlarged appendix in short axis with marked mural thickening (*short arrow*). At surgery, small periappendiceal abscess was noted adjacent to perforated appendiceal tip

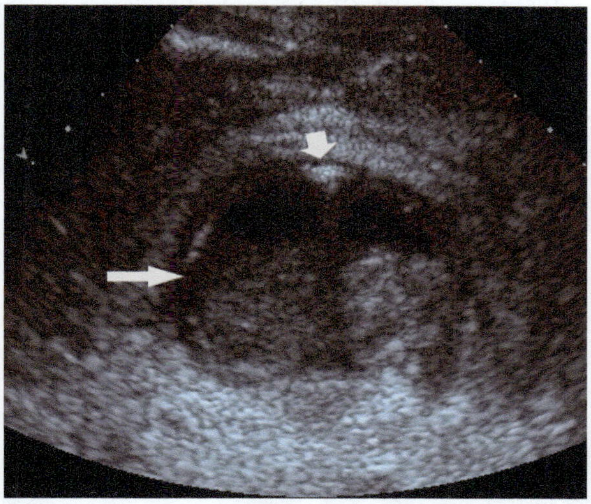

Fig. 13 Gas-forming periappendiceal abscess. Grayscale transverse sonogram of right lower quadrant demonstrates complex fluid collection (*long arrow*); note high-amplitude gas casting acoustic shadow within nondependent portion of abscess (*short arrow*). Appearance is nonspecific and could represent abscess from another etiology, but at surgery necrotic appendix was identified at cecal tip as cause for abscess

(Fig. 10). In areas of gangrenous necrosis there is absence of visualized color-Doppler flow within the wall, and there may be associated mural thickening of the cecum and adjacent terminal ileum (Borushok and Jeffrey 1990) (Fig. 11). Perforation may be identified

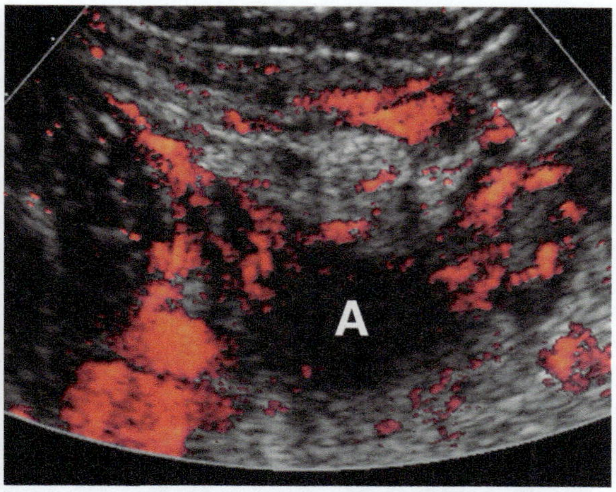

Fig. 14 Periappendiceal abscess as hypoechoic mass. Note hypoechoic mass representing abscess ("A") on transverse power-Doppler sonogram, surrounded by inflamed echogenic mesenteric and omental fat on power-Doppler sonogram. There is marked hyperemia within inflamed fat

on the basis of adjacent abscesses or gas collections. Sonographically, periappendiceal abscesses are typically hypoechoic masses with variable degrees of enhanced through-sound transmission as the proteinaceous fluid within the abscess cavity can attenuate sound (Quillin et al. 1992; Hayden et al. 1992) (Figs. 12, 13, 14, 15 and 16). In some instances, an extruded appendicolith identified as a highly echogenic structure with clean distal acoustic shadowing may be identified that can establish the fact that the abscess originated from the appendix. If there is complete disintegration and loss of the appendix, only an abscess with or without an appendicolith, may be present. An indurated inflammatory mass is the result of perforation (periappendiceal phlegmon) and is diagnosed when there is inflamed echogenic fat without an obvious fluid collection or abscess (Borushok and Jeffrey 1990) (Fig. 17). When perforation is suspected clinically, contrast-enhanced CT is often more accurate in differentiating an abscess from a phlegmon (Bixby et al. 2006).

6 Pitfalls in the Diagnosis of Appendicitis

As previously noted, it is important not to misconstrue the normal terminal ileum for an inflamed appendix. The terminal ileum does not end in a blind pouch, and

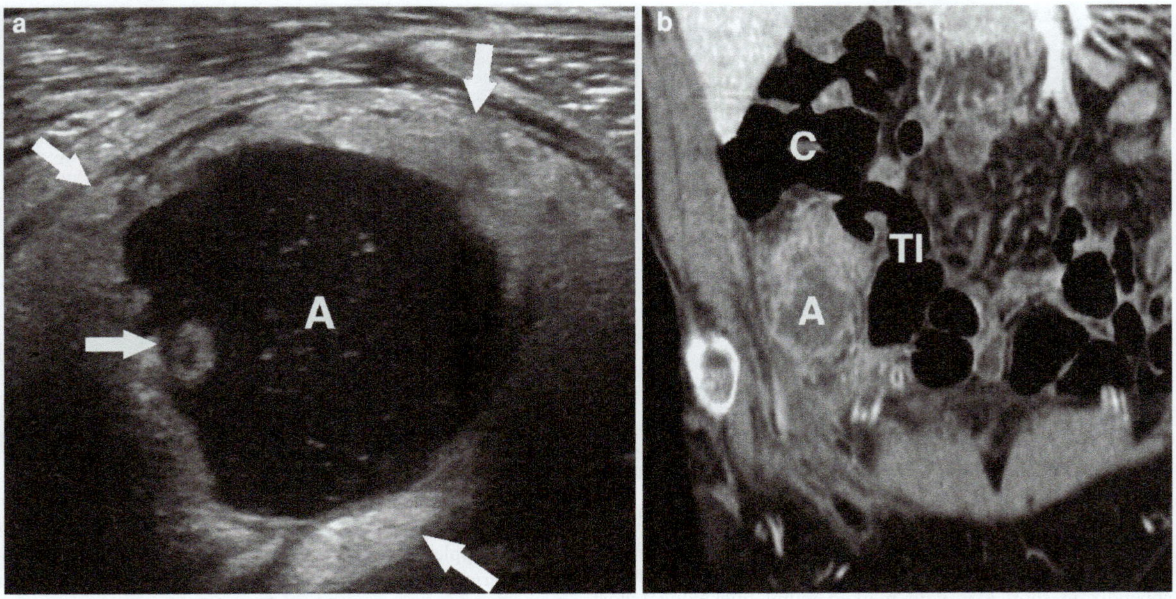

Fig. 15 **a, b** Periappendiceal abscess on ultrasound and CT. In **a**, transverse grayscale sonogram demonstrates complex fluid collection ("A") walled-off by surrounding echogenic fat (*black arrows*). Small residual of appendix is noted along lateral aspect of abscess cavity (*white arrow*), indicating origin of abscess. In **b**, coronal contrast-enhanced CT in same patient demonstrates liquefied abscess ("A") exerting mass effect on adjacent cecum ("C") and terminal ileum ("TI"). In absence of calcified appendicolith, CT cannot make definitive diagnosis of periappendiceal abscess

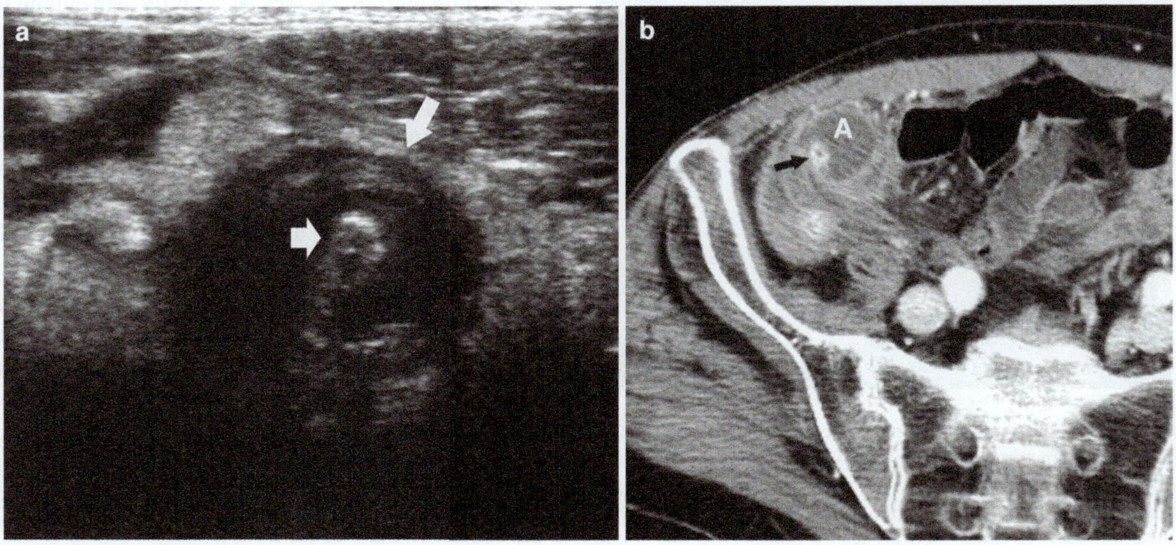

Fig. 16 **a, b** Periappendiceal abscess with calcified appendicolith. In **a**, transverse grayscale sonogram demonstrates appendicolith (*short arrow*) within complex fluid collection, representing periappendiceal abscess (*long white arrow*). **b** is contrast-enhanced CT in same patient; note calcified appendicolith (*arrow*) within periappendiceal abscess ("A")

will demonstrate peristalsis in real time (Jeffrey et al. 1994). Once the appendix has been identified, it is important to carefully evaluate the termination of the appendix. In some patients appendicitis may be confined to the distal tip (Nghiem and Jeffrey 1992; Lim et al. 1996) (Fig. 18).

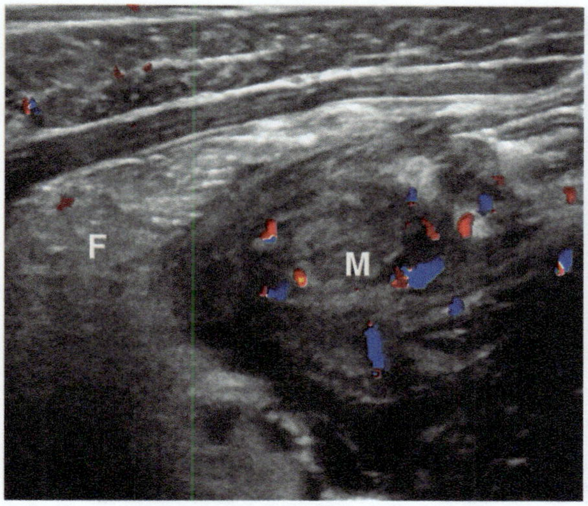

Fig. 17 Periappendiceal phlegmon. Note indurated soft-tissue mass containing internal flow on transverse color-Doppler sonogram, surrounded by inflamed echogenic fat ("F") in right lower quadrant. There was no liquefied pus for drainage

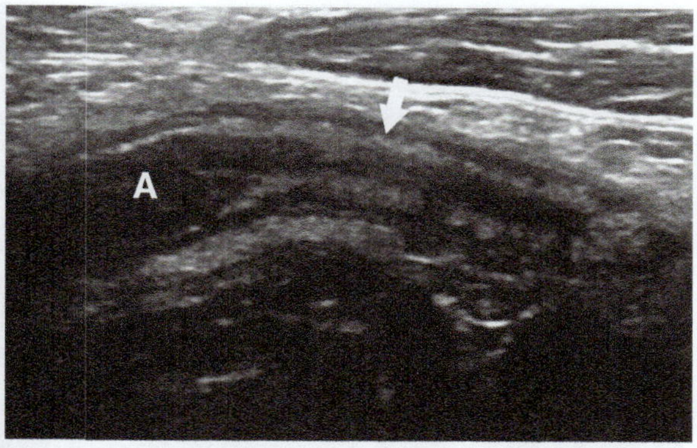

Fig. 19 Resolving appendicitis on sonography. Zero Grayscale sonogram through long axis of appendix demonstrates fluid distension of proximal appendix ("A"), and submucosal and mural thickening of distal appendix (*white arrow*). Findings were consistent with early acute appendicitis; however, patient's symptoms resolved at time of scanning and patient made uneventful recovery without surgery

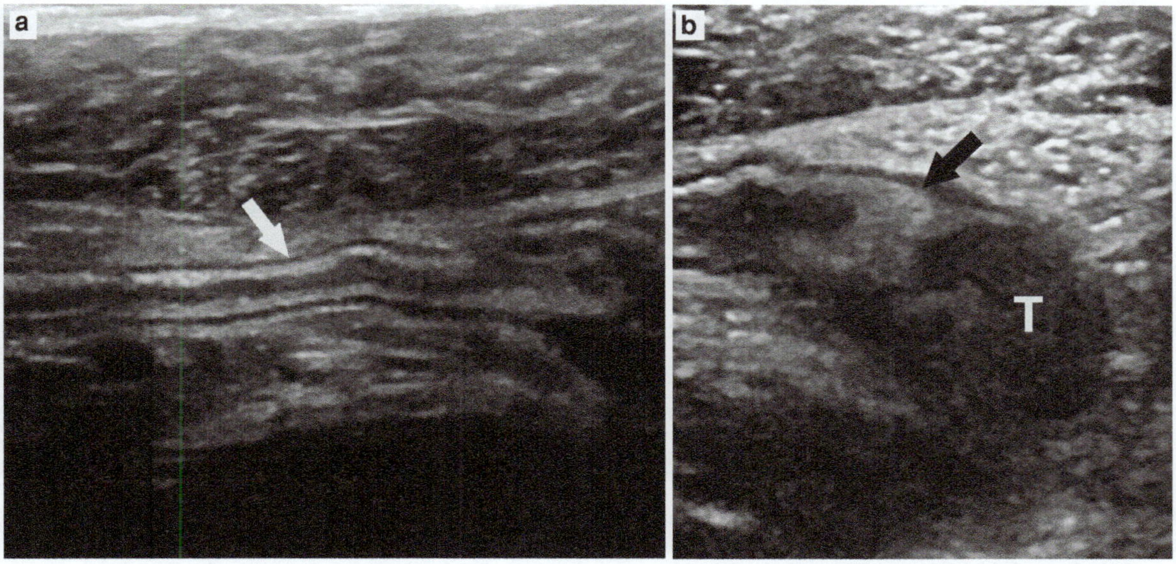

Fig. 18 **a, b** Tip appendicitis. **a** is long-axis grayscale sonogram demonstrating normal proximal appendix (*arrow*). **b** is long-axis grayscale sonogram through distal tip, demonstrating marked thickening of echogenic submucosal layer (*black arrow*) with loss of sonoreflectivity of submucosa in distal tip, consistent with gangrenous tip appendicitis

In a small subset of patients, clinical symptoms and right lower quadrant pain may spontaneously resolve, although there may still be imaging findings on sonography consistent with appendicitis (Cobben et al. 2000; Migraine et al. 1997). In these patients it is likely that there has been spontaneous resolution of the appendicitis (Fig. 19). Follow up may demonstrate interval decrease in size of the appendix; these patients are at risk for recurrence of the appendicitis, typically within a year, and therefore

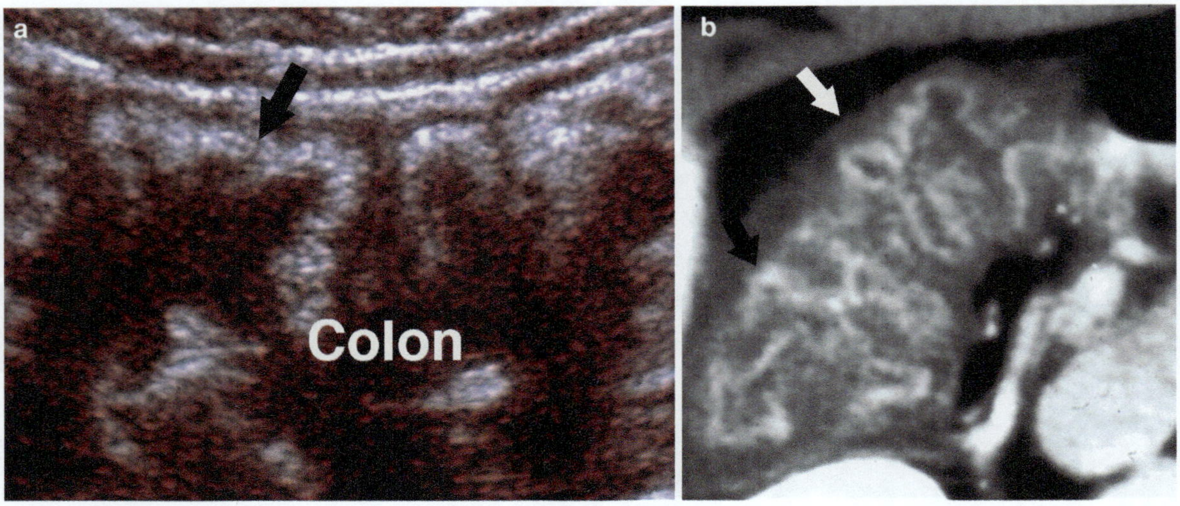

Fig. 20 **a, b** Pseudomembranous colitis mimicking appendicitis. In **a**, longitudinal grayscale sonogram of right colon, note marked mural thickening and prominence of echogenic submucosal layer, indicating submucosal edema (*white arrow*). **b** is contrast-enhanced CT in same patient demonstrating marked mucosal hyperemia (*black arrow*) and extensive submucosal edema (*white arrow*). Endoscopy and stool cultures were positive for Clostridium difficile organisms, diagnostic of pseudomembranous colitis

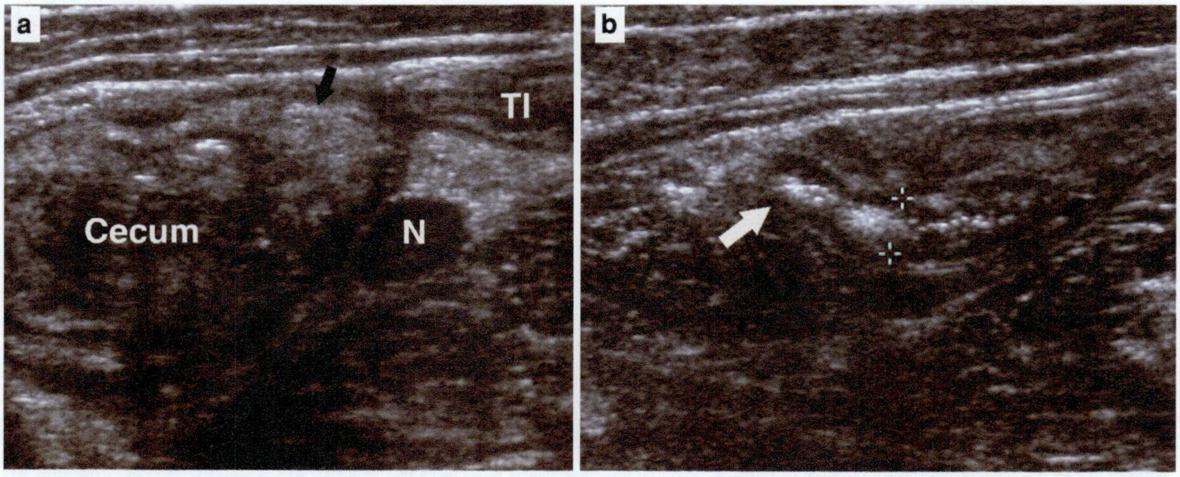

Fig. 21 **a, b** Camphylobacter ileocolitis mimicking appendicitis. **a** is transverse grayscale sonogram of cecum demonstrating marked mural thickening with increased echogenicity and thickening within submucosal layer (*black arrow*), indicating submucosal edema, note enlarged pericecal lymph node ("N"; TI = terminal ileum). **b** is transverse sonogram demonstrating normal appendix (calipers). Note gas in distal appendix (*white arrow*). Stool cultures were positive for Camphylobacter and patient made an uneventful recovery on antibiotics

close clinical observation is warranted (see also "Spontaneously Resolving and Chronic Appendicitis" by Cobben).

The retrocecal location of the appendix is a clearly recognized pitfall with sonography using only an anterior approach. As emphasized in the scanning portion of this review, if the appendix is not visualized using the standard anterior approach in the transverse plane, it is important to attempt to visualize the retrocecal area in a coronal approach by placing the patient in a left posterior oblique position and scanning in a more coronal plane to visualize the tissues behind the

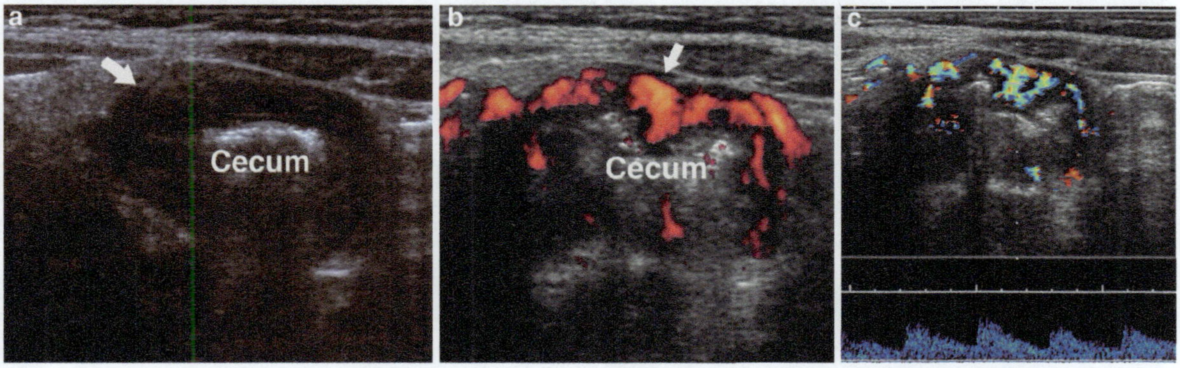

Fig. 22 a, b, c Cecal Crohn's disease mimicking appendicitis. In **a**, transverse grayscale sonogram of cecum demonstrates marked mural thickening (*white arrow*). **b** is power-Doppler image in same patient demonstrating marked mural hyperemia (*white arrow*). **c** is spectral Doppler tracing of cecum in same patient demonstrating prominent arterial intramural flow

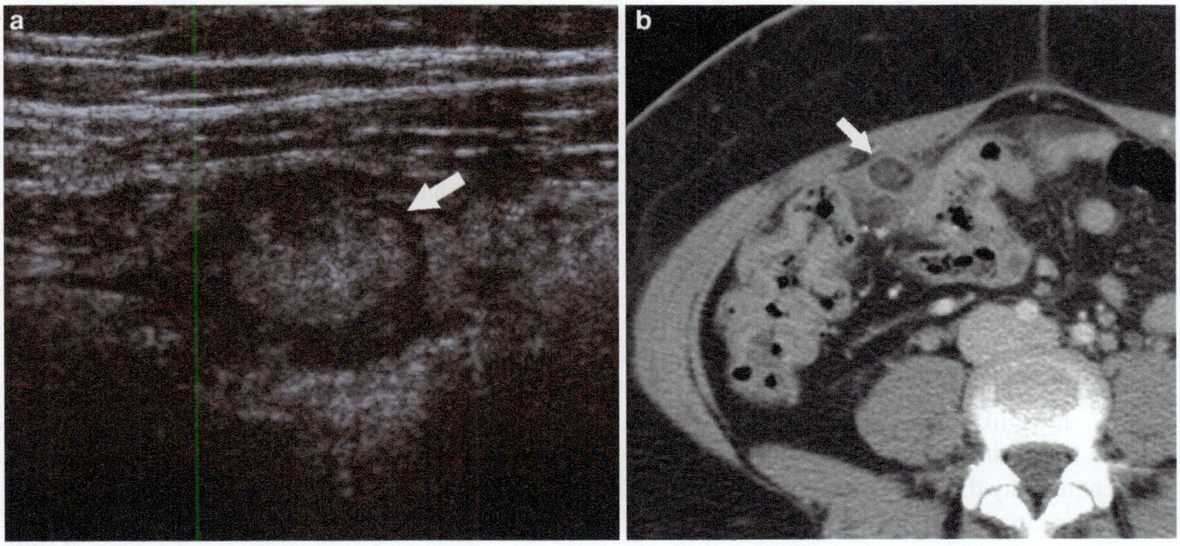

Fig. 23 a, b Epiploic appendagitis mimicking appendicitis. **a** is sagittal sonogram of right lower quadrant demonstrating rounded discrete echogenic structure representing infarcted epiploic appendage (*arrow*). **b** is contrast-enhanced CT scan demonstrating infarcted epiploic appendage involving right colon

cecum. The use of simultaneous posterior compression while scanning may also be of value to visualize retrocecal appendicitis (Lee et al. 2002).

The dilated fallopian tube on an endovaginal scan may on rare occasion be misconstrued for an appendix (Jeffrey et al. 1994). However, the appendix has an echogenic submucosal layer that the fallopian tube does not. The fallopian tube also has characteristic folds that are not present in the appendix. Similarly, the fallopian tube will not be seen to originate from the cecal tip.

Another potential pitfall is the development of "secondary" appendicitis due to pericecal inflammatory processes. Right lower quadrant abscesses from Crohn's disease, perforated diverticulitis, or even pelvic inflammatory disease may secondarily result in appendiceal serosal inflammation and thickening of the appendiceal wall.

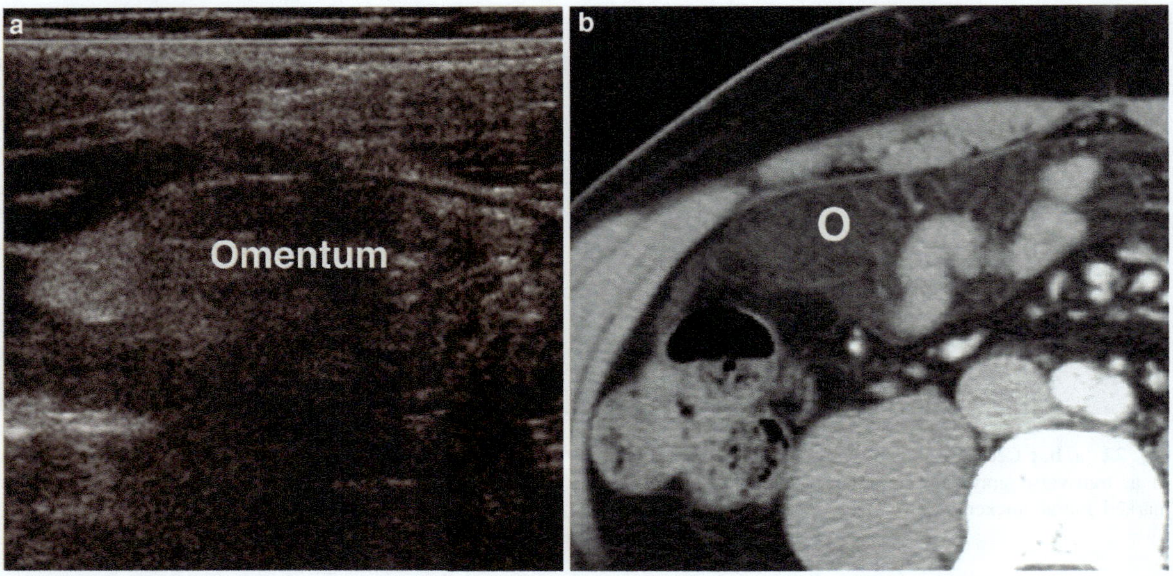

Fig. 24 **a, b** Omental infarction mimicking appendicitis. In **a**, transverse color-Doppler sonogram demonstrating echogenic omental mass with absent flow on color Doppler. **b** is contrast-enhanced CT demonstrating soft-tissue infiltration within area of omental infarction ("O")

7 Alternative Diagnoses

The majority of patients in most clinical series who are suspected of having acute appendicitis do not in fact have this diagnosis (Wagner et al. 1996). Many have benign, self-limited disorders that are never diagnosed pathologically and require no specific therapy. It is likely that the vast majority of the patients has various forms of viral gastroenteritis or transient motility disorders. However, in patients who have other intra-abdominal entities masquerading as appendicitis that require specific therapies, either medical or surgical, sonography and CT may be of considerable clinical value in suggesting an alternative diagnosis (van Breda Vriesman and Puylaert 2006; Jain et al. 1996; Townsend et al. 1989; Gaensler et al. 1989; Loh et al. 2005; Tarantino et al. 2003; Birnbaum 1998). It is important to re-emphasize that patient self-localization of the site of maximal pain may be an important clue to a site of alternative pathology (Chesbrough et al. 1993). While CT with contrast enhancement is often superior to sonography in the identification of some solid-organ parenchymal disorders such as small abscesses, sonography can diagnose a wide range of gastrointestinal and genitourinary abnormalities.

Inflammatory bowel disorders, either of infectious ileo-colitis or Crohn's disease, often result in mural thickening of the involved segments with increased echogenicity of the submucosal layer, indicating bowel wall edema (Frisoli et al. 2000) (Figs. 20, 21 and 22). Hyperemia of the thickened bowel wall in conjunction with inflamed fat adjacent to affected bowel loops is an important secondary clue. Cecal diverticulitis is well known to mimic appendicitis. Often the inflamed diverticulum is noted within a focal area of mural thickening and casts an acoustic shadow due to either a fecolith within the diverticulum or gas within an infected diverticulum (Townsend et al. 1989; Gaensler et al. 1989). There is invariably a degree of inflamed pericecal fat that is both echogenic on grayscale imaging and hyperemic on color Doppler. Crohn's disease often demonstrates striking findings, with sonography characterized by mural thickening and marked hyperemia. Hypoechoic sinus tracts into the mesentery may be identified, as well as adjacent abscesses in the iliac fossa. These enteric abscesses are often hypoechoic and demonstrate significant mass effect on adjacent bowel loops.

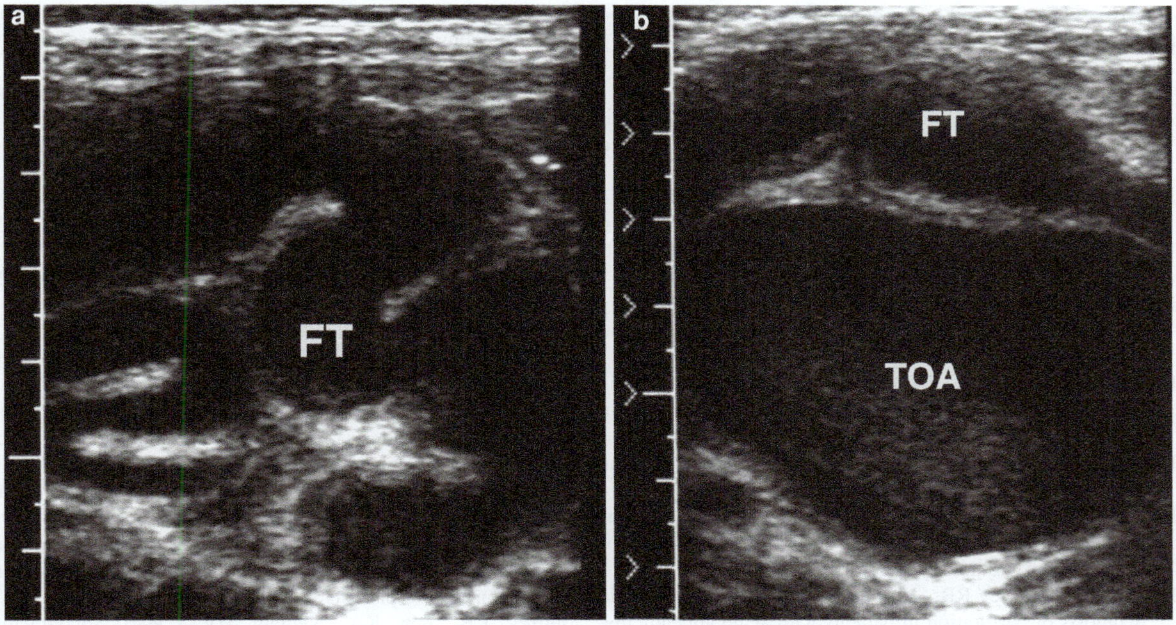

Fig. 25 **a, b** Pelvic inflammatory disease mimicking acute appendicitis. **a** is transverse sonogram of right lower quadrant demonstrating pyosalpinx with echogenic pus within dilated fallopian tube ("FT"). **b** is transverse scan of right lower quadrant demonstrating tubo-ovarian abscess ("TOA") adjacent to dilated fallopian tube ("FT")

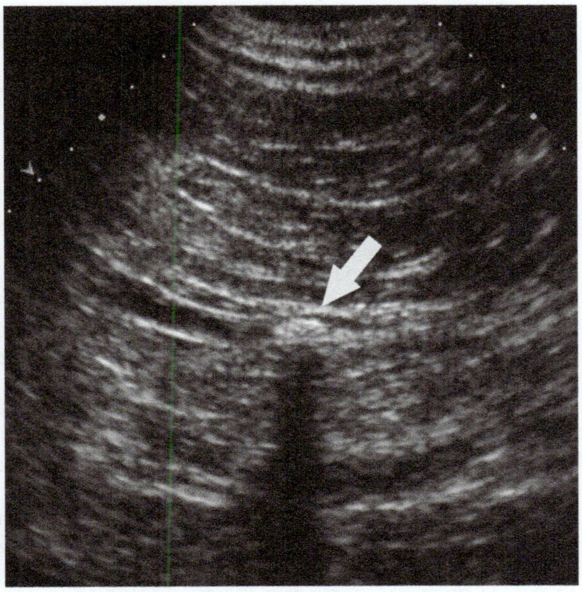

Fig. 26 Distal right ureteral calculus mimicking appendicitis. Sagittal sonogram of right lower quadrant demonstrates echogenic stone (*arrow*) within dilated right ureter

Omental infarction and epiploic appendagitis are two lesions involving fatty tissue in the right lower quadrant to mimic appendicitis (Jain et al. 1996; Loh et al. 2005; Garg and Singh 2008; Almeida et al. 2009; van Breda Vriesman and Puylaert 2002). Both are likely related to venous thrombosis and infarction, leading to identification of echogenic avascular masses on sonography. The edema within these areas of fatty infarction often results in fat stranding on CT (Garg and Singh 2008; Almeida et al. 2009; van Breda Vriesman and Puylaert 2002) (Figs. 23 and 24).

Finally, in the adult population ileal neoplasms including carcinoma or cecal lymphoma may cause right lower quadrant pain and clinically mimic appendicitis (Rubin and Jeffrey 1992). Colon neoplasms are typically hypoechoic masses that demonstrate minimal vascularity on color Doppler (Rubin and Jeffrey 1992). Of note is the fact that there is no thickening of the echogenic submucosal layer that is the hallmark of colonic inflammation.

Genitourinary abnormalities such as ureteral calculi, pelvic inflammatory disease, and ruptured ovarian cysts are all entities that may clinically mimic appendicitis (Figs. 25 and 26). As previously noted, the use of an endovaginal probe may help detect distal ureteral calculi. The endovaginal approach is also the imaging method of choice to diagnose adnexal pathology (Laing et al. 1994).

References

Addiss DG, Shaffer N, Fowler BS et al (1990) The epidemiology of appendicitis and appendectomy in the United States. Am J Epidemiol 132:910–925

Almeida AT, Melao L, Viamonte B et al (2009) Epiploic appendagitis: an entity frequently unknown to clinicians—diagnostic imaging, pitfalls, and look-alikes. Am J Roentgenol 193:1243–1251

Bendeck SE, Nino-Murcia M, Berry GJ et al (2002) Imaging for suspected appendicitis: Negative appendectomy and perforation rates. Radiology 225:131–136

Birnbaum BA, Jeffrey RB (1998) CT and sonographic evaluation of acute right lower quadrant abdominal pain. Am J Roentgenol 170:361–371. Review

Birnbaum BA, Wilson SR (2000) Appendicitis at the millennium. Radiology 215:337–348

Bixby SD, Lucey BC, Soto JA et al (2006) Perforated versus nonperforated acute appendicitis: accuracy of multidetector CT detection. Radiology 241:780–786

Borushok KF, Jeffrey RB, Laing FC et al (1990) Sonographic diagnosis of perforation in patients with acute appendicitis. Am J Roentgenol 154:275–278

Brody AS, Frush DP, Huda W et al (2007) American academy of pediatrics section on radiology. Radiation risk to children from computed tomography. Pediatrics 120:677–682

Chesbrough RM, Burkhard TK, Balsara ZN et al (1993) Self-localization in US of appendicitis: an addition to graded compression. Radiology 187:349–351

Cobben LP, de Van Otterloo AM, Puylaert JB (2000) Spontaneously resolving appendicitis: Frequency and natural history in 60 patients. Radiology 215:349–352

Coursey CA, Nelson RC, Patel MB et al (2010) Making the diagnosis of acute appendicitis: do more preoperative CT sans mean fewer negative appendectomies? A 10 year study. Radiology 254:460–468

de Dombal FT (1994) Acute abdominal pain in the elderly. J Clin Gastroenterol 19:331–335

Doria AS (2009) Optimizing the role of imaging in appendicitis. Pediatr Radiol 39 Suppl 2:S144–8. Review

Doria AS, Moineddin R, Kellenberger CJ et al (2006) US or CT for diagnosis of appendicitis in children and adults? A meta-analysis. Radiology 241:83–94

Fitz RH (1886) Perforating inflammation of the vermiform appendix, with special reference to its early diagnosis and treatment. Trans Assoc Am Physicians 1:107–144

Frisoli JK, Desser TS, Jeffrey RB (2000) Thickened submucosal layer: a sonographic sign of acute gastrointestinal abnormality representing submucosal edema or hemorrhage. 2000 ARRS Executive Council Award II. American Roentgen Ray Society. Am J Roentgenol 175:1595–1599

Gaensler EH, Jeffrey RB, Laing FC et al (1989) Sonography in patients with suspected acute appendicitis: Value in establishing alternative diagnoses. Am J Roentgenol 152:49–51

Gaitini D, Beck-Razi N, Mor-Yosef D et al (2008) Diagnosing acute appendicitis in adults: Accuracy of color Doppler sonography and MDCT compared with surgery and clinical follow-up. Am J Roentgenol 190:1300–1306

Garbutt JM, Soper NJ, Shannon WD et al (1999) Meta-analysis of randomized controlled trials comparing laparoscopic and open appendectomy. Surg Laparosc Endosc 9:17–26

Garg AG, Singh AK (2008) Inflammatory fatty masses of the abdomen. Semin Ultrasound CT MR 29:378–385

Hall EJ, Brenner DJ (2008) Cancer risks from diagnostic radiology. Br J Radiol 81:362–378

Hansen JB, Smithers BM, Schache D et al (1996) Laparoscopic versus open appendectomy: Prospective randomized trial. World J Surg 20:17–20

Hayden CK Jr, Kuchelmeister J, Lipscomb TS (1992) Sonography of acute appendicitis in childhood: Perforation versus nonperforation. J Ultrasound Med 11:209–216

Hermanz-Schulman M (2010) CT and US in the diagnosis of appendicitis: an argument for CT. Radiology 255:3–7

Jain KA, Ablin DS, Jeffrey RB et al (1996) Sonographic differential diagnosis of right lower quadrant pain other than appendicitis. Clin Imaging 20:12–16

Jeffrey RB (1989) Management of the periappendiceal inflammatory mass. Semin Ultrasound CT MR 10:341–7. Review

Jeffrey RB, Federle MP, Colentino CS (1988) Periappendiceal inflammatory masses: CT-directed management and clinical outcome in 70 patients. Radiology 167:13–16

Jeffrey RB, Jain KA, Nghiem HV (1994) Sonographic diagnosis of acute appendicitis: Interpretive pitfalls. Am J Roentgenol 162:55–59

Johansson EP, Rydh A, Riklund KA (2007) Ultrasound, computed tomography, and laboratory findings in the diagnosis of appendicitis. Acta Radiol 48:267–273

Kaiser S, Frenckner B, Jorulf HK (2002) Suspected appendicitis in children: US and CT–a prospective randomized study. Radiology 223:633–638

Keckler SJ, Tsao K, Sharp SW et al (2008) Resource utilization and outcomes from percutaneous drainage and interval appendectomy for perforated appendicitis with abscess. J Pediatr Surg 43:977–980

Laing FC, Benson CB, DiSalvo DN et al (1994) Distal ureteral calculi: Detection with vaginal US. Radiology 192:545–548

Lee JH (2003) Sonography of acute appendicitis. Semin Ultrasound CT MR 24:83–90. Review

Lee JH, Jeong YK, Hwang JC et al (2002) Graded compression sonography with adjuvant use of a posterior manual compression technique in the sonographic diagnosis of acute appendicitis. Am J Roentgenol 178:863–868

Lim HK, Lee WJ, Lee SJ et al (1996a) Focal appendicitis confined to the tip: Diagnosis at US. Radiology 200:799–801

Lim HK, Lee WJ, Kim TH et al (1996b) Appendicitis: Usefulness of color Doppler US. Radiology 201:221–225

Loh MH, Chui HC, Yap TL et al (2005) Omental infarction—a mimicker of acute appendicitis in children. J Pediatr Surg 40:1224–1226

McDonald GP, Pendarvis DP, Wilmoth R et al (2001) Influence of preoperative computed tomography on patients undergoing appendectomy. Am Surg 67:1017–1021

Migraine S, Atri M, Bret PM et al (1997) Spontaneously resolving cute appendicitis: Clinical and sonographic documentation. Radiology 205:55–58

Nghiem HV, Jeffrey RB (1992) Acute appendicitis confined to the appendiceal tip: Evaluation with graded compression sonography. J Ultrasound Med 11:205–207

Noguchi T, Yoshimitsu K, Yoshida M (2005) Periappendiceal hyperechoic structure on sonography: a sign of severe appendicitis. J Ultrasound Med 24:323–7; quiz 328–30
Oto A, Ernst RD, Ghulmiyyah LM et al (2009) MR imaging in the triage of pregnant patients with acute abdominal and pelvic pain. Abdom Imaging 34:243–250
Pokala N, Sadhasivam S, Kiran RP et al (2007) Complicated appendicitis—is the laparoscopic approach appropriate? A comparative study with the open approach: Outcome in a community hospital setting. Am Surg 73:737–741; discussion 741–2
Poljak A, Jeffrey RB, Kernberg ME (1991) The gas-containing appendix: Potential sonographic pitfall in the diagnosis of acute appendicitis. J Ultrasound Med 10:625–628
Poortman P, Oostvogel HJ, Bosma E et al (2009) Improving diagnosis of acute appendicitis: results of a diagnostic pathway with standard use of ultrasonography followed by selective use of CT. J Am Coll Surg 208:434–441
Puylaert JB (1986) Acute appendicitis: US evaluation using graded compression. Radiology 158:355–360
Puylaert JB (1988) Ultrasonography for diagnosing appendicitis. BMJ 297:740
Puylaert JB, Rutgers PH, Lalisang RI et al (1987) A prospective study of ultrasonography in the diagnosis of appendicitis. N Engl J Med 317:666–669
Quillin SP, Siegel MJ, Coffin CM (1992) Acute appendicitis in children: Value of sonography in detecting perforation. Am J Roentgenol 159:1265–1268
Raja AS, Wright C, Sodickson AD et al (2010) Negative appendectomy rate in the era of CT: an 18 year perspective. Radiology 256:460–465
Raval MV, Lautz T, Reynolds M et al (2010) Dollars and sense of interval appendectomy in children: a cost analysis. J Pediatr Surg 45:1817–1825
Rettenbacher T, Hollerweger A, Macheiner P et al (2001) Outer diameter of the vermiform appendix as a sign of acute appendicitis: Evaluation at US. Radiology 218:757–762
Rettenbacher T, Hollerweger A, Macheiner P et al (2003) Ovoid shape of the vermiform appendix: a criterion to exclude acute appendicitis–evaluation with US. Radiology 226:95–100
Rubin GD, Jeffrey RB (1992) Graded compression sonography of abdominal neoplasms mimicking acute appendicitis. Gastrointest Radiol 17:292–294
Rybkin AV, Thoeni RF (2007) Current concepts in imaging of appendicitis. Radiol Clin North Am 45:411–22, vii. Review
Singh A, Danrad R, Hahn PF et al (2007) MR imaging of the acute abdomen and pelvis: Acute appendicitis and beyond. Radiographics 27:1419–1431
Strouse PJ (2010) Pediatric appendicitis: an argument for US. Radiology 255:8–13
Tarantino L, Giorgio A, de Stefano G et al (2003) Acute appendicitis mimicking infectious enteritis: Diagnostic value of sonography. J Ultrasound Med 22:945–950
Townsend RR, Jeffrey RB, Laing FC (1989) Cecal diverticulitis differentiated from appendicitis using graded-compression sonography. Am J Roentgenol 152:1229–1230
van Breda Vriesman AC, Puylaert JB (2002) Epiploic appendagitis and omental infarction: Pitfalls and look-alikes. Abdom Imaging 27:20–28
van Breda Vriesman AC, Puylaert JB (2006) Mimics of appendicitis: Alternative nonsurgical diagnoses with sonography and CT. Am J Roentgenol 186:1103–1112
Wagner JM, McKinney P, Carpenter JL (1996) Does this patient have appendicitis? JAMA 276:1589–1594
Wan MJ, Krahn M, Ungar WJ et al (2009) Acute appendicitis in young children: Cost-effectiveness of US versus CT in diagnosis—a Markov decision analytic model. Radiology 250:378–386
Yacoe ME, Jeffrey RB (1994) Sonography of appendicitis and diverticulitis. Radiol Clin North Am 32:899–912. Review
Yau KK, Siu WT, Tang CN et al (2007) Laparoscopic versus open appendectomy for complicated appendicitis. J Am Coll Surg 205:60–65

Imaging of Acute Appendicitis in Adults: Computed Tomography

Caroline Keyzer and Pierre Alain Gevenois

Contents

C. Keyzer (✉) · P. A. Gevenois
Department of Radiology, Hôpital Erasme,
Université libre de Bruxelles,
Route de Lennik, 808,
1070 Brussels, Belgium
e-mail: caroline.keyzer@erasme.ulb.ac.be

Abstract

Computed Tomography (CT) examination of the entire abdomen and pelvis is more and more frequently performed in patients suspected of acute appendicitis but this examination can be obtained with various CT protocols. As there are still controversies regarding these protocols, this chapter will discuss their differences in terms of contrast material and anatomic coverage. This chapter will also review the CT features of acute appendicitis and the alternative diseases that can be detected at CT, including the impact of saving radiation dose on these features and alternative diagnoses.

Abbreviations

BMI	Body mass index
MPR	Multi-planar reformations
NPV	Negative predictive value
PPV	Positive predictive value
RLQ	Right lower quadrant

1 Introduction

Computed tomography (CT) is widely used for imaging the abdomen in various clinical circumstances including acute pain. This wide use is explained by the fact that this technique is highly reproducible, rapid, sensitive and specific, easy to perform, and causes little discomfort to the patient (Birnbaum and Wilson 2000; Wise et al. 2001). With multi-detector row CT (MDCT) scanners, rapid

C. Keyzer and P. A. Gevenois (eds.), *Imaging of Acute Appendicitis in Adults and Children*,
Medical Radiology. Diagnostic Imaging, DOI: 10.1007/174_2011_216, © Springer-Verlag Berlin Heidelberg 2011

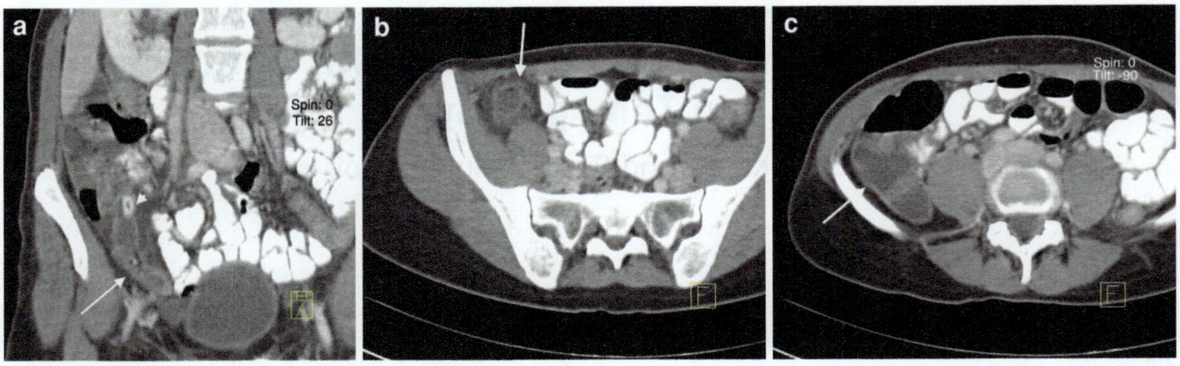

Fig. 1 Patient with acute appendicitis. **a** Coronal CT image obtained with IV and oral contrasts showing enlarged, enhancing, and fluid-filled appendix (*long arrow*) and appendicolith (*arrowhead*). **b** Transverse CT image obtained with IV and oral contrasts showing enlarged, enhancing, fluid-filled appendix, and moderate periappendiceal fat stranding (*long arrow*). **c** The cecum is not opacified by oral contrast administered one and a half hour before (*arrow*)

volume acquisition became possible and examination of the entire abdomen and pelvis is more and more frequently performed as a screening test in patients suspected of abdominal disorder, particularly in those with acute abdominal pain. Examination of the entire abdomen and pelvis is justified by the ability to detect alternative and/or additional diagnoses. Nevertheless, since the mean age of patients suspected of acute appendicitis is approximately 30 years, the delivered radiation dose is a particular concern. Strategies to reduce this dose have been developed and clinical investigations have shown that in several abdominal disorders, including acute appendicitis, the performance of CT is not decreased by dose reduction.

2 Acquisition Protocols

Depending on studies, sensitivities, specificities, positive, and negative predictive values of CT in the diagnosis of acute appendicitis range, respectively from 71 to 100%, from 83 to 98%, from 58 to 98%, and from 64 to 100% (Wise et al. 2001; Balthazar et al. 1994; Jacobs et al. 2001; Raman et al. 2002; Rao et al. 1997a, b; Wijetunga et al. 2001; Poortman et al. 2003; Funaki et al. 1998). These performances could be influenced by the type of CT scanners (helical vs. incremental) and by the acquisition protocol.

In fact there are still controversies regarding these protocols, including on the use of enteric and/or IV contrast, and on the anatomic coverage of the examination. In the United States, the most popular protocol, performed in up to 80% of patients suspected of acute appendicitis, is a single helical acquisition on the entire abdomen and pelvis with simultaneous oral and IV contrast administration (O'Malley et al. 2000; Johnson et al. 2006). This protocol has been showed to be very effective in terms of sensitivity and specificity (Jacobs et al. 2001; Hershko et al. 2007). The use of contrast agents induces, however, costs and risks inherent to iodined contrast materials, increases waiting time due to the ingestion of contrast material as well as patient's discomfort. As acute appendicitis is a potentially life-threatening condition, but treatable by simple and efficient surgical procedures, it is imperative that diagnostic tests should be highly sensitive with a high negative predictive value (NPV) (Krieg et al. 1975). Most importantly, unenhanced MDCT scans achieve sensitivities and NPV as high as 95% and even higher (Ege et al. 2002; Lane et al. 1999; Keyzer et al. 2004).

Oral contrast is administered in order to opacify the ileum, the cecum, and the appendix. Oral contrast is thought to increase the conspicuity of the appendix, whatever normal or not. The absence of benefit of oral contrast for diagnosing acute appendicitis has been advocated in a review article that has reported performance of CT without oral contrast as high—and even higher in terms of specificity, positive predictive value (PPV), and accuracy—without as with oral contrast (Anderson et al. 2005). This review article was, however, based on studies that were either retrospective or prospective and based on different CT acquisition protocols (with or without rectal and/or IV contrast, on

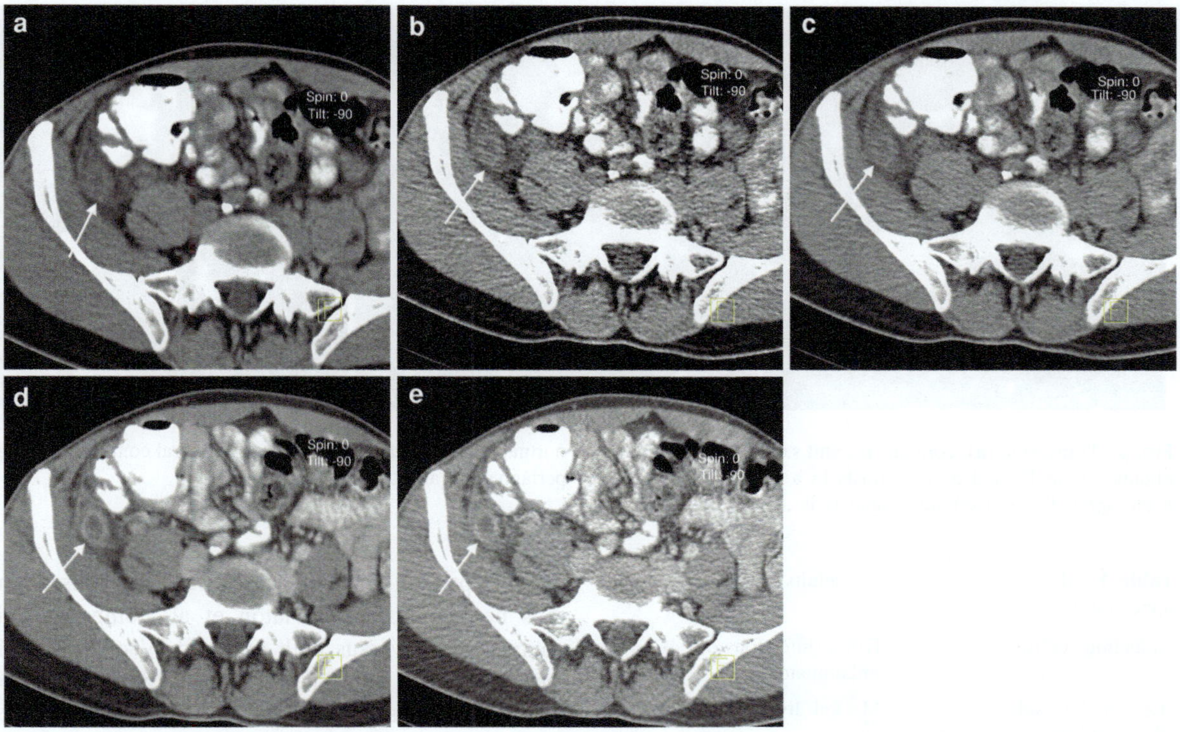

Fig. 2 Transverse CT images obtained for comparison with firstly oral contrast and secondly IV contrast in a patient (BMI = 22 kg m^2-1) with acute appendicitis. **a** Transverse CT image obtained at standard dose with oral contrast showing an enlarged, fluid-filled appendix, and moderate periappendiceal fat stranding. **b** Transverse CT image at simulated low-dose with oral contrast showing the same features than **a**. **c** Thick transverse MPR image (with reduced noise) at simulated low-dose with oral contrast. **d** Transverse CT image obtained at standard dose with oral and IV contrasts showing an enlarged, enhancing, fluid-filled appendix, and moderate periappendiceal fat stranding. **e** Transverse CT image obtained at simulated low-dose with oral and IV contrasts showing the same features than **d**. The appendix is visible and the diagnosis of acute appendicitis is obvious in all figures from **a** to **e**

helical single slice CT or MDCT, or even incremental CT). In addition, all but one study did not compare different CT protocols applied to the same study group (Jacobs et al. 2001; Anderson et al. 2005). With that in mind, randomized studies have been recently conducted in order to compare examinations performed with and without oral contrast with the same protocol regarding the administration of IV contrast and the anatomic coverage (Anderson et al. 2009; Keyzer et al. 2009). Globally, these more recent studies show that diagnostic performances of CT in diagnosing acute appendicitis are independent on oral contrast. Anderson et al. mentioned, however, that their study had a too low statistical power to detect any difference in terms of sensitivity. We showed that the correctness in diagnosing acute appendicitis as well as alternative diseases is far more predominantly influenced by the reader than by any contrast (oral and IV) (Keyzer et al. 2009). Furthermore, the studies by Anderson et al. (2009) and ours show that despite allowing 1–2 h between contrast ingestion and scanning, oral contrast reaches the colon level in 68–82% of patients only, with no appendix visualization impairment (diseased or not) (Keyzer et al. 2009). Finally, a study performed in patients who were not suspected of acute appendicitis and with a normal appendix, showed that 1 h after the contrast ingestion, it opacifies the appendiceal lumen in 24% of patients only (Tamburrini et al. 2005) (Fig. 1). This raises an important issue for practical organization of emergency rooms and the radiology departments that are stressed to reduce the length stay, are more and more busy, and for which eliminating the time required for oral contrast administration could be of major interest (Kim et al. 2008; Mun et al. 2006). All these studies did not reveal any influence of oral contrast on reader's concordance, confidence, and correctness in

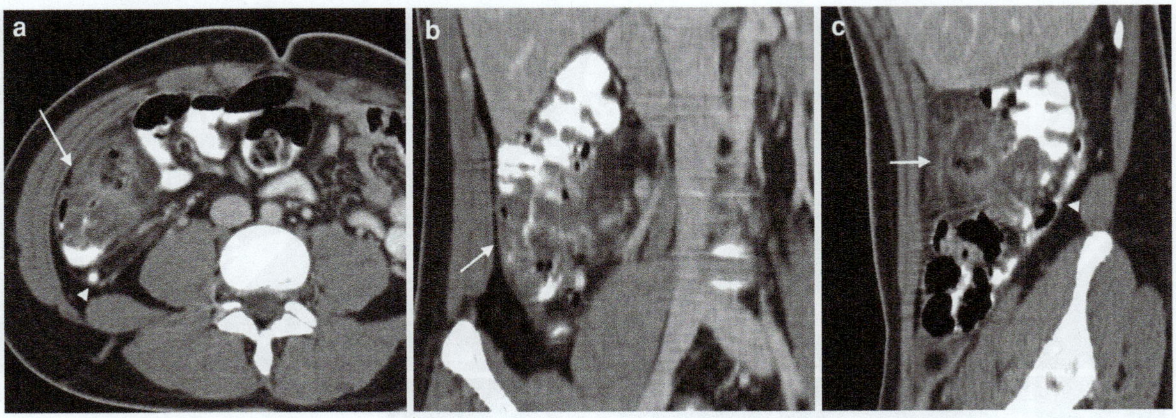

Fig. 3 Transverse (**a**), coronal (**b**), and sagittal (**c**) CT images obtained with IV and oral contrasts in a patient suspected of acute appendicitis. Definite diagnosis is a right colitis with a normal appendix (*arrowhead*) filled with oral contrast. Minimal periappendiceal fat stranding is visible (**a**)

Table 1 Alternative diagnoses in adults suspected of acute appendicitis

Infectious colitis	Ileitis (infectious or inflammatory)
Left or right-sided diverticulitis	Meckel diverticulitis
Pyelonephritis	Ileal occlusion
Right ureteral stone	Lower right lobe pneumonia
Acute cholecystitis	Cystitis
Acute pancreatitis	Ovarian diseases
Mesenteric panniculitis	Ovarian vein thrombosis
Mesenteric adenitis	Pelvic inflammatory disease
Epiploic appendagitis	Perforated gastric ulcus
Bowel intussusception	Right inguinal hernia
Cecal neoplasia	Prostatitis

diagnosing acute appendicitis, whatever the patient's BMI but their samples had a mean BMI corresponding to the overweight category (Keyzer et al. 2009; Anderson et al. 2010; Wolfe et al. 2006; No authors 1998). Therefore, further studies should be targeted on underweight patients in whom the paucity of intra-abdominal fat could impair the appendix detectability and could thus benefit from oral contrast.

Concerning IV contrast, the study by Jacobs et al. (2001) reported that IV contrast improves the performance of CT in diagnosing acute appendicitis, a result not confirmed by Wise et al. (2001). In these two discordant studies, the regions scanned with and without IV contrast were different in terms of extent and comparison between these two conditions might thus be inappropriate. Platon et al. compared oral contrast alone versus both oral and IV contrasts, all the acquisitions being performed on the entire abdomen and pelvis. These authors reported a higher sensitivity with both oral and IV contrasts, but without any information on statistical significance. It is important to note that these two acquisitions were obtained with different radiation doses, the acquisition with oral contrast alone being at lower dose than that with oral and IV contrasts, with subsequent possible bias (Platon et al. 2009). Finally, Seo et al. (2009) compared unenhanced low-dose CT with IV enhanced low-dose CT and did not elicit any difference in diagnostic performance even for the diagnosis of appendiceal perforation.

Two of our studies suggested that the visualization of the appendix, either normal or diseased, is not influenced by IV contrast injection although IV contrast is susceptible to increase reader's reproducibility in the identification of an anatomic structure as the appendix (Keyzer et al. 2009, 2008) (Fig. 2). This observation is, at least in part, in accordance with that by Jacobs et al. (2001) who reported that IV contrast does not impact on the rate of visualization of the normal appendix but of diseased appendices. On the other hand, it should be kept in mind that IV contrast can be necessary to diagnose or to confirm ischemic and inflammatory processes (Jacobs et al. 2001; Johnson et al. 2006; Macari and Balthazar 2003; Pinto Leite et al. 2005). IV enhanced CT could thus be recommended when unenhanced scans are not definitely conclusive (Keyzer et al. 2009;

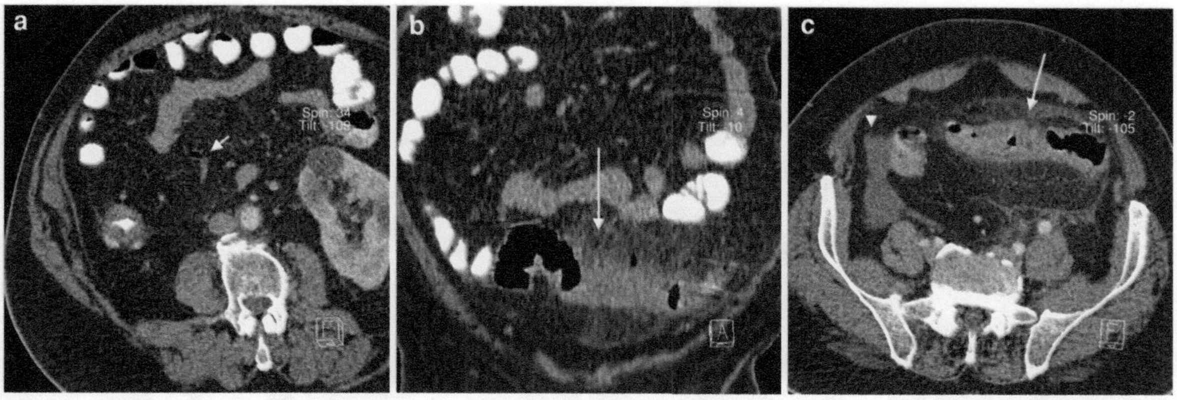

Fig. 4 CT images obtained with oral and IV contrast in a patient suspected of acute appendicitis with a definite diagnosis of acute sigmoid diverticulitis. **a** 3 mm oblique reformation image. The normal appendix is filled with air (*short arrow*) but not by oral contrast administered one and half hour before. **b** Coronal image demonstrates acute sigmoid diverticulitis (*long arrow*). **c** Transverse image demonstrates acute sigmoid diverticulitis (*long arrow*) and peritoneal effusion in the right iliac fossa (*arrowhead*)

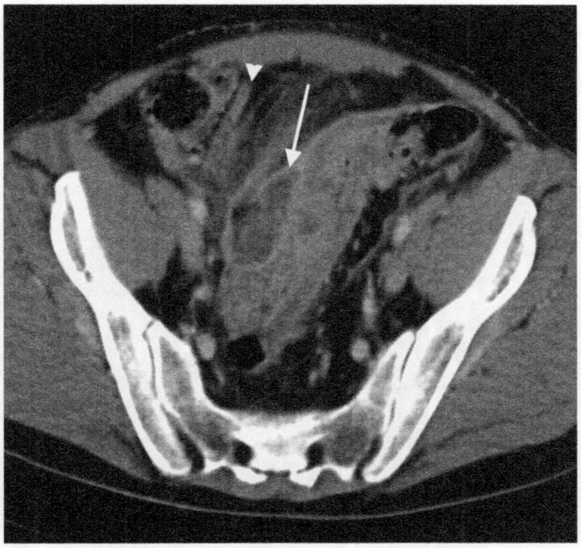

Fig. 5 Transverse CT image obtained with IV contrast only in a patient suspected of acute appendicitis with a definite diagnosis of high-grade acute sigmoid diverticulitis with abscess (*arrow*) and peritoneal stranding reaching the normal appendix (*arrowhead*)

Seo et al. 2009; Tamburrini et al. 2007; Paulson and Coursey 2009). Furthermore, IV contrast enables to detect a focal defect in the enhancing appendiceal wall that has been reported to be associated with perforation at surgery with, depending on studies, variable specificity (ranging from 80 to 100%) and sensitivity (ranging from 60 to 95%), and a lack of interobserver agreement (Bixby et al. 2006; Foley et al. 2005; Horrow et al. 2003; Tsuboi et al. 2008).

Rectal contrast is less frequently used than oral and IV contrasts in patients with acute abdominal pain, in particular in those with suspected acute appendicitis (O'Malley et al. 2000; Johnson et al. 2006). Rectal contrast administration enables a rapid opacification of the cecum and the normal appendix. However, such administration is quite uncomfortable for the patient and the rectal catheterization is not without risk particularly if the rectal wall is weakened by an inflammatory or ischemic process (Wise et al. 2001; Anderson et al. 2005; Pinto Leite et al. 2005; Dearing et al. 2008). Few studies have reported the high diagnostic performances of CT with rectal contrast alone, with sensitivity and NPV up to 98% (Rao et al. 1997b), but when compared with CT enhanced with both oral and IV contrast, rectal enhanced CT is not more accurate and has even lower sensitivity and NPV than dual enhanced CT for the diagnosis of acute appendicitis (Wise et al. 2001; Hershko et al. 2007).

It is important to remind that most studies with only rectal contrast were focused on the pelvis alone. Focused CT has the advantage to reduce the radiation dose but with MDCT scanners, rapid volume acquisition became possible and there is a clear trend to scan the entire abdomen and pelvis in all patients suspected of any abdominal disorder (O'Malley et al. 2000; Johnson et al. 2006). In addition, such examinations of the entire abdomen and pelvis are more effective than those focused on the pelvis, including their ability to detect alternative and/or additional diagnoses (some requiring even urgent surgical

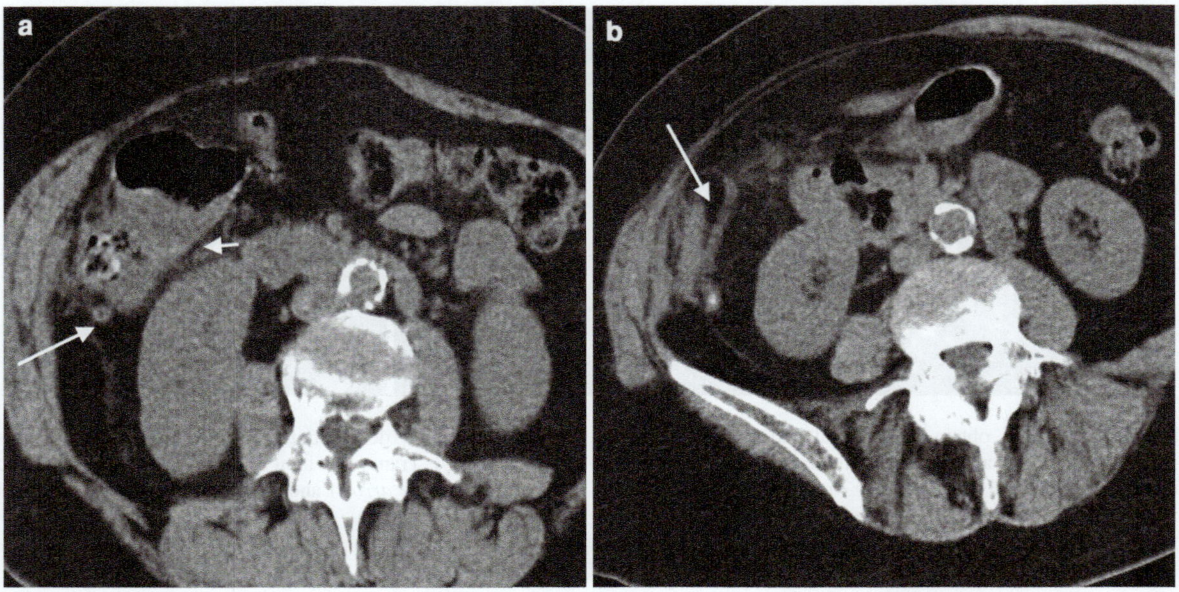

Fig. 6 **a**, **b** Transverse CT images obtained without any contrast (neither oral nor IV) in a patients suspected of acute appendicitis with a definite diagnosis of cecal neoplasia (*a short arrow*) with a normal appendix containing an appendicolith (*long arrows*) and minimal periappendiceal fat stranding

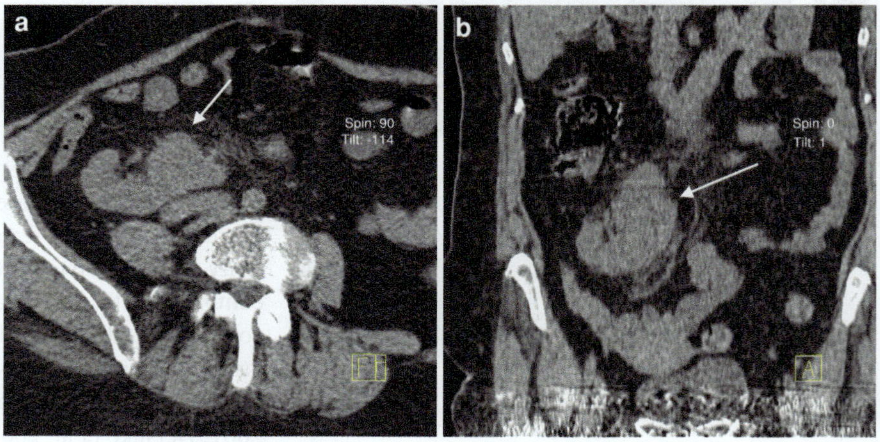

Fig. 7 Transverse (**a**) and coronal (**b**) CT images obtained without any contrast (neither oral nor IV) in a patient (BMI = 32 kg m^2-1) suspected of acute appendicitis. Definite diagnosis was acute pyelonephritis on a pelvic right kidney, diagnosed at CT without contrast and confirmed by microscopic urine examination

treatment) that could otherwise be missed in up to 7% of patients (Kamel et al. 2000). Another way to reduce the radiation dose is to decrease the tube current–time product and/or the tube potential. Several studies have showed that low-dose CT obtained by decreased tube current–time product (with subsequent effective dose ranging from 1.2 to 4.2 mSv, depending on the study and the patient's gender) has similar diagnostic performance than standard-dose CT for the diagnosis of acute appendicitis (Keyzer et al. 2004, 2009; Platon et al. 2009; Seo et al. 2009) (Fig. 2). Furthermore, none of these studies has been able to elicit any lower or upper threshold of BMI at which the diagnosis of acute appendicitis or the appendix visualization were hindered at low-dose (Keyzer et al. 2004, 2009; Seo et al. 2009). These observations should, however, be confirmed by studies focused on patients with extreme BMI categories (underweight and extremely obese patients) as their numbers were low in all these studies.

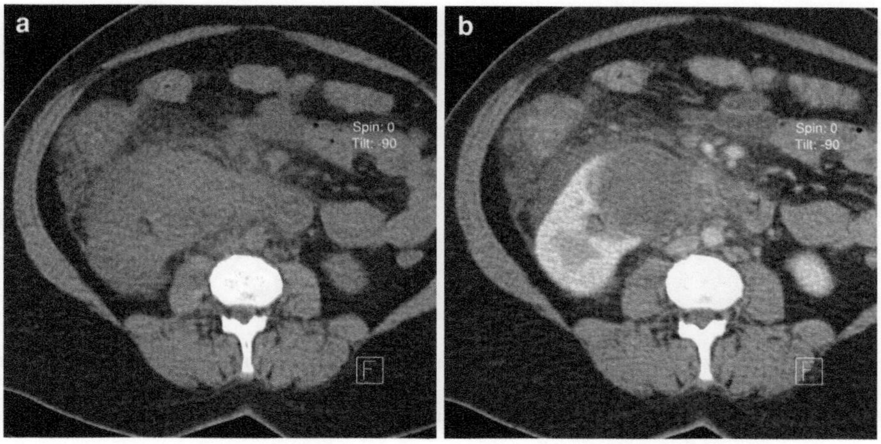

Fig. 8 Transverse CT images obtained a without and b with IV contrast in a patient suspected of acute appendicitis. Renal abscess with marked perirenal and pericolic fat stranding that can be depicted on unenhanced CT image (**a**) and clearly demonstrated on IV enhanced CT image (**b**)

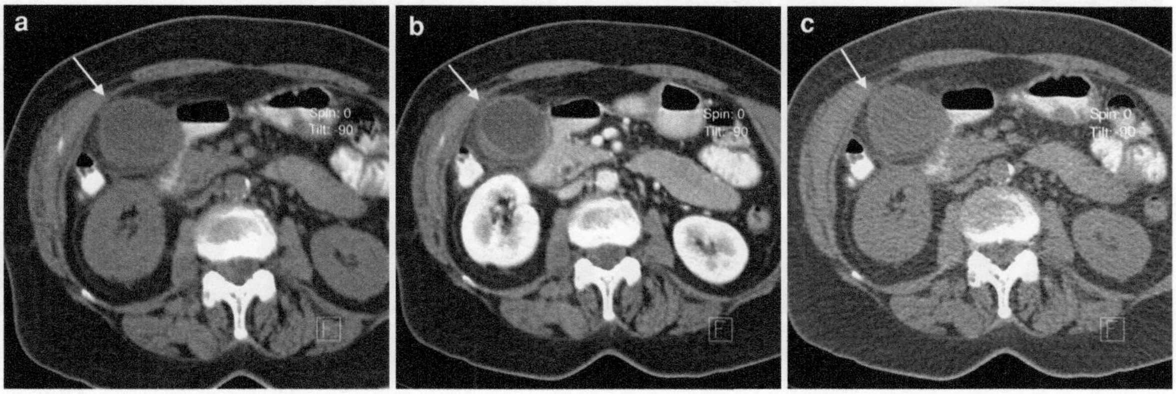

Fig. 9 Patient suspected of acute appendicitis and with a definite diagnosis of acute cholecystitis demonstrated on IV unenhanced CT image (**a**), IV enhanced CT image (**b**), and simulated low-dose IV unenhanced CT image (**c**)

In clinical practice and on the basis of the available literature, we recommend to perform an unenhanced low-dose CT on the entire abdomen and pelvis in adult patients suspected of acute appendicitis as a first step. If this unenhanced low-dose CT is inconclusive or if there is a need to confirm an alternative diagnosis, we recommend to perform an IV and/or oral enhanced low-dose CT, also on the entire abdomen and pelvis, as a second step (Keyzer et al. 2009; Seo et al. 2009; Tamburrini et al. 2007; Paulson and Coursey 2009). Such a protocol will globally reduce contrast material-related risks and examination costs without substantially increasing the radiation dose. Tips and tricks to reduce and optimize the radiation dose of abdominal CT in adults are extensively discussed in "Radiation Dose from MDCT Examinations for Suspected Acute Appendicitis" by D. Tack.

With MDCT, much attention has been focused on data set reconstruction and display, in particular, multi-planar reformations (MPR). It is now possible to scan the entire abdomen and pelvis within a single and comfortable breath hold at a spatial resolution less than 1 mm in the *x*-, *y*-, and *z*-axes. The obtained data sets allow MPR in any plane with a similar spatial resolution than in the transverse plane. It has been showed that coronal reformations improve the confidence in visualization of the appendix (whether normal or diseased) as well as for diagnosing or ruling out acute appendicitis (Kim et al. 2008; Paulson et al. 2005). Furthermore, it has been showed that performance of CT in the diagnosis of acute appendicitis is higher with 5 mm than with 10 mm thick CT sections and that the rate of appendiceal visualization and the reader confidence in his diagnosis are both increased

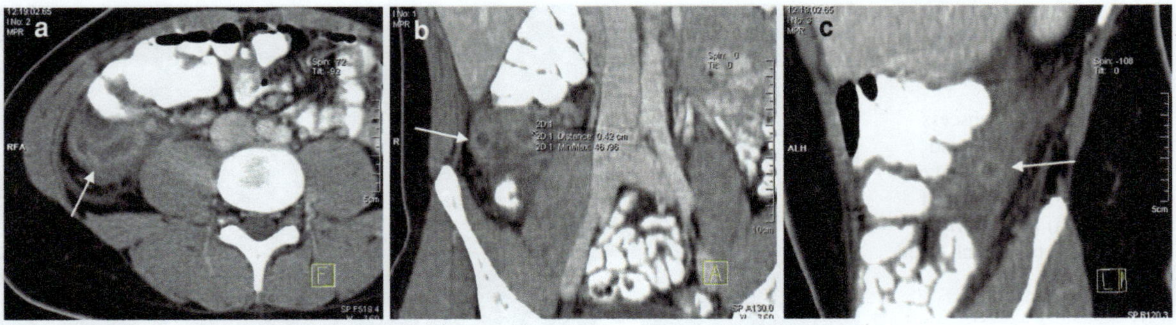

Fig. 10 Patient with definite diagnosis of acute appendicitis. Transverse (**a**), coronal (**b**) and sagittal (**c**) CT images obtained with oral and IV contrasts demonstrate an enlarged and enhancing appendix with parietal thickness of 4 mm (measured on figure **b**) and periappendiceal phlegmon

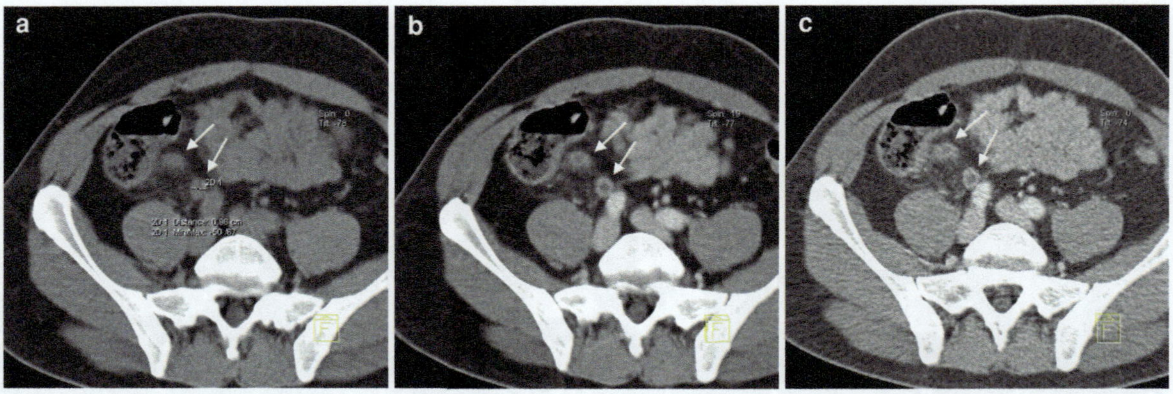

Fig. 11 CT images obtained without oral contrast in a patient with a definite diagnosis of acute appendicitis. **a** IV unenhanced standard dose CT image demonstrates enlarged appendix (*arrows*). **b** IV enhanced standard dose CT demonstrates enlarged appendix and abnormal enhancement of the appendiceal wall (*arrows*). **c** IV enhanced simulated low-dose CT demonstrates enlarged appendix and abnormal enhancement of the appendiceal wall (*arrows*). Minimal periappendiceal fat stranding is visible on all images

with slice thicknesses lower than 5 mm (i.e., 3 × 3 mm and 2 × 1 mm) (Weltman et al. 2000; Johnson et al. 2009).

3 CT Findings of Acute Appendicitis

CT findings of acute appendicitis are divided into appendiceal changes, cecal apical changes, and periappendiceal inflammatory changes (or right lower quadrant (RLQ) inflammatory changes) (Pinto Leite et al. 2005; Choi et al. 2003; Rao et al. 1997c). Many of these findings are also found in patients with alternative diseases mimicking acute appendicitis. Alternative diseases are numerous and listed in Table 1. Examples of these diagnoses, some of them with appendiceal and/or periappendiceal changes, are illustrated in Figs. 3, 4, 5, 6, 7, 8 and 9. The tumors of the appendix will be separately extensively described and illustrated in "Imaging of Primary Appendiceal Neoplasm" by Potretzke and Pickhardt.

3.1 Appendiceal Changes

Appendiceal changes consist in appendiceal enlargement, appendiceal wall thickening, appendicolith, and abnormal appendiceal wall enhancement after IV contrast injection (Figs. 1, 2, 10 and 11). Conversely, an appendiceal lumen completely—i.e., from its base to the tip—filled with gas and/or contrast material after oral or rectal contrast administration suggests the absence of acute appendicitis (Rao et al. 1997a, c).

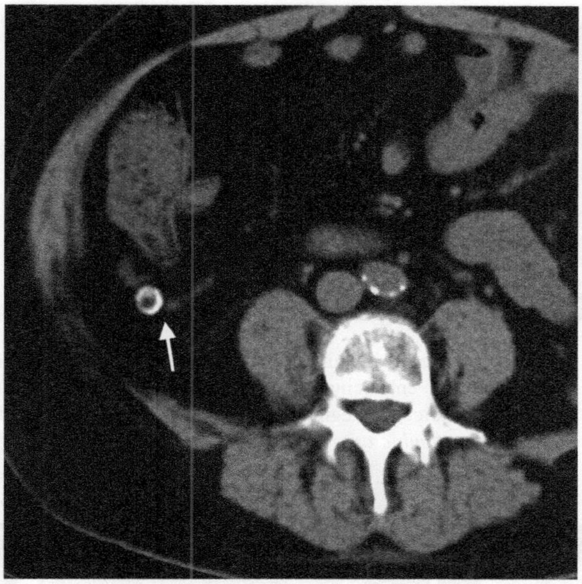

Fig. 12 Transverse unenhanced CT image demonstrates a normal appendix with a large appendicolith

There are controversies regarding the appendiceal diameter threshold suggesting acute appendicitis in adults. Such a threshold was first extrapolated from the sonography literature and was defined as an outer-wall-to-outer-wall transverse diameter larger than 6 mm (Funaki et al. 1998; Choi et al. 2003; Rao et al. 1997c; Raptopoulos et al. 2003). However, the diameter of the appendix at US is measured during graded compression of the RLQ which may produce smaller measures than at CT performed without compression (Pinto Leite et al. 2005). There are indeed normal appendices with a diameter larger than 6 mm (Pinto Leite et al. 2005; Paulson et al. 2005; Daly et al. 2005; Moteki and Horikoshi 2007). Facing these observations, higher thresholds (ranging from 8 to 10 mm) have been proposed and validated in the diagnosis of acute appendicitis, in particular if its content is not visualized and in the absence of periappendiceal changes (Keyzer et al. 2004; Benjaminov et al. 2002). The appendiceal diameter measured at CT from outer-wall-to-outer-wall depends on the appendiceal content. Therefore, it could be recommended to measure the appendiceal wall only, with a threshold of 3 mm if the lumen content is visible (Tamburrini et al. 2005; Pinto Leite et al. 2005; Benjaminov et al. 2002; Webb et al. 2010) (Fig. 10).

Appendicolith, when considered alone, is not a 100% specific sign of acute appendicitis as it can be seen in normal adults, the presence of appendicolith alone being associated with acute appendicitis in 10% of adult patients only (Lane et al. 1999; Daly et al. 2005) (Fig. 12).

At IV enhanced CT, abnormal appendiceal wall enhancement is one of the most suggestive findings of acute appendicitis (Choi et al. 2003). The thickened wall is usually homogeneously enhanced, but mural stratification can be seen (Pinto Leite et al. 2005; Choi et al. 2003). In addition it has been showed that a focal enhancement defect in the appendiceal wall is highly suggestive of appendiceal perforation (Fig. 13).

Concerning the features ruling out acute appendicitis, we must emphasize that intraluminal air can be seen in inflamed appendix as well and thus does not necessarily mean that the appendix is patent and normal (Choi et al. 2003) (Fig. 13 and 14).

3.2 Periappendiceal Inflammatory Changes

Periappendiceal inflammatory changes consist in periappendiceal fat stranding and/or extraluminal fluid, phlegmon, abscess, and lymphadenopathies (Figs. 1, 2, 10, 11, 13 and 14).

When associated with an appendiceal enlargement, periappendiceal fat stranding is highly suggestive of acute appendicitis (Keyzer et al. 2004; Choi et al. 2003; Rao et al. 1997c). However, with the increased use of CT in patients with acute appendicitis, patients undergo CT examination very early after the onset of their symptoms and the periappendiceal fat stranding can be lacking in patients who have a definite acute appendicitis but who are scanned very early (Raptopoulos et al. 2003).

Periappendiceal phlegmon and abscess are highly suggestive of appendiceal perforation with a specificity ranging from 95 to100%. The other CT signs suggesting the perforation are extraluminal air or extraluminal appendicolith, and focal enhancement defect in the appendiceal wall after IV contrast injection. When considered separately, these signs are highly specific but have a low sensitivity, the only one with a sensitivity higher than 60% being the focal enhancement defect (Bixby et al. 2006; Horrow et al. 2003; Tsuboi et al. 2008) (Figs. 10, 13).

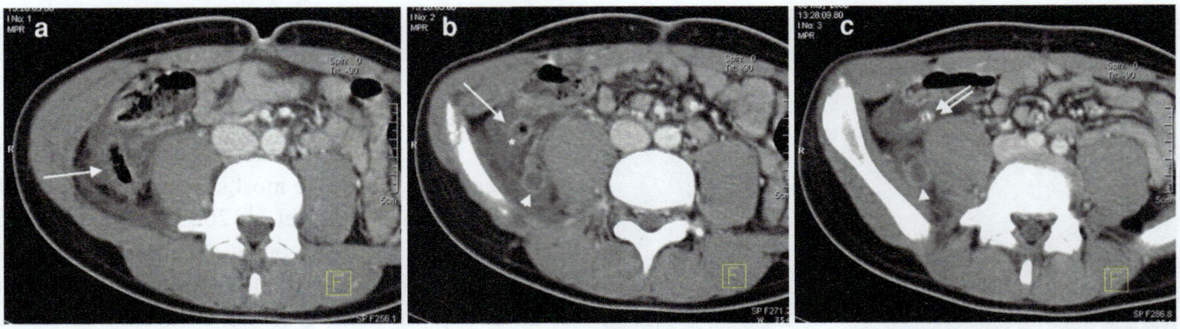

Fig. 13 **a**, **b**, **c** CT images obtained with IV contrast but without oral contrast in a patient with perforated acute appendicitis. **a** Presence of air in the enlarged appendix surrounded by a phlegmon (*arrow*) **b** Enlarged and enhancing appendix with focal enhancement defect in its wall (*star*). The appendix is filled with air (*arrow*) and liquid (*arrowhead*). **c** Enlarged and enhancing fluid-filled appendix (*arrowhead*) with periappendiceal phlegmon and appendicolith at the base of the appendix (*double arrow*)

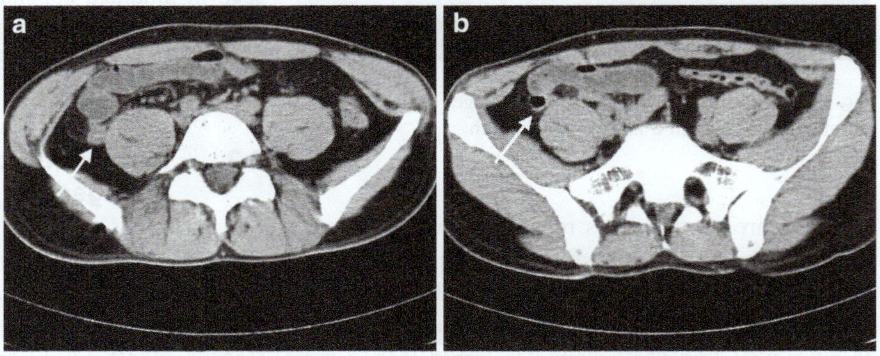

Fig. 14 **a**, **b** Patient with a definite diagnosis of acute appendicitis. Transverse CT images obtained without any contrast demonstrate an enlarged appendix with minimal periappendiceal fat stranding (**a**) and air at the tip of the appendix on an image obtained more inferiorly (**b**)

3.3 Cecal Apical Changes

Cecal apical changes consist in cecal apical thickening, and after enteric contrast administration, the so-called arrowhead sign and cecal bar sign (Rao et al. 1997a, b, d, e). The arrowhead sign is observed when cecal contrast material funnels in between each side of symmetric cecal apical thickening and targets to the point of appendiceal occlusion (Fig. 15). The cecal bar sign is observed when a proximal calcified appendicolith is separated from the cecal lumen containing dense cecal contrast material by inflamed soft tissue of the appendiceal base and the cecal apex.

3.4 Detection of the Normal Appendix

The detection of the normal appendix rules out the diagnosis of acute appendicitis (Balthazar et al. 1986; Ganguli et al. 2006; Nikolaidis et al. 2004). At CT, the rate of its visualization ranges from 43 to 91% depending on the study (patients included being symptomatic or asymptomatic, different anatomic coverage, various contrast administrations) (Balthazar et al. 1994; Benjaminov et al. 2002; Jan et al. 2005). The detection of the normal appendix strengthens the reader's confidence in a truly negative result, even if recent studies have reported that a non-visualized appendix at CT reliably excludes acute appendicitis if secondary inflammatory changes are also absent (Balthazar et al. 1986; Ganguli et al. 2006; Nikolaidis et al. 2004). We have, however, shown that the reproducibility in visualization of the normal appendix depends on the reader (Keyzer et al. 2008). This should make us cautious in considering rates of visualization of the appendix that are reported in studies based on the identification of a normal appendix on one hand, and in the confidence that the physician could have in his/her colleague radiologist when he/she states that the normal appendix is visualized on the other hand.

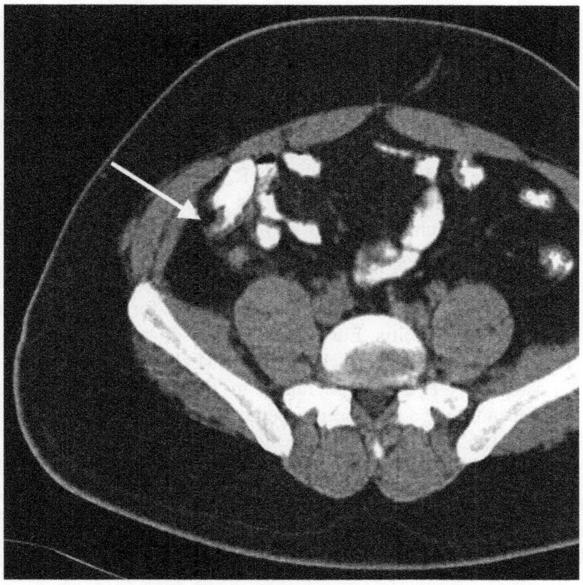

Fig. 15 CT image obtained with oral contrast in a patient with a definite diagnosis of acute appendicitis demonstrates the so-called *arrowhead sign* (*arrow*)

4 Conclusions

CT is extensively used in adult patients with acute appendicitis. Contrast, in particular oral contrast, is not mandatory to make or rule out the diagnosis of acute appendicitis in normal to obese adult patients. IV contrast could be reserved if there are doubts on the diagnosis of acute appendicitis or alternative disease. The radiation dose can be reduced at unenhanced as well as at enhanced CT. Further studies are still needed to investigate the appropriateness of these approaches in particular patients, i.e. without any contrast material in underweight patients as well as with reduced radiation dose in extremely obese patients.

References

Anderson BA, Salem L, Flum DR (2005) A systematic review of whether oral contrast is necessary for the computed tomography diagnosis of appendicitis in adults. Am J Surg 190:474–478

Anderson SW, Soto JA, Lucey BC et al (2009) Abdominal 64-MDCT for suspected appendicitis: the use of oral and IV contrast material versus IV contrast material only. Am J Roentgenol 193:1282–1288

Anderson SW, Rhea JT, Milch HN, Ozonoff A, Lucey BC, Soto JA (2010) Influence of body habitus and use of oral contrast on reader confidence in patients with suspected acute appendicitis using 64 MDCT. Emerg Radiol 17(6):445–453

Balthazar EJ, Megibow AJ, Hulnick D, Gordon RB, Naidich DP, Beranbaum ER (1986) CT of appendicitis. Am J Roentgenol 147:705–710

Balthazar EJ, Birnbaum BA, Yee J, Megibow AJ, Roshkow J, Gray C (1994) Acute appendicitis: CT and US correlation in 100 patients. Radiology 190:31–35

Benjaminov O, Atri M, Hamilton P, Rappaport D (2002) Frequency of visualization and thickness of normal appendix at non-enhanced helical CT. Radiology 225:400–406

Birnbaum BA, Wilson SR (2000) Appendicitis at the millennium. Radiology 215:337–348

Bixby SD, Lucey BC, Soto JA, Theysohn JM, Ozonoff A, Varghese JC (2006) Perforated versus non-perforated acute appendicitis: Accuracy of multi-detector CT detection. Radiology 241:780–786

Choi D, Park H, Lee YR et al (2003) The most useful findings for diagnosing acute appendicitis on contrast-enhanced helical CT. Acta Radiol 44:574–582

Daly CP, Cohan RH, Francis IR, Caoili EM, Ellis JH, Nan B (2005) Incidence of acute appendicitis in patients with equivocal CT findings. Am J Roentgenol 184:1813–1820

Dearing DD, Recabaren JA, Alexander M (2008) Can computed tomography scan be performed effectively in the diagnosis of acute appendicitis without the added morbidity of rectal contrast? Am Surg 74:917–920

Ege G, Akman H, Sahin A, Bugra D, Kuzucu K (2002) Diagnostic value of unenhanced helical CT in adult patients with suspected acute appendicitis. Br J Radiol 75:721–725

Foley TA, Earnest F, Nathan MA, Hough DM, Schiller HJ, Hoskin TL (2005) Differentiation of non-perforated from perforated appendicitis: Accuracy of CT diagnosis and relationship of CT findings to length of hospital stay. Radiology 235:89–96

Funaki B, Grosskreutz SR, Funaki CN (1998) Using unenhanced helical CT with enteric contrast material for suspected appendicitis in patients treated at a community hospital. Am J Roentgenol 171:997–1001

Ganguli S, Raptopoulos V, Komlos F, Siewert B, Kruskal JB (2006) Right lower quadrant pain: Value of the non-visualized appendix in patients at multi-detector CT. Radiology 241:175–180

Hershko DD, Awad N, Fischer D et al (2007) Focused helical CT using rectal contrast material only as the preferred technique for the diagnosis of suspected acute appendicitis: a prospective, randomized, controlled study comparing three different techniques. Dis Colon Rectum 50:1223–1229

Horrow MM, White DS, Horrow JC (2003) Differentiation of perforated from non-perforated appendicitis at CT. Radiology 227:46–51

Jacobs JE, Birnbaum BA, Macari M et al (2001) Acute appendicitis: Comparison of helical CT diagnosis focused technique with oral contrast material versus non-focused technique with oral and intravenous contrast material. Radiology 220:683–690

Jan YT, Yang FS, Huang JK (2005) Visualization rate and pattern of normal appendix on multi-detector computed tomography by using multi-planar reformation display. J Comput Assist Tomogr 29:446–451

Johnson PT, Horton KM, Mahesh M, Fishman EK (2006) Multidetector computed tomography for suspected appendicitis: Multi-institutional survey of 16-MDCT data acquisition protocols and review of pertinent literature. J Comput Assist Tomogr 30:758–764

Johnson PT, Horton KM, Kawamoto S et al (2009) MDCT for suspected appendicitis: Effect of reconstruction section thickness on diagnostic accuracy, rate of appendiceal visualization, and reader confidence using axial images. Am J Roentgenol 192:893–901

Kamel IR, Goldberg SN, Keogan MT, Rosen MP, Raptopoulos V (2000) Right lower quadrant pain and suspected appendicitis: Non-focused appendiceal CT–review of 100 cases. Radiology 217:159–163

Keyzer C, Tack D, De Maertelaer V, Bohy P, Gevenois PA, Van Gansbeke D (2004) Acute appendicitis: Comparison of low-dose and standard-dose unenhanced multi-detector row CT. Radiology 232:164–172

Keyzer C, Pargov S, Tack D et al (2008) Normal appendix in adults: Reproducibility of detection with unenhanced and contrast-enhanced MDCT. Am J Roentgenol 191:507–514

Keyzer C, Cullus P, Tack D, De Maertelaer V, Bohy P, Gevenois PA (2009) MDCT for suspected acute appendicitis in adults: Impact of oral and IV contrast media at standard-dose and simulated low-dose techniques. Am J Roentgenol 193:1272–1281

Kim HC, Yang DM, Jin W, Park SJ (2008) Added diagnostic value of multi-planar reformation of multi-detector CT data in patients with suspected appendicitis. Radiographics 28:393–405

Krieg AF, Gambino R, Galen RS (1975) Why are clinical laboratory tests performed? When are they valid? JAMA 233:76–78

Lane MJ, Liu DM, Huynh MD, Jeffrey RB Jr, Mindelzun RE, Katz DS (1999) Suspected acute appendicitis: Nonenhanced helical CT in 300 consecutive patients. Radiology 213:341–346

Macari M, Balthazar EJ (2003) The acute right lower quadrant: CT evaluation. Radiol Clin North Am 41:1117–1136

Moteki T, Horikoshi H (2007) New CT criterion for acute appendicitis: Maximum depth of intraluminal appendiceal fluid. Am J Roentgenol 188:1313–1319

Mun S, Ernst RD, Chen K, Oto A, Shah S, Mileski WJ (2006) Rapid CT diagnosis of acute appendicitis with IV contrast material. Emerg Radiol 12:99–102

Nikolaidis P, Hwang CM, Miller FH, Papanicolaou N (2004) The non-visualized appendix: Incidence of acute appendicitis when secondary inflammatory changes are absent. Am J Roentgenol 183:889–892

No authors (1998) Executive summary of the clinical guidelines on the identification, evaluation, and treatment of overweight and obesity in adults. Arch Intern Med 158:1855–1867

O'Malley ME, Halpern E, Mueller PR, Gazelle GS (2000) Helical CT protocols for the abdomen and pelvis: a survey. Am J Roentgenol 175:109–113

Paulson EK, Coursey CA (2009) CT protocols for acute appendicitis: Time for change. Am J Roentgenol 193:1268–1271

Paulson EK, Harris JP, Jaffe TA, Haugan PA, Nelson RC (2005) Acute appendicitis: Added diagnostic value of coronal reformations from isotropic voxels at multi-detector row CT. Radiology 235:879–885

Pinto Leite N, Pereira JM, Cunha R, Pinto P, Sirlin C (2005) CT evaluation of appendicitis and its complications: Imaging techniques and key diagnostic findings. Am J Roentgenol 185:406–417

Platon A, Jlassi H, Rutschmann OT et al (2009) Evaluation of a low-dose CT protocol with oral contrast for assessment of acute appendicitis. Eur Radiol 19:446–454

Poortman P, Lohle PN, Schoemaker CM et al (2003) Comparison of CT and sonography in the diagnosis of acute appendicitis: a blinded prospective study. Am J Roentgenol 181:1355–1359

Raman SS, Lu DS, Kadell BM, Vodopich DJ, Sayre J, Cryer H (2002) Accuracy of non-focused helical CT for the diagnosis of acute appendicitis: a 5 year review. Am J Roentgenol 178:1319–1325

Rao PM, Rhea JT, Novelline RA et al (1997a) Helical CT technique for the diagnosis of appendicitis: Prospective evaluation of a focused appendix CT examination. Radiology 202:139–144

Rao PM, Rhea JT, Novelline RA, Mostafavi AA, Lawrason JN, McCabe CJ (1997b) Helical CT combined with contrast material administered only through the colon for imaging of suspected appendicitis. Am J Roentgenol 169: 1275–1280

Rao PM, Rhea JT, Novelline RA (1997c) Sensitivity and specificity of the individual CT signs of appendicitis: Experience with 200 helical appendiceal CT examinations. J Comput Assist Tomogr 21:686–692

Rao PM, Wittenberg J, McDowell RK, Rhea JT, Novelline RA (1997d) Appendicitis: use of arrowhead sign for diagnosis at CT. Radiology 202:363–366

Rao PM, Rhea JT, Novelline RA (1997e) Helical computed tomographic incidence and characterization of appendoliths in 100 patients with appendicitis. Emerg Radiol 4:55–61

Raptopoulos V, Katsou G, Rosen MP, Siewert B, Goldberg SN, Kruskal JB (2003) Acute appendicitis: Effect of increased use of CT on selecting patients earlier. Radiology 226:521–526

Seo H, Lee KH, Kim HJ et al (2009) Diagnosis of acute appendicitis with sliding slab ray-sum interpretation of low-dose unenhanced CT and standard-dose i.v. contrast-enhanced CT scans. Am J Roentgenol 193:96–105

Tamburrini S, Brunetti A, Brown M, Sirlin CB, Casola G (2005) CT appearance of the normal appendix in adults. Eur Radiol 15:2096–2103

Tamburrini S, Brunetti A, Brown M, Sirlin C, Casola G (2007) Acute appendicitis: Diagnostic value of non-enhanced CT with selective use of contrast in routine clinical settings. Eur Radiol 17:2055–2061

Tsuboi M, Takase K, Kaneda I et al (2008) Perforated and non-perforated appendicitis: Defect in enhancing appendiceal wall–depiction with multi-detector row CT. Radiology 246:142–147

Webb EM, Wang ZJ, Coakley FV, Poder L, Westphalen AC, Yeh BM (2010) The equivocal appendix at CT: Prevalence in a control population. Emerg Radiol 17:57–61

Weltman DI, Yu J, Krumenacker J Jr, Huang S, Moh P (2000) Diagnosis of acute appendicitis: Comparison of 5 and 10 mm CT sections in the same patient. Radiology 216:172–177

Wijetunga R, Tan BS, Rouse JC, Bigg-Wither GW, Doust BD (2001) Diagnostic accuracy of focused appendiceal CT in clinically equivocal cases of acute appendicitis. Radiology 221:747–753

Wise SW, Labuski MR, Kasales CJ et al (2001) Comparative assessment of CT and sonographic techniques for appendiceal imaging. Am J Roentgenol 176:933–941

Wolfe JM, Smithline H, Lee S, Coughlin B, Polino J, Blank F (2006) The impact of body mass index on concordance in the interpretation of matched non-contrast and contrast abdominal pelvic computed tomographic scans in ED patients with non-traumatic abdominal pain. Am J Emerg Med 24:144–148

Ultrasonography Versus Computed Tomography: Evidence-Based Imaging

Caroline Keyzer and Pierre Alain Gevenois

Contents

C. Keyzer (✉) · P. A. Gevenois
Department of Radiology, Hôpital Erasme,
Université libre de Bruxelles, Route de Lennik 808,
1070 Brussels, Belgium
e-mail: caroline.keyzer@erasme.ulb.ac.be

Abstract

Multi-detector row CT (MDCT) and graded-compression ultrasonography (US), associated or not with color Doppler US, are highly accurate techniques for diagnosing acute appendicitis in adult patients. The choice between these two techniques is however challenging and only few studies have compared them in the same group of patients. Beyond their performances, the choice between these techniques depends on patient's characteristics (age, habitus, and gender), available techniques and expertise, practitioner's preference, concern in radiation issues, economical aspects, and cost-effectiveness ratio. This chapter will discuss and comment the few studies comparing these techniques, discuss the parameters that could influence the choice between them and their cost-effectiveness, and will propose an imaging strategy.

Abbreviations

BMI	Body mass index
MDCT	Multi-detector row CT
US	Ultrasonography

1 Introduction

Multi-detector row CT (MDCT) and graded-compression ultrasonography (US), associated or not with color Doppler US, are highly accurate techniques for diagnosing acute appendicitis in adult patients. The choice between these two techniques is, however challenging

C. Keyzer and P. A. Gevenois (eds.), *Imaging of Acute Appendicitis in Adults and Children*,
Medical Radiology. Diagnostic Imaging, DOI: 10.1007/174_2011_217, © Springer-Verlag Berlin Heidelberg 2011

and could depend, among others, on institutional preferences, available expertise, patient's age, gender, and body habitus (Birnbaum and Wilson 2000).

US is rapid, non-invasive (requiring neither ionizing radiation nor contrast material), and inexpensive, but believed to be dependent on observer's experience and furthermore is uncomfortable in painful patients even if information obtained during the examination about the degree of pain and location of maximal tenderness are very helpful (Hernanz-Schulman 2010; Wise et al. 2001; Vermeulen et al. 1999). On the other hand, CT is nowadays widely available, reproducible, and offers images that can be easily reread by radiologists and surgeons other than one who first obtained or read them.

2 Comparison Between Performances of US and CT

Many studies evaluating imaging techniques in patients suspected of acute appendicitis have evaluated one single technique but have not compared different techniques in the same patient study group, or have not evaluated the incremental added value of one technique on the other, or on the clinical diagnosis.

A meta-analysis by van Randen et al., based on the very few available prospective studies that compared graded-compression US and CT (with or without contrast) in the same adult study groups globally showed higher sensitivity and specificity of CT than US (van Randen et al. 2008). Studies comparing US and enhanced CT (i.e., with oral and/or IV contrast material) reported higher performance of CT than US in diagnosing acute appendicitis as well as alternative diseases, with a higher rate of visualization of the normal appendix and less patient discomfort at CT than at US (Wise et al. 2001; Balthazar et al. 1994; Horton et al. 2000; Wilson et al. 2001). When compared to unenhanced CT (i.e., without any contrast material) however, US has similar diagnostic performance than CT for diagnosing acute appendicitis as well as alternative diseases, whatever patient's age, gender, and body habitus estimated through his Body Mass Index (BMI) (Keyzer et al. 2005; Poortman et al. 2003). These apparently discordant results could be explained, at least in part, by differences between the methods used in the studies by Keyzer et al. and Poortman et al. on one hand, and in the other studies on the other hand. In these other studies indeed (1) US examinations were performed by sonographers and not by radiologists, did not investigated the entire abdomen and pelvis, and/or were not performed with the graded-compression technique as recommended by Puylaert (Wise et al. 2001; van Randen et al. 2008; Wilson et al. 2001; Puylaert 1986); and (2) CT examinations were obtained with IV and/or oral contrast (Wise et al. 2001; van Randen et al. 2008; Balthazar et al. 1994; Wilson et al. 2001). One of our studies and a very recent retrospective investigation by Gaitani et al. showed however that inconclusive examinations—i.e., without diagnosis and without visualization of the normal appendix—are more frequent at US than at CT, probably because the normal appendix is far more frequently seen at CT than at US (Hernanz-Schulman 2010; Wise et al. 2001; Keyzer et al. 2005; Gaitini et al. 2008). Furthermore, in 52 pregnant women with acute abdominal pain who had both US and CT examinations, 46 had a negative US examination but CT demonstrated, however important diagnostic information in 14 of them (with nine needing a surgical intervention) with a diagnosis of acute appendicitis in seven (appendicitis was diagnosed at US in only one of those with definite acute appendicitis) (Lazarus et al. 2007). Imaging acute appendicitis in pregnant women is extensively discussed by Jaffe in "Imaging of Acute Appendicitis in Adults: Current Practices in Pregnant Woman".

The choice between US and CT could depend on patient's body habitus. The small distance between the transducer on the skin and the appendix in slim patients is favorable to US. Conversely, the absence of intra-abdominal fat or its low amount in these patients could reduce the performance of unenhanced CT. Obesity, on the other hand, is susceptible to reduce the performance of both techniques because obesity reduces the visualization of intra-abdominal organs by excessive ultrasound beam attenuation at US while it reduces the signal/noise ratio at CT. The increase in incidence of obesity in Western countries could thus lead to a subsequent increased proportion of inconclusive examinations, particularly at US (Uppot et al. 2006). However, in one of our studies comparing US and unenhanced CT, the body habitus estimated through BMI did not influence the visualization of the appendix or the diagnostic performance of either MDCT or US, but our study group included only a small number of underweight and obese-to-extremely-obese patients, as classified according to the BMI categories recommended by the World Health Organization (Keyzer et al. 2005; No authors 1998). The absence of BMI effect on the diagnostic performance of either technique could be explained by limitations of US in obese patients being offset by limitations of CT in underweight patients. Further studies with large numbers of patients in these extreme BMI's categories should thus be conducted to confirm these preliminary observations.

The choice between US and CT could also depend on patient's gender. We showed that gender influences the diagnostic correctness at CT either with or without contrast, with higher correctness and reproducibility of diagnosis in men than in women, particularly in case of alternative disease (Keyzer et al. 2005, 2009). This can be explained by the incidence of gynecological diseases mimicking acute appendicitis in women and for the diagnosis of which CT has a lower performance than US. We indeed did not observe a gender influence at US on the diagnosis correctness. This gender influence at CT was not elicited in a previous study by Raman et al. in which there were only a small proportion of gynecological diseases (Raman et al. 2003).

A recent multicentric study has evaluated the added value of plain radiographs, US (using the graded-compression technique), and CT (on the entire abdomen and pelvis with IV contrast only) after clinical evaluation for making urgent diagnoses–defined as conditions needing a treatment within 24 h, including acute appendicitis which was the most frequent diagnosis—in adults presenting with acute abdominal pain (Lameris et al. 2009). These authors evaluated multiple imaging strategies, single (plain radiographs, US, or CT) or conditional (CT if US was negative or inconclusive, or inconclusive alone). They also investigated imaging strategies driven by patient's age, BMI, and location of pain. These authors showed that the clinical diagnosis with or without plain radiographs has high sensitivity but a lack of specificity. Compared with the clinical diagnosis, US reduces the number of false positive diagnoses but produces an unacceptably high number of missed urgent conditions (30%) with the lowest sensitivity of all investigated strategies as showed in Fig. 1 (Lameris et al. 2009). These findings are in accordance with those previously reported by Wise et al. (Wise et al. 2001), as US alone has a lower sensitivity than CT alone. Compared with clinical evaluation alone, these

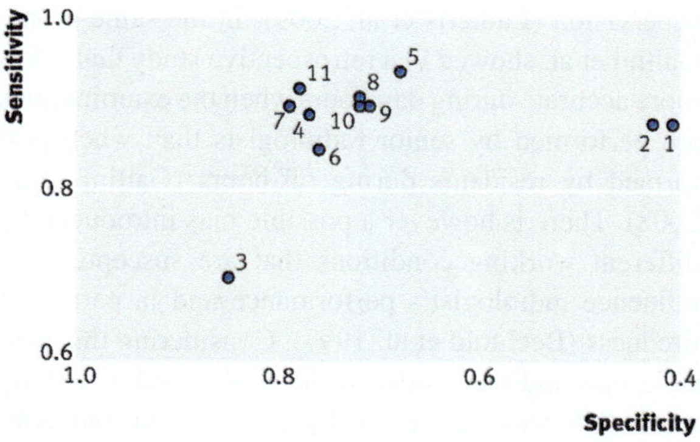

Fig. 1 Diagnostic performance of all imaging strategies presented in receiver operating characteristics space. Numbers correspond to strategies: (1) Clinical diagnosis, (2) Clinical diagnosis after plain radiographs, (3) Ultrasonography (US) in all patients, (4) Computed tomography (CT) in all patients, (5) US in all patients; CT if US negative or inconclusive, (6) US in all patients; CT if US inconclusive, (7) If age <45 then US and CT if US negative or inconclusive; if age ≥45 then CT, (8) If body mass index <30 then US and CT if US negative or inconclusive; if body mass index ≥30 then CT, (9) If body mass index <30 or age <45 then US and CT if US negative or inconclusive; CT in all other patients, (10) If tenderness in right upper quadrant then US; if tenderness in right lower quadrant, left upper quadrant, or left lower quadrant then CT; if diffuse tenderness then CT; CT in all other patients, (11) If tenderness in right upper quadrant or right lower quadrant then US; if tenderness in left lower quadrant or left upper quadrant then CT; if diffuse tenderness then CT; CT in all other patients. Reproduced from "Imaging strategies for detection of urgent conditions in patients with acute abdominal pain" by Lameris et al. 2009, with permission from BMJ Publishing Group Ltd

two techniques showed an increase in specificity but not in sensitivity when used as a single test. The use of conditional CT after negative or inconclusive US examinations had the highest sensitivity in these urgent conditions. In addition, with this conditional CT strategy, only one half of the patients require CT and the CT-related exposure would be the lowest even when compared to the strategies driven by patient's characteristics or location of pain (Lameris et al. 2009).

Finally, the choice between US and CT is susceptible to depend on the time of the examination. Interestingly, this multicentric study by Lameris et al. showed that the sensitivity of US performed after working hours by residents without supervision is lower than when performed by radiologists, but not during working hours when residents are supervised. However, there is no difference in specificity between radiologists and residents regardless of their supervision (Lameris et al. 2009). In the same scope, Gaitini et al. showed in a retrospective study that US is more accurate during day hours when the examinations are performed by senior radiologists than when performed by residents during off-hours (Gaitini et al. 2008). There is however a possible bias introduced by different working conditions that are susceptible to influence radiologist's performance and in particular tiredness (Bechtold et al. 1997). Considering this possible bias and the results we have obtained in a study where US was performed by experienced and non-experienced radiologists whatever the day time, we should not definitely conclude that US is influenced by radiologist's experience (Keyzer et al. 2005).

3 Imaging Strategy

There is not yet any consensus strategy for imaging adult patients suspected of acute appendicitis. In addition to scientific information, the care pathway could also be influenced by economic considerations and governmental or institutional allocation of health-care resources (i.e., availability of US all-around the clock, development of teleradiology that could potentially increase the use of CT, etc.), individual practitioner's experience or his/her preference in one technique (Frush et al. 2009). The care pathway could also be influenced by the practice environment as it could depend on the threshold of the surgeon at which he will consider acute appendicitis on one hand, and at which he will order imaging examinations on the other hand. This threshold is supposed to influence the added value of imaging by varying the pretest probability and thereby the posttest probability (van Randen et al. 2008). In their meta-analysis, van Randen et al. reported indeed a better differentiation of the disease at CT than at US at clinically relevant prevalences (prevalence of acute appendicitis was 50% in this meta-analysis), although at very low and very high prevalences, the difference in test performances between the imaging techniques was smaller (van Randen et al. 2008). Most importantly, these authors reported also a posttest probability at 9% after negative CT with a 50% prevalence of the disease. Thus, in a population with a high probability of acute appendicitis (depending on different factors as the proportion of women, ethnic-related differences, and referral practitioner), caution should be recommended after a negative CT examination in case of high clinical suspicion of acute appendicitis, and repeated clinical evaluation or diagnostic laparoscopy should be considered (van Randen et al. 2008). On the other hand, in a study based on 2,871 adult patients clinically suspected of acute appendicitis and with a prevalence of definite acute appendicitis approximating 20%, Pickhardt et al showed that the negative appendectomy rate would have been decreased from 7.5% to 4.1% if the patients with negative MDCT would not have undergo surgery (Pickhardt et al. 2011).

Each of the decision tree branches carries its own financial implications (Hernanz-Schulman 2010). Observation of patients without acute appendicitis can lead to unnecessary hospital days whereas prolonged observation of patients with acute appendicitis increases resources use if perforation occurs in addition to costs related to the observation itself. On the other hand, unnecessary surgery procedures increase also the costs and have their own possible complications. The use of imaging also influences the costs depending on its discriminating power with possible adverse effects (i.e., contrast material administration and/or radiation-induced effects at CT) (Wan et al. 2009). However, the theoretical increase in mortality related to radiation-induced malignancy should be weighted by the appendicitis-related mortality and its immediate consequences (i.e., unnecessary laparotomy, perforation, worsening of peritonitis) (Hernanz-Schulman 2010; McCollough et al. 2009). This balance should be carefully considered since the radiation dose can be dramatically reduced without impairment of the diagnostic performance of CT, whatever the use of contrast may be (Keyzer et al. 2004; Tack et al. 2003, 2005). The radiation dose reduction and optimization of abdominal CT in adults are extensively discussed in "Radiation Dose from MDCT Examinations for Suspected Acute Appendicitis" by Tack.

4 Conclusion

According to the currently available information, the following imaging strategy could be proposed in normal-weighted adult patients suspected of acute appendicitis. US examination should be performed first, particularly in young women in whom gynaecological diseases are common mimics of acute

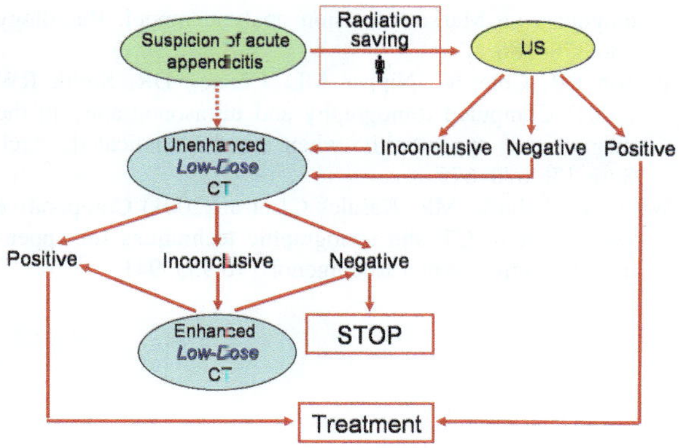

Fig. 2 Flow chart of the proposed imaging strategy in normal-weighted adults suspected of acute appendicitis

appendicitis. If US examination is negative or inconclusive, unenhanced MDCT should be recommended as a second step. If unenhanced MDCT is also inconclusive, enhanced MDCT with IV contrast alone or with both IV and oral contrasts should then be performed (Fig. 2). All these MDCT examinations should be done at reduced and optimized radiation dose. In underweight and overweight patients, currently available studies are insufficient to propose a definite strategy. In overweight patients, it could however be reasonable to skip US and to perform first unenhanced MDCT scan. In underweight patients on the other hand, it could be also reasonable to skip unenhanced CT and to perform IV and/or oral-enhanced CT only if US is inconclusive. Depending on the results of cost-effectiveness studies that should be conducted in adult patients as they were done in children, these strategies could nevertheless be modified in the next future.

References

Balthazar EJ, Birnbaum BA, Yee J, Megibow AJ, Roshkow J, Gray C (1994) Acute appendicitis: CT and US correlation in 100 patients. Radiology 190:31–35

Bechtold RE, Chen MY, Ott DJ et al (1997) Interpretation of abdominal CT: analysis of errors and their causes. J Comput Assist Tomogr 21:681–685

Birnbaum BA, Wilson SR (2000) Appendicitis at the millennium. Radiology 215:337–348

Frush DP, Frush KS, Oldham KT (2009) Imaging of acute appendicitis in children: EU versus U.S. or US versus CT? A North American Perspective. Pediatr Radiol 39: 500–505

Gaitini D, Beck-Razi N, Mor-Yosef D et al (2008) Diagnosing acute appendicitis in adults: accuracy of color Doppler sonography and MDCT compared with surgery and clinical follow-up. Am J Roentgenol 190:1300–1306

Hernanz-Schulman M (2010) CT and US in the diagnosis of appendicitis: an argument for CT. Radiology 255:3–7

Horton MD, Counter SF, Florence MG, Hart MJ (2000) A prospective trial of computed tomography and ultrasonography for diagnosing appendicitis in the atypical patient. Am J Surg 179:379–381

Keyzer C, Tack D, De Maertelaer V, Bohy P, Gevenois PA, Van Gansbeke D (2004) Acute appendicitis: comparison of low-dose and standard-dose unenhanced multi-detector row CT. Radiology 232:164–172

Keyzer C, Zalcman M, De Maertelaer V et al (2005) Comparison of US and unenhanced multi-detector row CT in patients suspected of having acute appendicitis. Radiology 236:527–534

Keyzer C, Cullus P, Tack D, De Maertelaer V, Bohy P, Gevenois PA (2009) MDCT for suspected acute appendicitis in adults: impact of oral and IV contrast media at standard-dose and simulated low-dose techniques. Am J Roentgenol 193:1272–1281

Lameris W, van Randen A, van Es HW et al (2009) Imaging strategies for detection of urgent conditions in patients with acute abdominal pain: diagnostic accuracy study. BMJ 338: b2431

Lazarus E, Mayo-Smith WW, Mainiero MB, Spencer PK (2007) CT in the evaluation of nontraumatic abdominal pain in pregnant women. Radiology 244:784–790

McCollough CH, Guimaraes L, Fletcher JG (2009) In defense of body CT. Am J Roentgenol 193:28–39

No authors (1998) Executive summary of the clinical guidelines on the identification, evaluation, and treatment of overweight and obesity in adults. Arch Intern Med 158: 1855–1867

Pickhardt PJ, Lawrence EM, Pooler BD, Bruce RJ (2011) Diagnostic performance of multidetector computed tomography for suspected acute appendicitis. Ann Intern Med 154:789–796.

Poortman P, Lohle PN, Schoemaker CM et al (2003) Comparison of CT and sonography in the diagnosis of acute appendicitis: a blinded prospective study. Am J Roentgenol 181:1355–1359

Puylaert JB (1986) Acute appendicitis: US evaluation using graded compression. Radiology 158:355–360

Raman SS, Kadell BM, Vodopich DJ, Sayer J, Cryer H, Lu DS (2003) Patient gender-related performance of nonfocused helical computed tomography in the diagnosis of acute appendicitis. J Comput Assist Tomogr 27:583–589

Tack D, Sourtzis S, Delpierre I, De Maertelaer V, Gevenois PA (2003) Low-dose unenhanced multi-detector CT of patients with suspected renal colic. Am J Roentgenol 180: 305–311

Tack D, Bohy P, Perlot I et al (2005) Suspected acute colon diverticulitis: imaging with low-dose unenhanced multi-detector row CT. Radiology 237:189–196

Uppot RN, Sahani DV, Hahn PF, Kalra MK, Saini SS, Mueller PR (2006) Effect of obesity on image quality: fifteen-year longitudinal study for evaluation of dictated radiology reports. Radiology 240:435–439

van Randen A, Bipat S, Zwinderman AH, Ubbink DT, Stoker J, Boermeester MA (2008) Acute appendicitis: meta-analysis of diagnostic performance of CT and graded compression US related to prevalence of disease. Radiology 249:97–106
Vermeulen B, Morabia A, Unger PF et al (1999) Acute appendicitis: influence of early pain relief on the accuracy of clinical and US findings in the decision to operate—a randomized trial. Radiology 210:639–643
Wan MJ, Krahn M, Ungar WJ et al (2009) Acute appendicitis in young children: cost-effectiveness of US versus CT in diagnosis—a Markov decision analytic model. Radiology 250:378–386
Wilson EB, Cole JC, Nipper ML, Cooney DR, Smith RW (2001) Computed tomography and ultrasonography in the diagnosis of appendicitis: when are they indicated? Arch Surg 136:670–675
Wise SW, Labuski MR, Kasales CJ et al (2001) Comparative assessment of CT and sonographic techniques for appendiceal imaging. Am J Roentgenol 176:933–941

Imaging of Acute Appendicitis in Adults: MRI

Christine Schmid-Tannwald and Aytekin Oto

Contents

C. Schmid-Tannwald · A. Oto (✉)
Department of Radiology, University of Chicago, 5841 S. Maryland Avenue, MC 2026, Chicago, IL 60637, USA
e-mail: aoto@radiology.bsd.uchicago.edu

Abstract

MR imaging provides systemic, multi-planar evaluation of the entire abdomen with excellent anatomic resolution and allows identification of the etiology for acute abdominal pain without exposing the patient to ionizing radiation and without the necessity of administration of intravenous contrast agents. Therefore, MR imaging is a valuable alternative to CT when US findings are inconclusive, especially in patients with higher risk for radiation exposure such as pregnant and pediatric patients. In this chapter, the role of MR imaging in diagnosis of acute appendicitis will be reviewed. Imaging protocols, MR-imaging features of the normal appendix, acute appendicitis and other causes of right-lower quadrant pain mimicking appendicitis will be described. Indications for MR imaging (with a special emphasis in pregnant patients) and safety issues will also be reviewed.

1 Introduction

Rapid and accurate diagnosis of acute appendicitis is essential for appropriate management. The diagnostic algorithm is based on clinical presentation, physical examination and laboratory findings but imaging has become an important part of diagnostic algorithm. Especially, patients with atypical clinical presentation may benefit from radiologic evaluation with cross-sectional imaging modalities. Ultrasonography (US) and computed tomography (CT) traditionally have been the dominant cross-sectional imaging modalities for the evaluation of patients with suspected acute

C. Keyzer and P. A. Gevenois (eds.), *Imaging of Acute Appendicitis in Adults and Children*,
Medical Radiology. Diagnostic Imaging, DOI: 10.1007/174_2011_218, © Springer-Verlag Berlin Heidelberg 2011

appendicitis (Abu Yousel et al. 1987; Balthazar et al. 1991; Balthazar et al. 1994; Foley et al. 1993; Incesu et al. 1997; Malone et al. 1993). In this setting, magnetic resonance imaging (MRI) plays only a secondary role, since CT is readily available in the emergency setting and provides the detection and evaluation of the appendix with a high accuracy, sensitivity and specificity. The major advantages of US are the lack of ionizing radiation exposure, widespread availability and its low cost. CT is increasingly used and advantages over US include a better accuracy (Stoker et al. 2009; van Randen et al. 2009) and enhanced ability to detect appendicoliths, retrocoecal appendicitis, perforation and other complications of acute appendicitis (Albiston 2002). However, both modalities have limitations. US may be limited due to overlying gas or obesity and quality of examination is dependent on the experience of the operator. CT results in considerable ionizing radiation exposure and relies on the use of iodinated contrast material, which is less desirable in pregnant patients and patients who have risk factors for contrast material.

Recent advances in sequences, gradient amplitudes, multichannel coils and parallel imaging make MRI an increasingly attractive option for evaluating acute abdominal and pelvic conditions. MR imaging provides systemic, multi-planar evaluation of the entire abdomen with excellent anatomic resolution and allows identification of the etiology for acute abdominal pain without exposing the patient to ionizing radiation (Levine et al. 2006; Pedrosa et al. 2007; Singh et al. 2007; Stoker et al. 2009; Tkacz et al. 2009). In addition, the administration of intravenous contrast agents is often not necessary due to the inherent high soft tissue contrast resolution of MRI. Recently, studies describing MR evaluation of acute abdominal pain during pregnancy and pediatric population have increased in number, reflecting the increased use of MR in this challenging clinical setting (Birchard et al. 2005; Cobben et al. 2004; Hörmann et al. 2002; Oto et al. 2005; Levine et al. 2006). In this chapter, we will review the role of MR imaging in diagnosis of acute appendicitis. Imaging protocols, MR-imaging features of the normal appendix, acute appendicitis and other causes of right-lower quadrant pain mimicking appendicitis will be described. Indications for MR imaging (with a special emphasis in pregnant patients) and safety issues will also be reviewed.

2 The Role of MRI for Diagnosis of Acute Appendicitis

Currently MRI is mainly used in evaluation of pregnant patients and children with acute abdominal pain. In 2007, the American College of Radiology (ACR) guidelines for MR-imaging practices recommended that MR imaging be used when the risk–benefit ratio warrants the study (Kanal et al. 2007). According to the ACR Appropriateness Criteria, MRI of the abdomen and pelvis without contrast should be considered in pregnant patients with right-lower quadrant pain, fever and leukocytosis when ultrasound findings are negative or equivocal. MR imaging is rated as the most appropriate imaging modality following US in this setting (American College of Radiology). In a series of pediatric patients, accurate diagnosis of acute appendicitis could be made even without administration of intravenous contrast material (Hörmann et al. 1998). MRI in children suspected of acute appendicitis is further discussed in "Imaging of Acute Appendicitis in Children: MRI" by Hörmann. MRI was shown to improve diagnosis of appendicitis and decrease the negative exploration rate in patients with suspected appendicitis (Cobben et al. 2004, 2009; Pedrosa et al. 2009). Its negative predictive value is very high and can save the patients from unnecessary appendectomies (Oto et al. 2009a). In a recent study by Cobben et al. 2009, MRI was also found to be a cost-effective tool in the workup of patients clinically suspected of having appendicitis.

The major advantages of MRI are the lack of ionizing radiation exposure and the generally accepted safety of the currently used intravenous contrast agents. MRI provides a high intrinsic contrast resolution with excellent characterization of pathologic tissue obviating the need for intravenous contrast medium. Its multi-planar imaging capability is also useful for determining the origin of the lesion or inflammatory process. On the other hand MRI is time-consuming and more expensive. Its lack of around-the-clock availability is still a logistic problem at many institutions. Referring physicians are not familiar with the imaging features of MRI in patients with acute abdominal and pelvic conditions. Other limitations include the poor spatial resolution in comparison to CT and its increased sensitivity for motion-related artifacts.

3 Technique and Protocol

3.1 Technique

According to the ACR practice guidelines, pregnant patients should be informed of the risk/benefit ratio and written informed consent regarding should be obtained before undergoing MRI examination. It should be documented that information cannot be acquired by other diagnostic modalities and that the evaluation of the MR examination has the potential to affect the care of the patient and the test cannot wait until pregnancy is over.

The current protocol in our institution does not require any specific patient preparation. Pedrosa et al. recommend administration of negative oral contrast [combination of ferumoxsil (Gastromark, Mallickrodt Medical, St. Lois, Missouri) and dilute barium sulfate (Readi-Cat 2; E-Z-Em Canada, Westbury, New York)] which may lead to an improved depiction of bowel on T1- and T2-weighted images without causing susceptibility artifacts (Pedrosa and Rofsky 2003). Phased-array coils should be used whenever possible, since they provide superior signal-to-noise ratio, but towards the end of pregnancy and in larger patients a body coil may be necessary. Often patients can be imaged in supine position. However, during the late second and third trimester of pregnancy, imaging in lateral decubitus position can be necessary to avoid impairing venous return from the pelvis and lower extremities. To prevent compression of the inferior vena cava by the gravid uterus, left lateral decubitus positioning is preferred over right (Leyendecker et al. 2004).

Gadolinium-based intravenous contrast media is routinely used in adults and may be helpful in increasing the diagnostic confidence and accuracy (Lam et al. 2008). However, the use of gadolinium may be contraindicated in patients with severe renal failure due to the risk of nephrogenic systemic fibrosis (NSF). Gadolinium is a class C drug (FDA classification) and in pregnant patients, it should be used highly selectively, in the second and third trimester when the benefits outweigh the risk (Brown et al. 2005). It is recommended that use of gadolinium in pregnant patients is only decided when unenanhanced MR images are inconclusive. At that point, radiologist and the referring physician should assess the risk and benefit of gadolinium administration and reach a mutual decision. Non-enhanced MRI can provide adequate information in most of the cases precluding the need for intravenous contrast (Chabanova et al. 2010; Inci et al. 2010a, b).

3.2 Protocol

In patients with acute abdominal pain, the MR-imaging protocol should be tailored to their clinical condition and image acquisition time should be minimized. Scanning protocols include T2-weighted imaging with and without fat saturation, axial T1-weighted images before and if needed after intravenous contrast administration. In addition to these routine sequences, axial 2D time of flight (TOF) images, steady-state free-precession sequences and diffusion-weighted images can be obtained. The detailed MR protocol is provided in Table 1.

T2-weighted imaging in three orthogonal planes with single-shot fast spin echo (SSFSE) or half-Fourier acquisition single-shot spin echo (HASTE) (TR = infinite, TE = 90 ms) forms the backbone of the MR protocol. SSFSE T2-weighted images have high spatial resolution and can be obtained during limited breath-hold and should be preferred over other fast-spin echo sequences. T2-weighted imaging with fat saturation is performed to improve the detection of inflammation or characterization of fat-containing adnexal lesions. The resolution of T1-weighted FSE sequence is superior to the gradient-echo version and can help to detect small structures such as a normal appendix.

In pregnant patients, TOF gradient echo (GRE) T2*-weighted images are helpful to differentiate the appendix from dilated venous tributaries and evaluate venous thrombosis. Steady-state free-precession sequences can provide motion free images of the abdomen, nicely depicting the outline of the bowel segments and vessels. Diffusion-weighted images may potentially improve the conspicuity of the inflamed appendix (Inci et al. 2010a, b) found that in 78/79 surgically proven appendicitis, inflamed appendix were hyperintense on DWI and addition of DWI facilitated the diagnosis of acute appendicitis. T1-weighted in-phase and opposed-phase GRE images can be used to define fat-containing lesions and hemorrhagic collections. Blooming artefacts due

Table 1 MR protocol for suspected acute appendicitis

	MR sequences
Routine protocol	1. Single-shot fast spin echo (SSFSE) or Half-Fourier acquisition single-shot spin echo (HASTE) (axial, coronal, sagittal)
	2. T2-weighted sequence with fat saturation (SSFSE, HASTE or FSE) (axial and coronal)
	3. T1-weighted sequence (breath-hold spoiled gradient echo or Respiratory gated fast spin echo) (axial)
Not part of the routine protocol for pregnant patients	4. Post-contrast imaging: 2D or 3D GRE T1-weighted images
Optional	2D time-of-flight sequence (axial)
	Steady-state free-precession sequences (FIESTA, true FISP, balanced FFE)
	Diffusion-weighted images

to air, metallic objects, or hemosiderin and calcium are more visible on in-phase images and they can help to locate the appendix, when it is air-filled (Pedrosa et al. 2007; Singh et al. 2007; Tkacz et al. 2009).

4 MR Findings

4.1 Normal Appendix

The normal appendix is a blind-ending tubular structure which measures circa 10 cm in length, arises from the posteromedial wall of the cecum, approximately 3 cm below the ileocoecal valve (Birnbaum and Wilson 2000; Buschard and Kjaeldfaard 1973; Stoker et al. 2009). The normal appendiceal wall typically measures less than 2 mm in thickness and diameter of its lumen is usually less than 7 mm. The normal appendix can be filled with air, fluid or contrast media or can be totally collapsed. The appendiceal wall has a low to intermediate signal on T1- and T2-weighted images similar to the signal intensity of the bowel wall (Fig. 1). The appearance of its lumen is dependent on filling: Air or iron-based oral contrast medium within the lumen can cause blooming artifacts which can be recognized on T1-weighted in-phase images and TOF GRE images and help in exclusion of acute appendicitis (Pedrosa et al. 2007).

During pregnancy, there is a gradual upward displacement of the appendix and cecum so the appendix may be located in the right mid abdomen or right upper quadrant during the second and third trimester (Oto et al. 2006). In a recent study by Oto et al. while the appendix was well below the iliac crest in the first trimester, it rose to the level of the iliac crest in the second trimester and further progressed superiorly with a mean of 2.6 cm above the iliac crest in the third trimester. Also the cecum elevates progressively during the course of pregnancy and demonstrates a tilted orientation, where the base of the cecum is anteriorly and outwardly displaced (Nagayama et al. 2002). Since the cecum is a larger and more recognizable anatomic structure, its localization may help to localize the appendix. In a study with 146 pregnant patients, Lee et al. (2008) showed that the cecal tilt angle was useful for localizing the appendix in pregnant patients and helps to predict the location of the appendix within the right upper quadrant of the abdomen regardless of gestational age with a high specificity.

Nikolaidis et al. evaluated the incidence of visualization of the normal appendix on MRI in adults and compared the yield of commonly used sequences (Nikolaidis et al. 2006). A normal appendix was definitively visualized in 55 of 71 patients on T1 spin-echo (SE) sequences (78%) and T2 SE sequence provided the highest rate of appendiceal visualization. The second best rate of appendiceal visualization was seen on SSFSE sequences. The appendix was seen on 25 of 42 (60%) patients on T2-weighted SSFSE images. Visualization rates were 42% on pre-gadolinium T1 FS GRE, 54% on post-gadolinium T1 fat-suppressed gradient echo and 17% of short tau

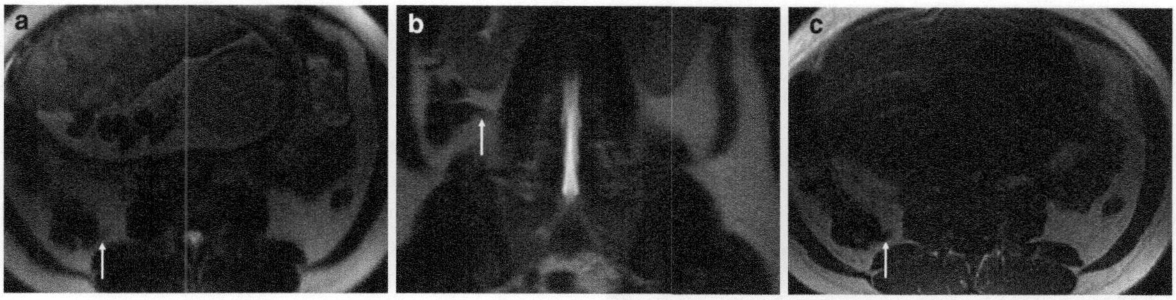

Fig. 1 Normal appendix in a 28-year-old pregnant woman. Axial (**a**) and coronal (**b**) T2-weighted single-shot fast spin-echo image and T1-weighted gradient-echo image (**c**) show a hypointense, blind ending tubular structure (*arrow*) arising from the cecum. The diameter of its lumen is less than 7 mm consistent with a normal appendix

inversion recovery sequences. In smaller series performed in pregnant patients, normal appendix is seen at MR imaging between 83 and 89% of pregnant patients (Hörmann et al. 2002; Nitta et al. 2005; Oto et al. 2005; Levine et al. 2006; Pedrosa et al. 2007). Similar to CT, coronal images are helpful in depiction of the normal and inflamed appendix.

4.2 Acute Appendicitis

In acute appendicitis, increased intraluminal pressure and intraluminal dilatation leads to venous engorgement, arterial compromise and tissue ischemia with transmural inflammation. In severe cases, continued tissue ischemia results in appendiceal infarction and perforation (Birnbaum and Wilson 2000). The MRI-criteria for the diagnosis of appendicitis are similar to the criteria of CT (Levine et al. 2006; Rybkin and Thoeni 2007; Singh et al. 2007): An enlarged appendix with a diameter of more than 7 mm, wall thickening of the appendix and signs of inflammation in the periappendiceal fat, depending on the severity of acute appendicitis. In patients with initial, mild appendicitis, the appendix may be only minimally distended and fluid-filled and the surrounding mesentery may not show inflammatory changes (Fig. 2). Incesu et al. (1997) reported that an inflamed appendix demonstrates marked wall enhancement with slight distention. In a series of pediatric patients, accurate diagnosis of acute appendicitis could be made even without administration of intravenous contrast material (Hörmann et al. 1998). Edematous wall thickening of the appendix leads to an increased intramural signal on T2-weighted images and hypointense signal on T1-weighted images (Hammond et al. 2008; Nitta et al. 2005). After contrast administration, the wall enhances abnormally. The appendix is fluid-filled and therefore, its lumen appears hyperintense on T2-weighted images. In coronal images, wall thickening and inflammation in the wall can be seen along the entire length of the appendix. In the gangrenous type of appendicitis, however, it may be difficult to visualize the wall in its entire length (Nitta et al. 2005). Periappendiceal inflammatory changes such as fat stranding or local fascial thickening appear as hypointense on T1-weighted images and hyperintense on T2-weighted fat suppressed images. Periappendiceal inflammatory changes can be especially helpful when the appendix itself is not visualized. They have to be actively and carefully sought for since they can be the only findings of acute appendicitis. Other findings include thickening of the upper cecal wall (Birnbaum and Wilson 2000). The presence of an appendicolith in association with periappendiceal inflammation indicates acute appendicitis (Birnbaum and Wilson 2000). An appendicolith is difficult to identify on MR images but may sometimes be seen as a focal hypointense area on all sequences (Pedrosa et al. 2007).

Perforated appendicitis is usually accompanied by increased inflammation, extraluminal gas, pericecal phlegmon, abscess formation and peritonitis. Local and diffuse fluid collections, lymphadenopathy and small bowel obstruction are associated findings (Birnbaum and Wilson 2000; Incesu et al. 1997; Stoker et al. 2009). Periappendiceal phlegmon appears as an ill-defined, heterogenous, moderately high signal on T2-weighted images and dark signal on the background of bright fat on non-fat saturated T1-

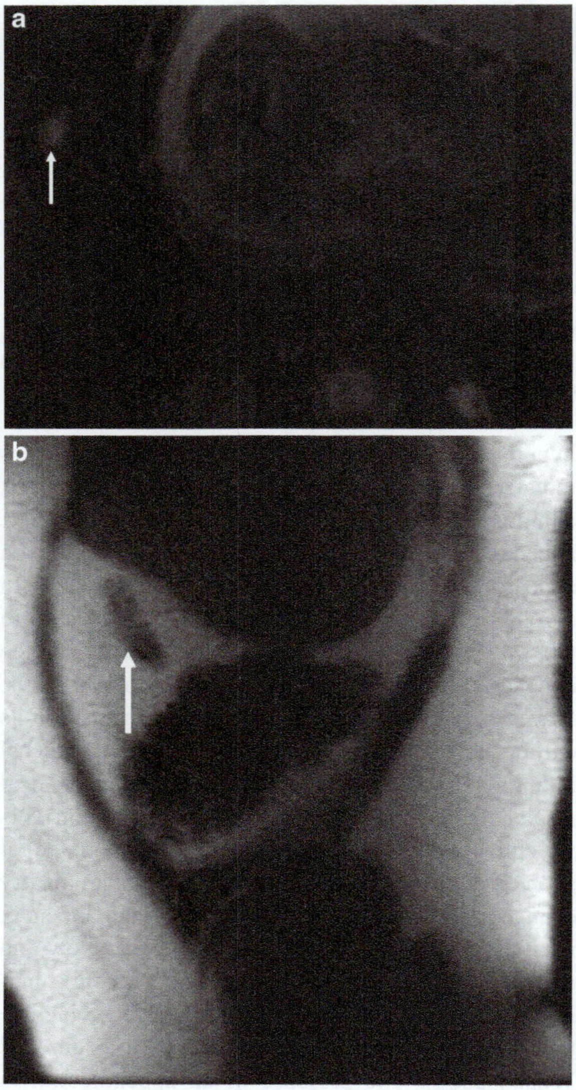

Fig. 2 Mild appendicitis in a 29-year-old pregnant woman. Axial short inversion time inversion-recovery image (**a**) shows dilated, fluid-filled structure (*arrow*) with thickened wall and fat stranding, consistent with acute appendicitis. Coronal T2-weighted single-shot fast spin-echo image (**b**) shows the dilated, thick walled appendix with increased intramural signal (*arrow*)

weighted images (Pedrosa et al. 2007). In cases complicated by a periappendiceal abscess, its cavity appears hyperintense on T2-weighted images and demonstrates significant wall enhancement following intravenous contrast administration (Martin et al. 2005; Pedrosa et al. 2007) (Fig. 3).

MRI is shown to be superior to US (Albiston 2002; Hörmann et al. 1998; Incesu et al. 1997) with high reported sensitivity (97–100%), specificity (92–93%) and accuracy (92–94%) for the diagnosis of acute appendicitis (Levine et al. 2006). According to a recent study by Cobben et al. (2009), even unenhanced MRI has a high accuracy in detecting and excluding appendicitis and can be a valuable and cost-effective tool in the management of patients with clinically suspected appendicitis. In addition, Inci et al. (2010a) found out that unenhanced MRI provides the detection of acute appendicitis even in cases with low Alvarado scores. A recently published meta-analysis concluded that MRI has excellent diagnostic capabilities in the diagnosis of appendicitis (Barger and Nandalur 2010).

5 MRI and Acute Appendicitis During Pregnancy

Acute appendicitis is the most common cause of acute abdomen in pregnancy and occurs in approximately 1 in 1500 deliveries (Sharp 2002). Its management in a pregnant woman implies unique diagnostic and therapeutic challenges. Anatomical and physiological changes during pregnancy confound the clinical evaluation. In pregnant patients, localization of pain is not specific for the diagnosis of acute appendicitis, as the appendix migrates upwards during pregnancy. It is also important to realize that there is a physiologic increase in the white blood cell count in pregnancy. These difficulties can lead to a delay in diagnosis which can be associated with serious complications. The incidence of fetal loss ranges between 3 and 5% without rupture and increases to 30% with ruptured appendicitis (Sharp 2002). On the other hand, higher false-negative laparotomy rate in pregnant patients compared with that of the general population results from the lack of specificity in clinical and laboratory findings (Levine et al. 2006): In 48–80% of pregnant patients who underwent appendectomy, the diagnosis of acute appendicitis can be confirmed (Hee and Viktrup 1999). Unnecessary surgeries are not free from risk and preterm contractions are common in as many as 83% of pregnant patients who undergo appendectomy (Firstenberg and Malangoni 1998). Therefore, there is a need for an accurate and safe non-invasive imaging tool to evaluate pregnant patients with acute appendicitis. The current practices in imaging pregnant women by MRI, as well as by

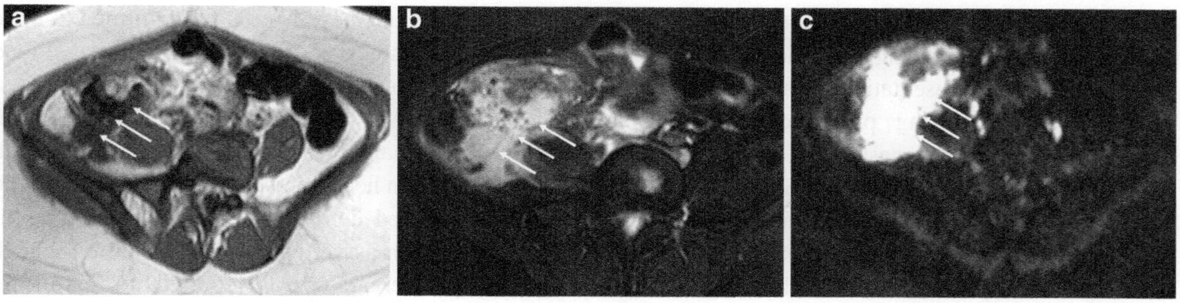

Fig. 3 Perforated appendicitis in a 18-year-old pregnant woman. T1-weighted gradient-echo image (**a**) shows inflammatory mass (*arrows*) in the right-lower quadrant with low signal intensity. T2-weighted single-shot fast spin-echo image with fat saturation (**b**) inflammatory mass (*arrows*) has high signal abnormality and is compatible with a periappendiceal abscess from ruptured appendicitis. Inflammatory changes (*arrows*) show bright signal on diffusion-weighted image at b-value of 800 mm^2/s (**c**)

other imaging techniques (ultrasonography and CT), is also extensively discussed by Jaffe in "Imaging of Acute Appendicitis in Adults: Current Practices in Pregnant Women".

5.1 Role and Performance of MRI

US with a graded compression technique is the first-line investigation in pregnant patients presenting with right-lower quadrant pain. However, identification of normal or inflamed appendix is more difficult in pregnant patients due to the enlarged uterus, especially in the advancing gestational age. Several papers from different centers investigating the role of MR imaging for evaluation of acute appendicitis specifically in pregnant patients have been published within the last couple of years (Birchard et al. 2005; Cobben et al. 2004; Israel et al. 2008; Oto et al. 2005; Oto et al. 2009a). In their small series of 12 patients, Cobben et al. (2004) concluded that MR imaging may be a good alternative to CT in pregnant patients with indeterminate sonographic findings. The two other series with relatively larger study populations ($n = 23$ and $n = 29$) showed that MR can enable the diagnosis of acute appendicitis and other causes of right-sided abdominal pain, such as ovarian torsion, pelvic abscesses, ureteral stones or biliary obstruction by providing a systematic evaluation of abdominal and pelvic organs (Birchard et al. 2005; Oto et al. 2005). In another series of 50 patients, the overall sensitivity, specificity and accuracy for MR imaging in diagnosis of acute appendicitis was reported as 100, 93.6 and 94% respectively (Levine et al. 2006). Intravenous contrast was not administered in the majority of the patients included in these series. MR can also show the normal appendix, helping to exclude the diagnosis of acute appendicitis and saving the pregnant patients from unnecessary appendectomies. In a study of pregnant patients, normal appendix could be detected in 83% of 47 patients (Levine et al. 2006). In a series of 148 pregnant patients, clinically suspected of having acute appendicitis, use of MR imaging yielded favorable combinations of negative laparotomy rate (30%) and perforation rate (21%) compared with previously reported values. The radiation exposure associated with CT examination can be avoided in most cases. In comparison to US, MRI showed an improved detection rate for appendicitis (100 vs. 36%) (Pedrosa et al. 2009). Israel et al. (2008) also found MRI superior to US in detection of both normal and inflamed appendix. The sensitivity, specificity, positive predictive value (PPV) and negative predictive value for the diagnosis of appendicitis on MRI was 100% for all parameters whereas the sensitivity, specificity, PPV and NPV on US was 50, 100, 100 and 66%, respectively. MR imaging can be an excellent modality in pregnant women who present with acute abdominal pain and in whom a normal appendix is not visualized at US (Levine et al. 2006).

An important difference between appendicitis in pregnant and non-pregnant patients is the anatomical alterations during pregnancy, which are visible on MRI: Oto et al. (2006) confirmed the gradual upward displacement of the appendix during the pregnancy on MRI in a study with 72 pregnant patients. The visualization of anatomical changes is not only crucial for the detection and evaluation of the appendix but it can be a helpful tool for the choice of appendectomy incision. Due to the changes in the location of the appendix, clinical presentation of acute appendicitis can also change during pregnancy and pregnant patients with advancing gestational age may present with right upper quadrant pain (Sharp 2002). MR imaging can demonstrate other etiologies of acute abdominal pain and is an excellent modality for diagnosis of acute appendicitis and exclusion of diseases requiring surgical/interventional treatment. Therefore, MR imaging is useful for triage of pregnant patients with acute abdominal and pelvic pain. (Oto et al. 2009a). The sensitivity, specificity, accuracy, positive predictive value and negative predictive value of MR imaging for diagnosis of etiology of acute abdominal pain requiring surgical/interventional treatment was 88.9, 95.0, 94.1, 76.2 and 97.9%, respectively.

5.2 MR-Safety

Ultrasound is safe technique for the fetus but limited in performance during pregnancy. When CT is performed as an alternative to US to evaluate abdominopelvic pathologies, fetus is included in the field of view and exposed to an estimated dose between 12.5 and 35 mSV (El-Khoury et al. 2003; Leyendecker et al. 2004). MRI does not expose the mother or fetus to ionizing radiation and unenhanced MR images are often diagnostic (Leyendecker et al. 2004). No studies have demonstrated a clear risk to unborn human fetuses from MRI, but the safety of MR imaging with respect to the fetus has not been definitively established. In 1991, the safety Committee of the Society for Magnetic Resonance Imaging stated that "MR imaging may be used in pregnant women if other non-ionizing forms of diagnostic imaging are inadequate or if the examination provides important information that would otherwise require exposure to ionizing radiation" (Shellock and Kanal 1991). MR imaging utilizes the static, time-varying and radio-frequency electromagnetic fields, and all of these fields can potentially cause adverse effects on the fetus. Animal studies on the safety of fetal MR are not conclusive and sometimes conflicting (De Wilde et al. 2005). However, a small number of studies in human fetuses using regular MR-imaging protocols have not revealed any harmful effects on the fetus (Baker et al. 1994; Clements et al. 2000; Kok et al. 2004; Myers et al. 1998). Baker et al. (1994) performed a three year follow-up study of children imaged in utero and found no demonstrable increase in disease or disability related to in utero MR exposure. Schenck et al. reviewed the safety of high-static magnetic field effects on human health and concluded that there is no firmly-established detrimental effect except for sensory effects such as vertigo or metallic taste (Schenk 2000). Myers et al. (1998) reported no significant reduction in fetal growth versus matched controls in 74 volunteer subjects exposed in utero to echo-planar MRI performed at 0.5-Tesla. A survey of reproductive health among 280 pregnant MR health care professionals performed by Kanal et al. (2007) showed no substantial increase in common adverse reproductive outcomes.

Thermal heating is a potential result of pulsed radio-frequency (RF) (De Wilde et al. 2005). Heats on embryo or fetus can potentially result in a range of deformities of the central nervous system and there is a particular vulnerability during organogenesis (Edwards et al. 2003). The amount of energy deposited in a patient as a result of a MR examination is referred to as the specific abortion rate (SAR), which is regulated in the United States by the Food and Drug Administration. So far, different limits have not been accepted for pregnant patients. Increasing static magnetic field strength, flip angle, number and spacing of radiofrequency pulses lead to higher SAR values. Therefore, there are sequences with higher SAR values such as fast spin-echo-based while gradient-echo sequences, which do not depend on radiofrequency refocusing, are associated with relatively low SAR values (De Wilde et al. 2005; Leyendecker et al. 2004). But even there is the potential that long echo trains cause fetal heating, single-shot echo train spin-echo sequences is commonly used in maternal and fetal imaging and unlikely result in significant temperature changes (Leyendecker et al. 2004; Levine et al. 2001). Due to lack of conclusive data, MR imaging of pregnant women should be used when the benefits outweigh the theoretical risks, and extra caution should be exercised in the first trimester (US Food and Drug Administration 1988).

5.2.1 First-Trimester Imaging

The first trimester is the period of active organogenesis and the absolute safety during this period is difficult to establish. MR imaging is to be avoided in this period even there is no scientific evidence in humans to suggest an increased risk to the fetus from a routine MR examination. MR examination should thus be only performed if the potential benefits justify the theoretical risks.

5.2.2 Intravenous Contrast Media

Gadolinium is a class C drug and its safety in humans is not proven. Therefore, it is suggested that in pregnant patients, gadolinium-based agents can be only used in the second and third trimester when the benefits outweigh the risk (Brown et al. 2005). In animal studies, Gadolinium-based contrast agents cross the placenta and have been shown to cause retarded fetal development and skeletal malformation at higher doses. Although gadolinium crosses the placenta, no direct toxic effect has been reported in a small number of human studies (Webb et al. 2005). Especially in the advanced staging of pregnancy, fetal kidney may also clear some of the injected gadolinium. Consequently, the Committee on Drugs and Contrast Media recommends that radiologists confer with the referring physician and discuss the potential clinical benefit of MR imaging over that of other modalities and the necessity of gadolinium for diagnosis (MRIsafety.com Web site 2010; Webb et al. 2005).

5.2.2.1 Field Strengths

During the last decade, 3 T MRI scanners have been widely available and started to be utilized in body imaging. Main advantages of 3.0 T MR, compared to 1.5 T MR, are increased signal-to-noise ratio and higher spatial and temporal resolution. In addition, contrast effects are more pronounced using 3.0 T MR. On the other hand, 3.0 T MR leads to increased field inhomogeneity, standing wave artifacts, chemical shift and susceptibility artifacts. Altered relaxation times, especially prolonged T1 relaxation time, lead to a reduction of contrast on T1-weighted images, which necessitate an increase in TR and acquisition time.

For more than 20 years MR imaging has been used to evaluate obstetric, placental and fetal abnormalities and many investigations have been conducted in laboratory and clinical settings to determine the effects of MR imaging during pregnancy (Prasad et al. 1990; Tyndall and Sulik 1991; Yip et al. 1995). However, most of these studies were performed at field strengths of less than 3.0 T, and these results should not be directly applied to 3.0 T or higher field strengths scanners (Barth et al. 2007). Further research is necessary to draw more certain conclusions about the safety of higher field strength scanners and lower field strength (up to 1.5 T) should be preferred for pregnant patients.

6 Differential Diagnoses and Pitfalls

Acute right-lower quadrant pain may be caused by a myriad of diagnosis including inflammatory processes involving the small and large bowel, obstetric and gynaecologic disorders or urinary tract disorders. Rapid and accurate diagnosis is essential for the appropriate treatment of these acute conditions. Imaging protocols should be tailored to the specific clinical question that needs to be answered and patient's clinical condition with emphasis on minimizing scan duration and motion-related artifacts. MR imaging has particular advantages over CT for assessing pelvic and biliary abnormalities.

6.1 Biliary System

6.1.1 Acute Cholecystitis

Acute cholecystitis is the third most common non-obstretric surgical emergency during pregnancy. Increased cholesterol synthesis by estrogen and impaired gallbladder motility lead to bile lithogenicity and sludge formation during the pregnancy (van Bodegraven et al. 1998). US is the imaging modality of choice but MR imaging with single-shot turbo spin-echo sequences is an excellent modality to evaluate acute biliary pain and is comparable to US in the preoperative management of acute cholecystitis (Regan et al. 1998). Findings of acute cholecystitis on MR imaging include wall thickening of the gall bladder, distended gallbladder with the presence of gallstones and increased pericholecystic signal on T2-weighted images (Adusumilli and Siegelman 2002). In a series of 18 pregnant patients who underwent MRCP and US, biliary dilatation was detected in eight patients by ultrasound, but the cause of biliary dilatation could not be determined by ultrasound in seven patients. MRCP demonstrated the etiology in four of these patients (choledocholithiasis ($n = 1$), Mirizzi syndrome ($n = 1$),

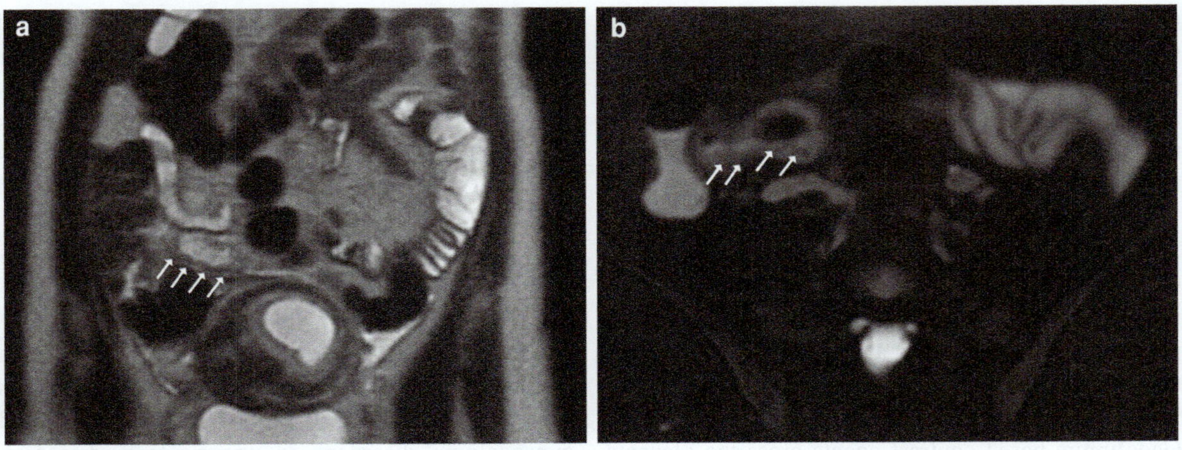

Fig. 4 Ileitis in a 31-year-old pregnant woman. Coronal T2-weighted single-shot fast spin-echo image (**a**) shows wall thickening of the terminal ileum (*arrows*) consistent with ileitis. T2-weighted fat saturated fast spin-echo image (**b**) reveals edematous wall thickening leads to intramural high signal intensity (*arrows*)

choledochal cyst ($n = 1$) and intrahepatic biliary stones ($n = 1$) and excluded obstructive pathology in the other four patients. Especially when ultrasound shows biliary dilatation, MRCP can determine the etiology and save the patient from unnecessary endoscopic retrograde cholangiopancreatography by excluding a biliary pathology (Oto et al. 2009b).

6.2 Inflammatory Processes Involving the Small and Large Bowel

6.2.1 Right-Sided Acute Diverticulitis

Acute colonic diverticulitis is the second most common cause of acute abdominal pain, usually affecting the left colon. If the right colon is involved, it can mimic acute appendicitis. Contrast-enhanced CT is the imaging modality of choice but is limited in patients with renal failure and in pregnant patients due to fetal safety issues. MRI allows the diagnosis of acute diverticulitis (Hammond et al. 2008; Heverhagen et al. 2001). Imaging features include inflammatory changes in the bowel wall with thickening, fluid and enema with high signal intensity on T2-weighted images in the inflamed mesenteric fat surrounding the inflamed diverticulum. The inflamed diverticulum shows enhancement on post-contrast T1-weighted images outpouching of the colon. Diverticular abscesses show a peripheral rim-enhancement with central low signal on T1-weighted images and high signal on T2-weighted images.

6.2.2 Inflammatory Bowel Disease

Patients with inflammatory bowel disease (e.g., Crohn's disease and ulcerative colitis) can be evaluated with high sensitivity with MR imaging (Sinha et al. 2009). The peak age of incidence of inflammatory bowel disease and acute appendicitis is very similar and acute flare of Crohn's disease may mimic acute appendicitis. In patients with acute flare of Crohn's disease, MRI may demonstrate of a normal appendix and inflamed terminal ileum and other small bowel segments. Edematous bowel thickening at the acute phase is seen as hyperintense intramural signal on T2-weighted images and enhancement after contrast administration suggest inflamed, abnormal bowel (Fig. 4). Furthermore MRI provides the detection of complications such as fistulas and abscesses. In some cases, appendix may also be diffusely inflamed due to involvement by Crohn's disease. These cases should be differentiated from acute appendicitis cases requiring immediate surgical treatment.

6.3 Obstretic and Gynecologic Disorders

6.3.1 Adnexal Torsion

Ovarian torsion is a gynecologic emergency which is a result of twisting of the ovary around its vascular pedicle. It most commonly occurs in the first three decades of life and frequently involves the ovary and corresponding fallopian tube. Initially, torsion compromises venous return from the ovary and ovarian

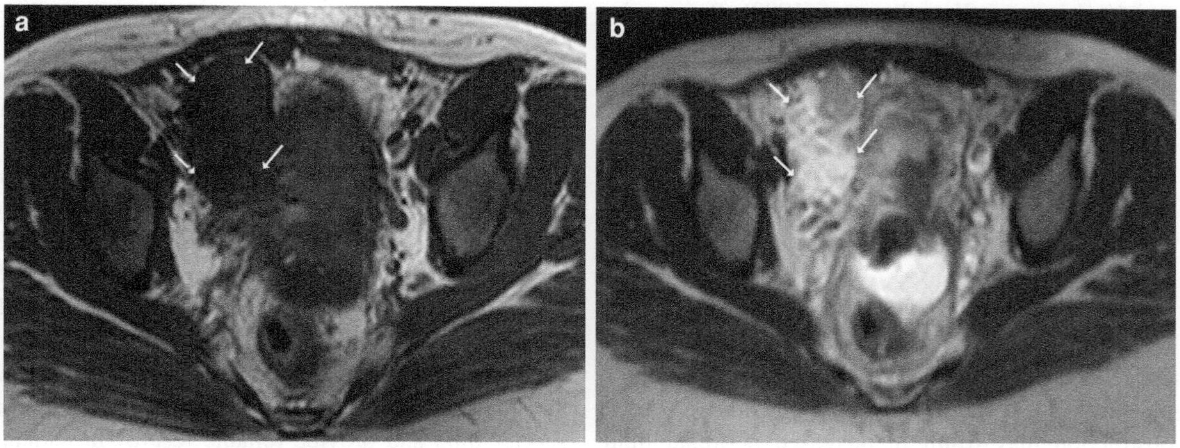

Fig. 5 Adnexal torsion in an 18-year-old pregnant woman. Axial T1-weighted gradient-echo image (**a**) shows enlarged, hypointense right adnexa (*arrows*) containing multiple peripherally located follicles. The right enlarged adnexa (*arrows*) has a high-signal intensity on T2-weighted single-shot fast spin-echo image (**b**) and the follicles appear as circumscribed low signal intensity areas

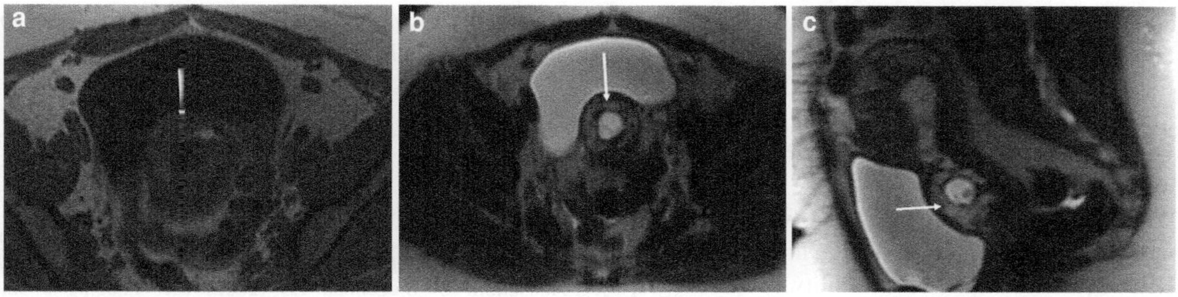

Fig. 6 Ectopic pregnancy in a 40-year-old pregnant woman. Axial T1-weighted gradient-echo image (**a**) shows a well-defined, hypointense, cystic structure (*arrow*) at the anterior-inferior aspect of the uterus. Axial T2-weighted single-shot fast spin-echo image (**b**) reveals the ectopic positioning gestational sac (*arrow*) just above the level of the cervix and posterior bladder. Sagittal T2-weighted single-shot fast spin-echo image (**c**) shows the uterine contour appears posterior to the gestational sac (*arrow*) and no viable myometrium is seen anterior to the gestational sac

enlargement because stromal edema is noted. On T2-weighted images ovarian edema leads to an increased signal (Fig. 5). A greater degree of torsion results in arterial insufficiency with hemorrhagic infarction and necrosis. The signal intensity of the ovary on MRI is variable and decreased on T1- and T2-weighted images at presence of hemorrhagic infarction. Other MR findings include tubal thickening, deviation of the uterus to the torsed side, a twisted vascular pedicle and inflammatory fluid in the cul-de-sac (Bennett et al. 2002; Chiou et al. 2007; Ghosain et al. 2004; Pedrosa et al. 2007; Vijayaraghavan et al. 2009). T1-weighted images with fat saturation provide the detection of hemorrhagic tube or hemorrhage within the twisted adnexal mass or hemoperitoneum as high signal intensity (Rha et al. 2002). In some cases, an associated ovarian cyst or benign neoplasm may be seen (Singh et al. 2007).

6.3.2 Ectopic Pregnancy

Ectopic pregnancy refers to implantation and growth of a fertilized ovum in a location outside the cavity of the uterus. Potentially, rupture at the extrauterine site may result in massive hemorrhage or occasional death. Laboratory findings and transvaginal US remain the gold standard of care in the evaluation and MR imaging is proposed in patients where US findings are inconclusive. The most common finding is a tubal hematoma which appears as intermediate signal on T1-weighted images and low signal on T2-

weighted images (Kataoka et al. 1999). Paraovarian gestional sac-like structure in the adnexa may be identified (Fig. 6). Free fluid of intermediate signal intensity, greater than that of urine is characteristic for hemoperitoneum.

6.4 Urinary Tract Disorders

6.4.1 Urolithiasis

Even if the urinary tract is commonly evaluated by US and CT, MRI can be helpful in patients with contra-indications for contrast media or radiation. Acute obstruction may result in increased perirenal fluid, which is best seen on T2-weighted images as high-signal intensity. Dilated ureter is suspicious for the presence of ureterolithiasis and stones may be seen as filling defects on T2-weighted images (Pedrosa et al. 2007). Unenhanced MR urography is a valuable and well-tolerated investigation for evaluation of painful hydronephrosis during pregnancy and its differentiation from obstruction by stones (Roy et al. 1996; Spencer et al. 2004). Spencer et al. (2004) described the MR findings of physiological hydronephrosis as extrinsic compression of the middle third of the ureter with a collapsed distal ureter and without any filling defect. Thin slice, high resolution highly T2-weighted FSE sequences improves the ability of MR urography for detection of small stones. Care should be taken not to mistake air, clot or flow artifacts for a stone.

6.5 Pitfalls

One of the pitfalls is the mistaking of the terminal ileum and appendix for each other. Therefore, a fluid-filled terminal ileum or terminal ileitis might lead to false-positive diagnosis. Further conditions which can lead to false-positive results include right sided inflammatory changes such as right sided diverticulitis, cholecystitis or fluid in the right lower quadrant (e.g., ascites, abscess) which may be read as associated findings with acute appendicitis. In pregnant patients, it may be difficult to locate the appendix and differentiate it from engorged adnexal vessels. On the other hand, false-negative MR diagnosis of acute appendicitis may result if a distended appendix is mistaken for the terminal ileum or if ascites obscures periappendiceal inflammation.

7 Conclusion

MR imaging enables a systemic, multiplanar evaluation of the entire abdomen and allows diagnosis of a variety of diseases presenting as acute abdominal pain. It is proven to be an useful alternative imaging technique for the diagnosis of acute appendicitis. MR imaging is a valuable alternative to CT when US findings are inconclusive, especially in patients with higher risk for radiation exposure such as pregnant and pediatric patients. With the recent technical advantages, MR examinations can be performed in a shorter time and provide reliable results. In patients with acute abdominal pain, MR-imaging protocol should be tailored to their clinical condition and imaging should be completed in the shortest possible duration. As MR imaging is being increasingly used for acute settings, it is important for the radiologists to recognize the MR appearance of common causes of acute abdominal pain during pregnancy.

References

Abu Yousel MM, Bleicher JJ, Maher JW et al (1987) High-resolution sonography of acute appendicitis. AJR 149:53–58

Adusumilli S, Siegelman ES (2002) MR imaging of the gallbladder. Magn Reson Imaging Clin N Am 10:165–184

Albiston E (2002) The role of radiological imaging in the diagnosis of acute appendicitis. Can J Gastroenterol 16:451–463

American College of Radiology. ACR appropriateness criteria. Available at: http://www.acr.org/SecondaryMainMenuCategories/quality_safety/app_criteria/pdf/ExpertPanelonGastrointestinalImaging/RightLowerQuadrantPainDoc12.aspx

Baker PN, Johnson IR, Harvey P et al (1994) A three year follow-up of children imaged in utero with echo-planar magnetic resonance imaging. Amer J Obstet Gynecol 170: 32–33

Balthazar EJ, Megibow AJ, Siegel SE et al (1991) Appendicitis: prospective evaluation with high-resolution CT. Radiology 180:21–24

Balthazar EJ, Birnbaum BA, Yee J et al (1994) Acute appendicitis: CT and US correlation in 100 patients. Radiology 190:31–35

Barger RL, Nandalur KR (2010) Diagnostic performance of magnetic resonance imaging in the detection of appendicitis in adults: a meta-analysis. Acad Radiol 17:1211–1216

Barth MM, Smith MP, Pedrosa I et al (2007) Body MR Imaging at 3.0 T: understanding the opportunities and challenges. RadioGraphics 27:1445–1464

Bennett G, Slywotzky C, Giovanniello G et al (2002) Gynecological causes of acute pelvic pain: spectrum of CT findings. RadioGraphics 22:785–801

Birchard KR, Brown MA, Hyslop WB et al (2005) MRI of acute abdominal and pelvic pain in pregnant patients. AJR 184:452–458

Birnbaum BA, Wilson SR (2000) Appendicitis at the millennium. Radiology 215:337–348

Brown MA, Birchard KB, Semelka RC et al (2005) MR evaluation of pregnant patients with acute abdominal pain. Semin Ultrasound CT MRI 26:206–211

Buschard K, Kjaeldfaard A (1973) Investigation and analysis of the position, fixation, length and embryology of the vermiform appendix. Acta Chir Scan 139:293–298

Chabanova E, Balslev I, Achiam M et al (2010) Unenhanced MR imaging in adults with clinically suspected acute appendicitis. Eur J Radiol. doi:10.1016/j.ejrad.2010.03.007

Chiou SY, Lev-Toaff AS, Emi Masuda E et al (2007) Adnexal torsion. New clinical and imaging observations by sonography, computed tomography and magnetic resonance imaging. J Ultrasound Me 26:1289–1301

Clements H, Duncan KR, Fielding K et al (2000) Infants exposed to MRI in utero have a normal paediatric assessment at 9 months of age. Br J Radiol 73:190–194

Cobben LP, Groot I, Haans L et al (2004) MRI for clinically suspected appendicitis during pregnancy. AJR 183:671–675

Cobben LP, Bakker OJ, Puylaert JB et al (2009) Imaging of patients with clinically suspected appendicitis in the Netherlands: conclusion of a survey. Br J Radiology 82:482–485

De Wilde JP, Rivers AW, Price DL (2005) A review of the current use of magnetic resonance imaging in pregnancy and safety implications for the fetus. Prog Biophys Mol Biol 87:335–353

Edwards MJ, Saunders RD, Shiota K (2003) Effects of heat on embryos and foetuses. Int J Hyperthermia 19:295–324

El-Khoury GY, Madsen MT, Blake ME et al (2003) A new pregnancy policy for a new era. AJR Am J Roentgenol 181:335–340

Firstenberg MS, Malangoni MA (1998) Gastrointestinal surgery during pregnancy. Gastroenterol Clin North Am 27:73–88

Foley CR, Latimer RG, Rimkus DS (1993) Detection of acute appendicitis by technetium 99 HMPAO scanning. Am Surg 58:761–765

Ghosain MA, Hachem K, Buy JN et al (2004) Adnexal torsion: magnetic resonance findings in the viable adnexa with emphasis on stromal ovarian appearance. J Magn Reson Imaging 20:451–462

Hammond NA, Miller FH, Yaghmai V et al (2008) MR imaging of acute bowel pathology: a pictorial review. Emerg Radiol 15:99–104

Hee P, Viktrup L (1999) The diagnosis of appendicitis during pregnancy and maternal and fetal outcome after appendectomy. Int J Gynaecol Obstet 65:129–135

Heverhagen J, Ishaque N, Zielke A et al (2001) Feasibility of MRI in the diagnosis of acute diverticulitis: initial results. Magma 12:4–8

Hörmann M, Paya K, Eibenberger K et al (1998) MR imaging in children with nonperforated acute appendicitis: value of unenhanced MR imaging in sonographically selected cases. AJR Am J Roentgenol 171:467–470

Hörmann M, Puig S, Prokesch SR et al (2002) MR imaging of the normal appendix in children. Eur Radiol 12:2313–2316

Incesu L, Coskun A, Selcuk MB et al (1997) Acute appendicitis: MR imaging and sonographic correlation. AJR Am J Roentgenol 168:669–674

Inci E, Hocaoglu E, Aydin S et al (2010a) Efficiency of unenhanced MRI in the diagnosis of acute appendicitis: comparison with Alvarado scoring system and histopathological results. Eur J Radiol. doi:10.1016/j.e.rad.2010.06.037

Inci E, Kilickesmez O, Hocaoglu E et al (2010b) Utility of diffusion-weighted imaging in the diagnosis of acute appendicitis. Eur Radiol. doi: 10.1007/s00330-010-1981-6

Israel GM, Malguria N, McCarthy S et al (2008) MRI vs. ultrasound for suspected appendicitis during pregnancy. J Magn Reson Imaging 28:428–433

Kanal E, Barkovich AJ, Borgstede JP et al (2007) ACR guidance document for safe MR practices: 2007. AJR 188:1–27

Kataoka ML, Togashi K, Kobayashi H et al (1999) Evaluation of ectopic pregnancy by magnetic resonance imaging. Hum Reprod 14:2644–2650

Kok RD, de Vries MM, Heerschap A et al (2004) Absence of harmful effects of magnetic resonance exposure at 1.5 T in utero during the third trimester of pregnancy: a follow-up study. Magn Reson Imaging 22:851–854

Lam M, Singh A, Kaewlai R et al (2008) Magnetic resonance of acute appendicitis: pearls and pitfalls. Curr Probl Diagn Radiol 37:57–66

Lee KS, Rofsky NM, Pedrosa I (2008) Localization of the appendix at MR imaging during pregnancy: utility of the cecal tilt angle. Radiology 249:134–141

Levine D, Zuo C, Faro CB et al (2001) Potential heating effect in the gravid uterus during MR HASTE imaging. J Magn Reson Imaging 13:856–861

Levine Pedrosa I, Eyvazzadeh AD et al (2006) MR imaging evaluation of acute appendicitis in pregnancy. Radiology 238:891–899

Leyendecker JR, Gorengaut V, Brown JJ (2004) MR Imaging of maternal diseases of the abdomen and pelvis during pregnancy and the immediate postpartum period. RadioGraphics 24:1301–1316

Malone AJ, Wolf CR, Malmed AS et al (1993) Diagnosis of acute appendicitis: value of unenhanced CT. AJR 160:763–766

Martin DR, Danrad R, Herrmann K (2005) Magnetic resonance imaging of the gastrointestinal tract. Top Magn Reson Imaging 16:77–98

MRIsafety.com Web site (2010) http://www.mrisafety.com. Accessed 2009–2010

Myers C, Duncan KR, Gowland PA (1998) Failure to detect intrauterine growth restriction following in utero exposure to MRI. Br J Radiol 71:549–551

Nagayama M, Watanabe Y, Okumura A et al (2002) Fast MR imaging in obstetrics. RadioGraphics 22:563–580

Nikolaidis P, Hammond N, Marko J et al (2006) Incidence of visualization of the normal appendix on different MRI sequences. Emerg Radiol 12:223–226

Nitta N, Takahashi M, Furukawa A et al (2005) MR imaging of normal appendix and acute appendicitis. J Magn Reson Imaging 21:156–165

Oto A, Ernst RD, Shah R et al (2005) Right-lower-quadrant pain and suspected appendicitis in pregnant women: evaluation with MR imaging-initial experience. Radiology 234:445–451

Oto A, Ernst RD et al (2006) Revisiting MRI for appendix location during pregnancy. AJR; 186:883–887

Oto A, Ernst RD, Ghulmiyyah L et al (2009a) MR imaging in the triage of pregnant patients with acute abdominal and pelvic pain. Abdom Imaging 34:243–250

Oto A, Ernst R, Ghulmiyyah L et al (2009b) The role of MR cholangiopancreatography in the evaluation of pregnant patients with acute pancreaticobiliary disease. Br J Radiol 82:279–285

Pedrosa I, Rofsky NM (2003) MR imaging in abdominal emergencies. Radiol Clin North Am 41:1243–1273

Pedrosa I, Zeikus EA, Levine D et al (2007) MR imaging of acute right lower quadrant pain in pregnant and nonpregnant patients. RadioGraphics 27:721–753

Pedrosa I, Lafornara M, Pandharipande PV et al (2009) Pregnant patients suspected of having acute appendicitis: effect of MR imaging on negative laparotomy rate and appendiceal perforation rate. Radiology 250:749–757

Prasad N, Wright DA, Ford JJ et al (1990) Safety of 4-T MR imaging: study of effects on developing frogs embryos. Radiology 174:251–253

Regan F, Schaefer DC, Smith DP et al (1998) The diagnostic utility of HASTE MRI in the evaluation of acute cholecystitis. Half Fourier acquisition single-shot turbo SE. J Comput Assist Tomogr 22:638–642

Rha SE, Byun JY, Jung SE et al (2002) CT and MR imaging features of adnexal torsion. RadioGraphics 22:283–294

Roy C, Saussine C, Le Bras Y et al (1996) Assessment of painful ureterohydronephrosis during pregnancy by MR urography. Eur Radiol 6:334–338

Rybkin A, Thoeni R (2007) Current concepts in imaging of appendicitis. Radiol Clin North Am 45:411–422

Schenk JF (2000) Safety of strong, static magnetic fields. J Magn Reson Imaging 12:2–19

Sharp HT (2002) The acute abdomen during pregnancy. Clin Obstet Gynecol 45:405–413

Shellock FG, Kanal E (1991) Policies, guidelines, and recommendations for MR imaging safety and patient management. SMRI safety committee. J Magn Reson Imaging 1:97–101

Singh A, Danrad R, Hahn PF et al (2007) MR imaging of acute abdomen and pelvis: acute appendicitis and beyond. RadioGraphics 27:1419–1431

Sinha R, Murphy P, Hawker P et al (2009) Role of MRI in Crohn's disease. Clin Radiol 64:341–352

Spencer JA, Chahal R, Kelly A et al (2004) Evaluation of painful hydronephrosis in pregnancy: magnetic resonance urographic patterns in physiological dilatation versus calculous obstruction. J Urol 171:256–260

Stoker J, van Randen A, Laméris W et al (2009) Imaging patients with acute abdominal pain. Radiology 253: 31–46

Tkacz JN, Anderson SA, Soto J (2009) MR imaging in gastrointestinal emergencies. RadioGraphics 29:1767–1780

Tyndall DA, Sulik KK (1991) Effects of magnetic resonance imaging on eye development in the C57BL/6 J mouse. Teratology 43:263–275

US Food and Drug Administration (1988) Magnetic resonance diagnostic device: panel recommendation and report on petitions for MR classification. Fed Reg 53:7575–7579

van Bodegraven AA, Bohmer CJ, Manoliu RA et al (1998) Gallbladder contents and fasting gallbladder volumes during and after pregnancy. Scand J Gastroenterol 33: 993–997

van Randen A, Lameris W, Bossuyt PM et al (2009) Comparison of accuracy of ultrasonography and computed tomography in patients with acute abdominal pain at the emergency department (abstr). In: Radiological Society of North America scientific assembly and annual meeting program. Oak Brook, III: Radiological Society of North America: 519

Vijayaraghavan G, Kurup D, Singh A (2009) Imaging of acute abdomen and pelvic: common acute pathologies. Semin Roentgenol 44:221–227

Webb JA, Thomsen HS, Morcos SK (2005) Members of contrast media safety committee of european society of urogenital radiology (ESUR). The use of iodinated and gadolinium contrast media during pregnancy and lactation. Eur Radiol 15:1234–1240

Yip YP, Capriotti C, Yip JW (1995) Effects of MR exposure on axonal outgrowth in the sympathetic nervous system of the chick. J Magn Reson Imaging 5:457–462

Imaging of Acute Appendicitis in Adults: Current Practices in Pregnant Women

Tracy A. Jaffe

Contents

Abstract

Appendicitis is the most common non-obstetric surgical diagnosis made during pregnancy and is the most frequent indication for emergency surgical intervention. Swift and accurate diagnosis of appendicitis greatly impacts these pregnancy outcomes. For these reasons, imaging has become central to the diagnosis of appendicitis in the pregnant patient. Current recommendations for evaluation of appendicitis in pregnant women involve initial imaging with ultrasound. Ultrasound is known to be safe in pregnancy and is routinely used as the first line imaging modality to identify the source of abdominal pain in the pregnant patient. If the diagnosis remains inconclusive, a thoughtful conference with referring clinicians should help guide the radiologist's next imaging modality of choice. MRI is preferable to CT given radiation concerns. The MR findings of appendicitis include a dilated, thick walled blind-ending tubular structure measuring >7 mm with periappendiceal stranding and inflammation. Periappendiceal inflammatory changes, best seen on T2-weighted imaging, correspond to edema surrounding the inflamed appendix. The use of gadolinium should be avoided in pregnancy. If MRI is unavailable, CT may be used although radiologists should make all efforts to reduce dose during this examination. Dose reduction recommendations include reduction of kilovoltage for smaller patients, decreasing milliamperage, increasing allowable noise, and taking care to limit the field of view and avoid multiple phases.

T. A. Jaffe (✉)
Department of Radiology,
Duke University Medical Center,
PO Box 3808, Durham, NC 27710, USA
e-mail: tracy.jaffe@duke.edu

C. Keyzer and P. A. Gevenois (eds.), *Imaging of Acute Appendicitis in Adults and Children*,
Medical Radiology. Diagnostic Imaging, DOI: 10.1007/174_2011_219, © Springer-Verlag Berlin Heidelberg 2011

1 Introduction

Appendicitis is the most common non-obstetric surgical diagnosis made during pregnancy and is the most frequent indication for emergency surgical intervention. The incidence of appendicitis in pregnancy is between 1:1,500 and 1:200 pregnancies (Dietrich et al. 2008). Pregnant women are not at greater risk of developing appendicitis, but because appendicitis is a disease of young adults, it is not uncommon for women of reproductive age to be affected.

The incidence of perforated appendicitis in the pregnant patient is 43%, well above that of the non-pregnant patient (Dietrich et al. 2008). Morbidity and mortality increase with delayed diagnosis and perforation and maternal mortality increases with advancing gestational age of the fetus. These rates have declined in the recent era of improved surgical intervention and techniques as well as superior antibiotic regimens. Fetal morbidity and mortality still exist, and perforated appendicitis is the number one surgical cause of fetal loss during pregnancy with mortality rates between 2 and 6% (McGory et al. 2007; Cappell and Friedel 2003; Parangi et al. 2007). Preterm delivery is the most common factor influencing fetal morbidity, with preterm delivery rates ranging from 4 to 37% (Dietrich et al. 2008; McGory et al. 2007). Swift and accurate diagnosis of appendicitis greatly impacts these pregnancy outcomes. For these reasons, imaging has become central to the diagnosis of appendicitis in the pregnant patient.

During the first trimester, the appendix resides in the right lower quadrant and in the setting of appendicitis there is localized peritoneal irritation to this region. By 24 weeks gestation, however, the appendix will have shifted above the right iliac crest and the tip of the appendix will have rotated medially toward the uterus (Parangi et al. 2007). By late in the pregnancy, the appendix may move closer to the gallbladder within the right upper quadrant. As there is increased separation of the visceral and parietal peritoneum during pregnancy, there is decreased somatic sensation of pain and ability to localize pain on examination. Pain become less localized and abdominal guarding and rebound tenderness become less reliable signs of appendiceal inflammation. A more diffuse peritonitis may be seen as the enlarging uterus may

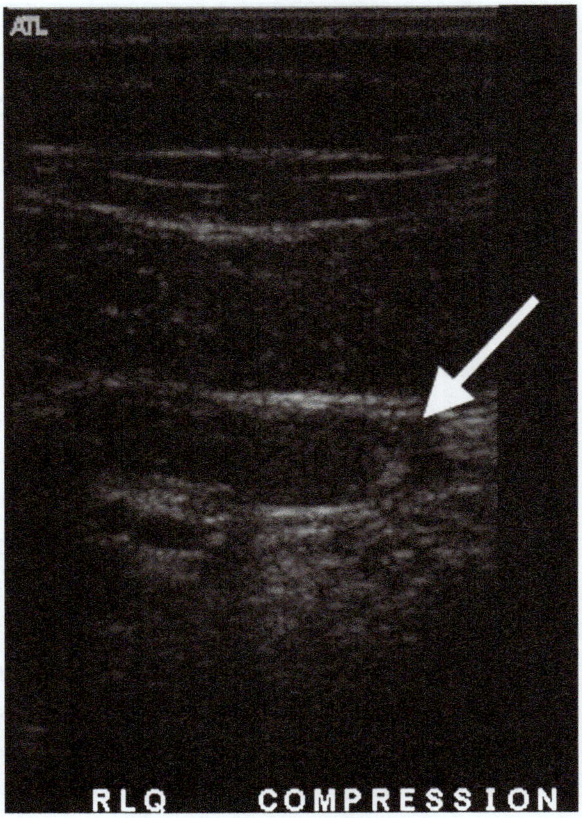

Fig. 1 Ultrasound of 8-week patient with right lower quadrant pain, rule out acute appendicitis. Longitudinal image of a dilated appendix in the right lower quadrant with an appendicolith (*white arrow*)

interfere in the ability of the omentum and bowel to wall-off appendiceal inflammation (Dietrich et al. 2008). To further confound the issue, pyrexia may be absent in the pregnant patient. Additionally, pregnant women have a physiologic leukocytosis that may confuse the presentation of appendicitis. Abdominal pain related to gestation (including nausea and vomiting as well as anorexia) may confound presenting symptomatology of appendicitis. The differential diagnosis of appendicitis in this patient population includes routine pregnancy pains (ligamentalgia, etc.), obstetrical conditions including ectopic pregnancy, placental abnormalities, and ovarian lesions/torsion. Finally, non-obstetrical conditions including pulmonary embolus, pancreatitis, pyelonephritis, urolithiasis, or biliary tract disease can present with similar symptoms to appendiceal inflammation (Dietrich et al. 2008).

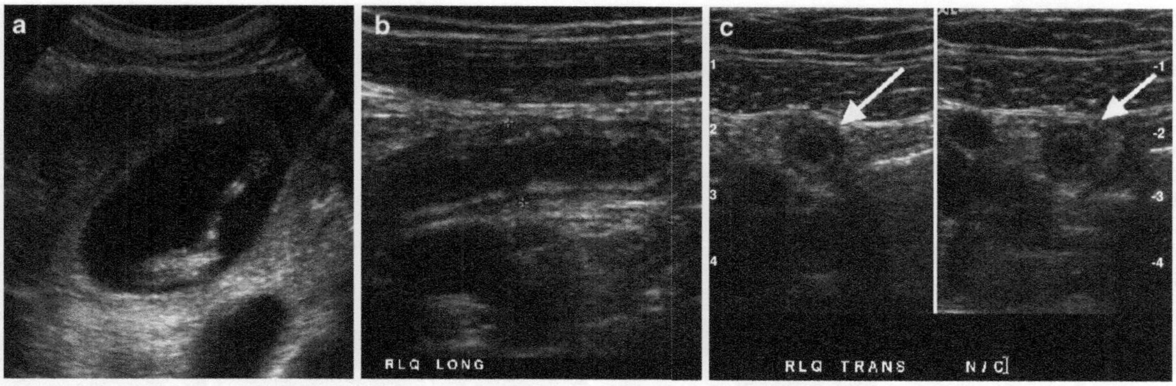

Fig. 2 Ultrasound of 13-week pregnant patient with right lower quadrant pain, rule out acute appendicitis. **a** Ultrasound image of uterus shows intrauterine pregnancy, **b** Longitudinal image in the right lower quadrant shows a dilated appendix with caliper measurement of 9 mm, **c** Transverse image of the appendix with (*left*) and without compression (*right*). The appendix does not change with compression

2 Ultrasound

While physical examination is the starting point for detection of appendicitis in pregnancy, a confirmative imaging modality is often required to rule out other potential diagnoses. Ultrasound is known to be safe in pregnancy and is routinely used as the first line imaging modality to identify the source of abdominal pain in the pregnant patient. The ultrasound diagnosis of appendicitis requires the identification of a dilated, aperistaltic, noncompressible, blind-ending tubular structure arising from the cecum. Additional findings including appendiceal wall thickening, appendicoliths, hyperechoic surrounding fat, or hypoechoic free fluid may also be seen in the setting of acute appendicitis (Figs. 1, 2) (see also chapter "Ultrasonography" by Jeffrey). Ultrasound is highly operator-dependent with sensitivity and specificity ranging from 50–100 to 33–95%, respectively (Barloon et al. 1995; Woodfield et al. 2010; Lim et al. 1992). The elevated or retrocecal appendix complicates the sonographic examination and negative ultrasound does not exclude the diagnosis of appendicitis. If the suspicion of appendicitis remains high, further imaging should be undertaken.

3 MRI

When available, MRI is the preferred method of imaging the pregnant patient in the setting of non-traumatic abdominal pain. In a 2007 survey of practice patterns in academic centers, Jaffe et al. (2007) found that 94% of respondents prefer MRI in the evaluation of right lower quadrant pain in a pregnant patient. Based on ACR Appropriateness Criteria, MRI is favored over CT for use in pregnant patients with symptomatology related to the right lower quadrant (American College of Radiology 2008). Furthermore, recent recommendations from a meta-analysis of the data available in imaging pregnant patients with abdominal pain suggest that MRI should be the preferred imaging modality (Long et al. 2011). The MRI examination should be short and tailored to identify inflammation. While there is no data to suggest that there is risk to the fetus at 1.5 T magnet strength, safety at higher field strength has not been adequately assessed. The use of oral contrast material is optional. The appendicitis MRI protocol typically includes axial, sagittal, and coronal T2-weighted imaging with single-shot fast spin echo (SSFSE or HASTE) and true fast imaging with steady state precession (TrueFISP, FIESTA, and balanced fast field echo). T2-weighted SSFSE images allow evaluation of bowel in a relatively motionless state and the multi-planar imaging allows identification of the appendix in multiple planes. The true FISP imaging helps to differentiate high signal intensity vessels from low signal intensity normal appendix. It is important for the radiologist to confirm adequate MRI coverage in an effort to limit excessive repetitive imaging.

The normal appendix can be seen on MRI imaging in approximately 52–87% of patients (Fig. 3) (Singh et al. 2007; Pedrosa et al. 2009; Israel et al. 2008; Oto et al. 2006). The MRI findings of appendicitis include

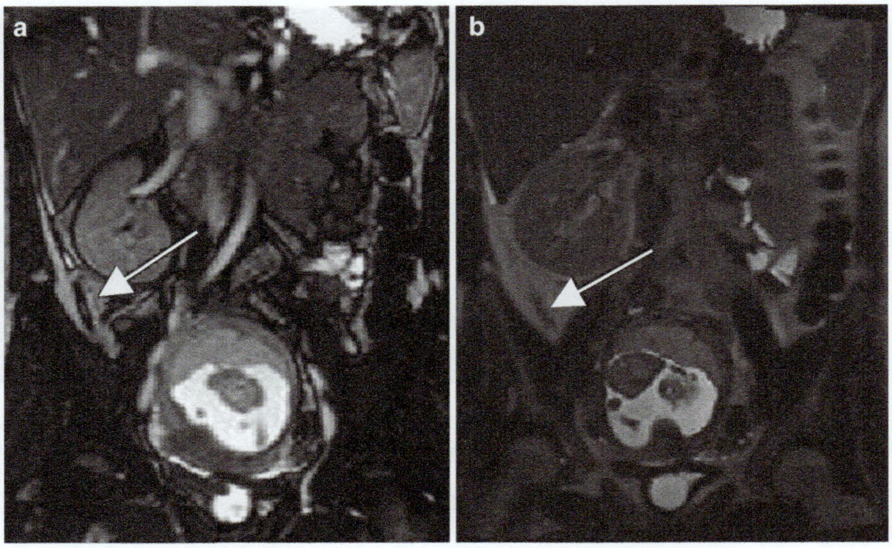

Fig. 3 MRI of 17-week pregnant patient with abdominal pain. **a** Coronal True-FISP MR image without contrast shows normal appendix in the right lower quadrant (*white arrow*), **b** Coronal HASTE MRI image again identifies a normal appendix in the right lower quadrant (*white arrow*)

a dilated, thick walled blind-ending tubular structure measuring >7 mm with periappendiceal stranding and inflammation (Fig. 4). Periappendiceal inflammatory changes, best seen on T2-weighted imaging, correspond to edema surrounding the inflamed appendix (Fig. 5). MRI findings of acute appendicitis are also discussed in chapter "MRI" by Schmid-Tannwald and Oto. There is a range of reported sensitivity and specificity of MRI in the diagnosis of appendicitis in the pregnant patient as well. A meta-analysis of available data reports MRI sensitivity and specificity ranging from 91 to 95 and 99%, respectively (Blumenfeld et al. 2010). Other data is less optimistic, with sensitivities and specificities ranging from 50–80 to 93–100%, respectively (Pedrosa et al. 2009; Israel et al. 2008; Vu et al. 2009; Pedrosa et al. 2006).

Gadolinium-based contrast materials are classified as FDA Pregnancy Class C medications, as defined by the following: either studies in animals have revealed adverse effects on the fetus and there are no controlled studies in women or studies in women are not available. Gadolinium given in a chelated form is nontoxic, however, as seen in animal studies, gadolinium crosses the placenta, and is retained in the repetitive fetal circulation and accumulates in the amniotic fluid where it may dissociate from the chelating agent (Cacheris et al. 1990). There is concern that free or unbound gadolinium in the amniotic fluid may have a teratogenic effect. The ACR Manual on Contrast Media 7 states, "gadolinium chelates should not be routinely used in pregnant patients" (American College of Radiology 2010). ESUR guidelines allow for the use of gadolinium in pregnancy when there is a very strong indication for contrast media to ensure

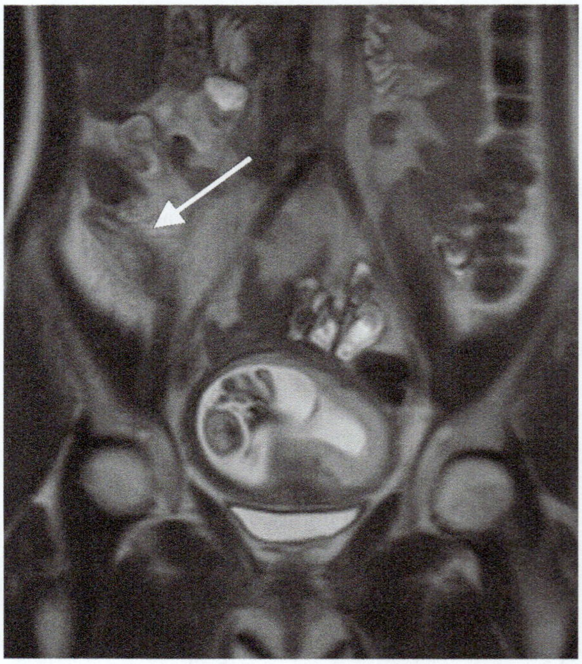

Fig. 4 MRI of 18-week pregnant patient with abdominal pain. Coronal HASTE MRI image without contrast shows a dilated appendix (*white arrow*) with mild periappendiceal inflammation. The patient went to the operating room for acute appendicitis

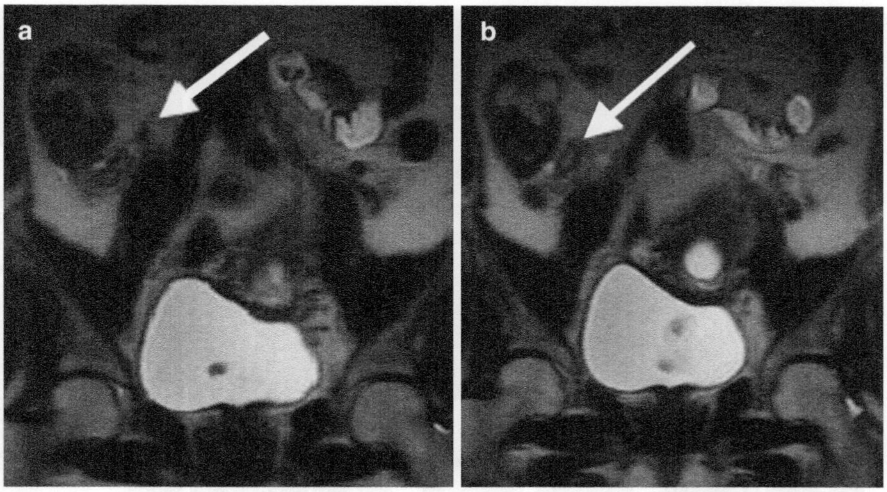

Fig. 5 **a, b** MRI of 22-week pregnant patient with abdominal pain. **a** Sequential coronal HASTE MRI images without contrast show a dilated, fluid-filled appendix (*white arrow*) with mild periappendiceal inflammation. **b** Tip of appendix with inflammation acute appendicitis was found in the pathologic specimen

diagnostic accuracy during pregnancy. In general, it advisable to avoid administration of gadolinium-based contrast media during pregnancy.

4 CT

Unfortunately, the detection of appendicitis in a pregnant patient may be limited by availability of imaging modalities. There are instances where ultrasound is inconclusive and MRI is not available. In this case, multidetector CT (MDCT) imaging may be a better than a delay in diagnosis. CT is routinely accessible and the examination carries with it sensitivity and specificity for diagnosis of appendicitis of 96 and 95%, respectively (Paulson et al. 2005). CT has been shown to be equally accurate for appendicitis in the pregnant woman, with reported sensitivities ranging from 92 to 100 and a specificity of 99% (Lazarus et al. 2007; Shetty et al. 2010). If the appendix can be identified and is normal in size and without periappendiceal inflammation, appendicitis can be excluded (Figs. 6, 7). CT findings of appendicitis in the pregnant patient are the same as those of the non-gravid patient: inflammation and enlargement of the appendix to >7 mm with wall thickening, stranding in the periappendiceal fat, and if perforated, air or fluid surrounds the inflamed appendix (Fig. 3). In a recent study of 400 non-pregnant patients with abdominal pain, Ganguli et al. (2006) concluded that nonvisualization of the appendix on MDCT reliably excludes appendicitis. While the identification of the appendix is more complex in the setting of a gravid uterus, if the appendix location is unclear and there is no evidence of inflammation at the base of the cecum, the diagnosis of appendicitis may be excluded.

The main limitation of CT in the pregnant patient is radiation exposure. While the existing language in the available literature varies as to suggested guidelines for the imaging of abdominal pain in the pregnant patient, the overarching message is that of the judicious use of CT when the benefit to patient outweighs the risk to the fetus. The American College of Radiology has issued recommendations regarding CT imaging in the pregnant patient which can be found in the ACR practice guideline for imaging pregnant or potentially pregnant adolescents and women with ionizing radiation: resolution 26 (American College of Radiology 2008). These guidelines include conference with the referring physician and documentation of the necessity for the examination, including the urgency of the examination. Recommendations from the Health Protection Agency, Royal College of Radiology, and College of Radiographers suggest that exposure of pregnant women to higher dose radiation procedures, including CT, should be avoided but if clinically justified, termination of the pregnancy would not be justified solely on radiation risk to the unborn child (Wall et al. 2009). ICRP guidelines suggest that all medical practices should be justified where the benefit will outweigh the risks and, if possible, for pregnant patients, the medical procedures should be tailored to reduce fetal dose (Valentin 2000). Finally, the American College of Obstetrics and Gynecology suggests that other imaging procedures

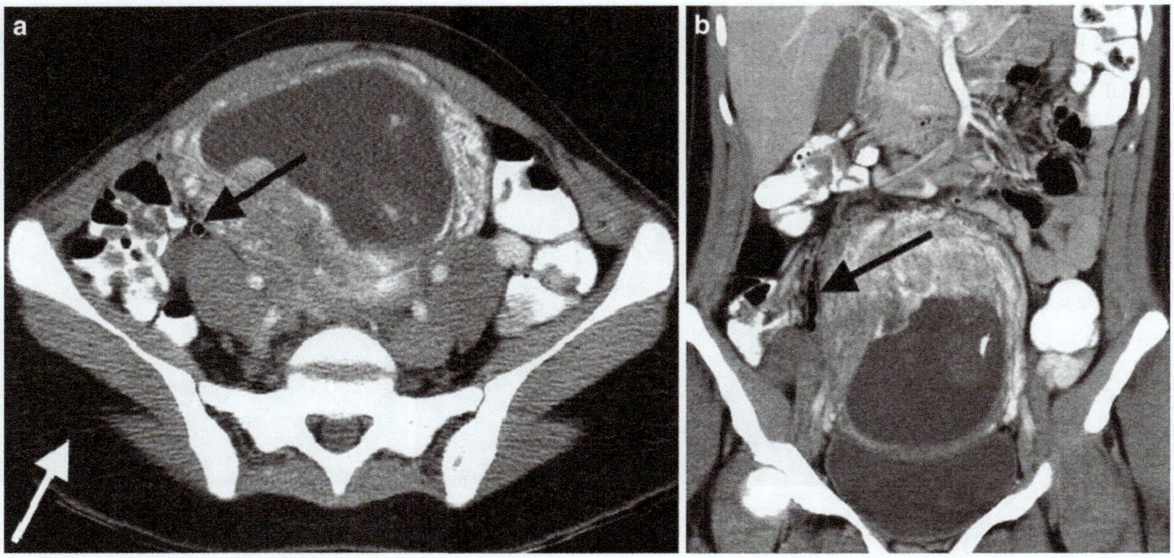

Fig. 6 CT of 20-week pregnant patient with abdominal pain. **a** Axial CT image with intravenous and oral contrast shows a normal air-filled appendix (*black arrow*). The CT was performed without tube current modulation and a reduction of tube current by 30%. The resultant increase in noise is most easily seen in the subcutaneous tissues (*white arrow*), **b** Coronal image with intravenous and oral contrast shows a normal air-filled appendix (*black arrow*)

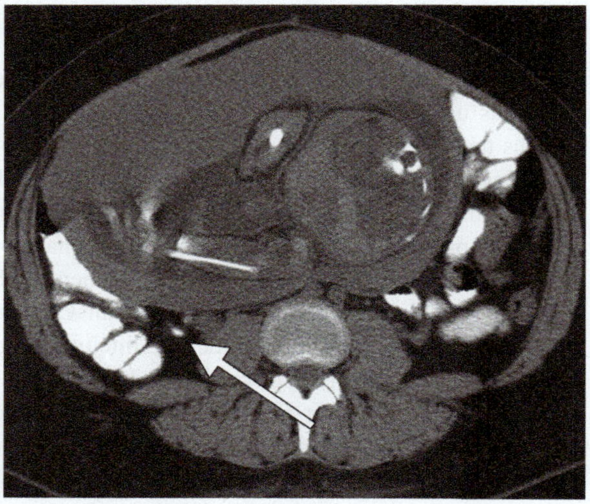

Fig. 7 CT of 30-week pregnant patient with abdominal pain. Axial CT image with oral contrast shows a normal appendix filled with oral contrast (*white arrow*). The tube current was reduced by 30% for this acquisition

without ionizing radiation be considered when appropriate (American College of Obstetrics and Gynecology 2004).

Fetal dose from an abdomen/pelvis MDCT scan in the first trimester ranges from 9.5 to 36, depending on the scanning parameters used, with lower doses seen using automated tube current modulation and lower kV (Jaffe et al. 2008, 2009). Fetal doses for MDCT during the second and third trimester are less well understood. It has been suggested in phantom data that fetal dose correlates with maternal perimeter and fetal depth and that normalized fetal doses decreases linearly with increasing maternal perimeter (Angel et al. 2008).

Although absorbed fetal dose during abdominal CT falls below the threshold for teratogenesis (50 mGy) (American College of Radiology 2008; Annals of the ICRP 2003), there is little human data regarding the carcinogenic effects of CT dose exposure in utero. Estimates from the International Commission on Radiological Protection Publication 90 suggests that the overall risk of childhood cancer for a fetus receiving 3.0 cGy (the fetal dose reported by Hurwitz et al. 2006 for an appendicitis protocol) is double that of the general population, an increase from 1 in 600 to 2 in 600 (Annals of the ICRP 2003). The excess risk of developing a childhood cancer has been estimated to be approximately 0.28 at 1 mGy in the first trimester, 0.03 in the third trimester, and 0.037 overall during the pregnancy (Annals of the ICRP 2003).

All efforts should be undertaken to modify CT protocols in the pregnant patient to allow for the lowest tolerable dose for diagnostic accuracy. To date, there is debate about the role of automated tube current modulation and fetal dose. While automated tube current

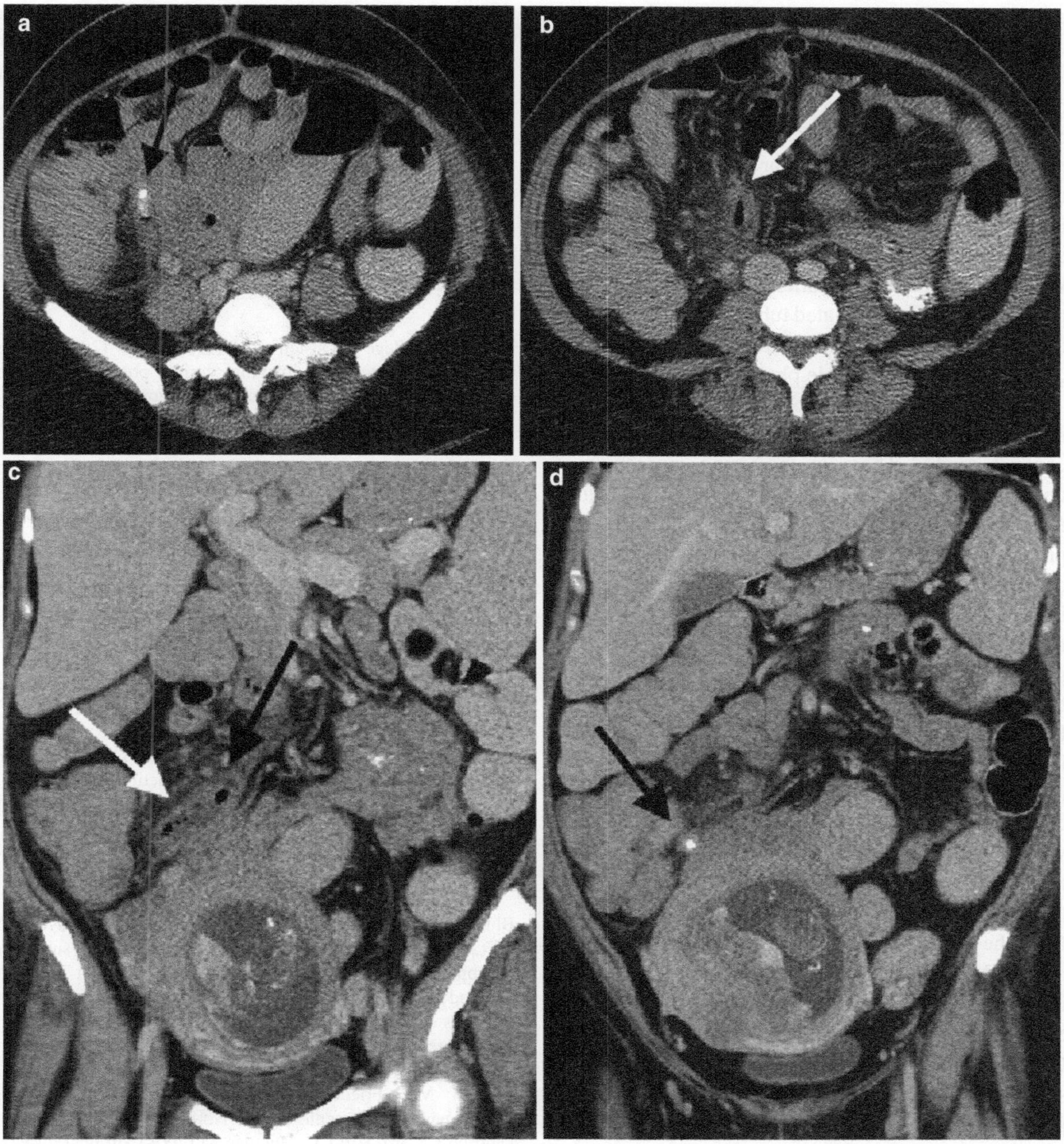

Fig. 8 CT of 17-week pregnant patient with abdominal pain. Surgeons insisted on CT imaging. **a** Transverse image with intravenous and oral contrast shows a dilated enflamed appendix containing appendicoliths (*black arrow*). The tube current was reduced by 30% for this acquisition, **b** Transverse image in the same patient shows a periappendiceal inflammation and fat stranding (*white arrow*), **c** Coronal image in the same patient shows a dilated enflamed appendix (*black arrow*) and periappendiceal fat (*white arrow*), **d** Coronal image in the same patient shows appendicoliths (*black arrow*). The patient was taken to the operating room for acute appendicitis. The fetus did not survive

modulation (ATCM) has been shown to decrease fetal dose in the first trimester, data regarding the later trimesters is scarce. ATCM settings are derived by the scanogram (CT projection radiography). As maternal girth increases, so will tube current increase to maintain the same level of image noise. This model has not been tested in the pregnant patient, where increases in abdominal size include displacement of maternal organs in a cephalad direction and increasing size of the developing fetus. Caution should be undertaken in the application of ATCM in imaging of the abdomen and pelvis in the pregnant woman. Either modification of the CT protocol using ATCM to increase allowable noise, and thus reduce dose, or application of a fixed and lower tube current should be applied if CT is to be undertaken in pregnancy. Dose reduction recommendations from Wieseler et al. (2010) include decreasing kilovoltage for smaller patients, decreasing milliamperage, and using automated tube current modulations, increasing the pitch >1, and taking care to limit the field of view and avoid multiple phases.

A discussion of CT protocols for imaging the pregnant patient would be incomplete without addressing contrast media. There is increasing momentum to abandon both oral and intravenous contrast media in the evaluation of appendicitis. A recent review of imaging protocols suggests that sensitivity and specificity for detection of appendicitis are not altered in the absence of intravenous contrast (Paulson and Coursey 2009) although the studies have not been performed in the pregnant patient. In contrast to gadolinium-based contrast agents, iodinated contrast is classified as a U.S. Food and Drug Administration (FDA) Class B drug, as in vivo tests in animals have shown no evidence of either mutagenic or teratogenic effects with low-osmomolality contrast media (LOCM), however, no adequate and well-controlled teratogenic studies of the effects of these media in pregnant women have been performed (American College of Radiology 2010). Guidelines from the American College of Radiology (2010) recommend documenting informed consent in the use of iodinated contrast in the pregnant patient. The European Society of Urogenital Radiology (ESUR) Guidelines on Contrast Media suggest that in exceptional circumstances, iodinated contrast may be administered to the pregnant female (ESUR Contrast Media Safety Committee 2007). Although the ESUR guidelines advise surveillance of thyroid function in the neonate during the first week of life, recent data suggests that this may not be necessary (Atwell et al. 2008).

5 Conclusion

Current recommendations for evaluation of appendicitis in pregnant women involve initial imaging with ultrasound. If the diagnosis remains inconclusive, a thoughtful conference with referring clinicians should help guide the radiologist's next imaging modality of choice. MRI is preferable to CT given radiation concerns, and gadolinium should be avoided. If MRI is unavailable, CT may be used although radiologists should make all efforts to reduce dose during this examination.

References

American College of Obstetrics and Gynecology (2004) Guidelines for diagnostic imaging during pregnancy. Obstet Gynecol 104:647–651 Committee opinion number 299

American College of Radiology (2008) ACR practice guideline for imaging pregnant or potentially pregnant adolescents and women with ionizing radiation: resolution 26. American College of Radiation, Reston

American College of Radiology (2010) ACR manual on contrast media v7. Radiology ACo, Reston

Angel E, Wellnitz CV, Goodsitt MM et al (2008) Radiation dose to the fetus for pregnant patients undergoing multidetector CT imaging: Monte Carlo simulations estimating fetal dose for a range of gestational age and patient size. Radiology 249:220–227

Annals of the ICRP (2003) Biological effects after prenatal radiation (embryo and fetus). Pergamon Press, New York ICRP publication 90

Atwell TD, Lteif AN, Brown DL, McCann M, Townsend JE, Leroy AJ (2008) Neonatal thyroid function after administration of IV iodinated contrast agent to 21 pregnant patients. AJR Am J Roentgenol 191:268–271

Barloon TJ, Brown BP, Abu-Yousef MM, Warnock N, Berbaum KS (1995) Sonography of acute appendicitis in pregnancy. Abdom Imaging 20:149–151

Blumenfeld YJ, Wong AE, Jafari A, Barth RA, El-Sayed YY (2011) MR imaging in cases of antenatal suspected appendicitis - a meta-analysis. J Matern Fetal Neonatal Med 24:485–488

Cacheris WP, Quay SC, Rocklage SM (1990) The relationship between thermodynamics and the toxicity of gadolinium complexes. Magn Reson Imaging 8:467–481

Cappell MS, Friedel D (2003) Abdominal pain during pregnancy. Gastroenterol Clin North Am 32:1–58

Dietrich CS 3rd, Hill CC, Hueman M (2008) Surgical diseases presenting in pregnancy. Surg Clin North Am 88:403–419 vii–viii

ESUR Contrast Media Safety Committee (2007) ESUR guidelines on contrast media, version 6. In: http://www.esur.org/fileadmin/Guidelines/ESUR_2007_Guideline_6_Kern_Ubersicht.pdf

Ganguli S, Raptopoulos V, Komlos F, Siewert B, Kruskal JB (2006) Right lower quadrant pain: value of the nonvisualized appendix in patients at multidetector CT. Radiology 241:175–180

Hurwitz LM, Yoshizumi T, Reiman RE et al (2006) Radiation dose to the fetus from body MDCT during early gestation. AJR Am J Roentgenol 186:871–876

Israel GM, Malguria N, McCarthy S, Copel J, Weinreb J (2008) MRI vs. ultrasound for suspected appendicitis during pregnancy. J Magn Reson Imaging 28:428–433
Jaffe TA, Miller CM, Merkle EM (2007) Practice patterns in imaging of the pregnant patient with abdominal pain: a survey of academic centers. AJR Am J Roentgenol 189: 1128–1134
Jaffe TA, Yoshizumi TT, Toncheva GI, Nguyen G, Hurwitz LM, Nelson RC (2008) Early first-trimester fetal radiation dose estimation in 16-MDCT without and with automated tube current modulation. AJR Am J Roentgenol 190: 860–864
Jaffe TA, Neville AM, Anderson-Evans C et al (2009) Early first trimester fetal dose estimation method in a multivendor study of 16- and 64-MDCT scanners and low-dose imaging protocols. AJR Am J Roentgenol 193: 1019–1024
Lazarus E, Mayo-Smith WW, Mainiero MB, Spencer PK (2007) CT in the evaluation of nontraumatic abdominal pain in pregnant women. Radiology 244:784–790
Lim HK, Bae SH, Seo GS (1992) Diagnosis of acute appendicitis in pregnant women: value of sonography. AJR Am J Roentgenol 159:539–542
Long SS, Long C, Lai H, Macura KJ (2011) Imaging strategies for right lower quadrant pain in pregnancy. AJR Am J Roentgenol 196:4–12
McGory ML, Zingmond DS, Tillou A, Hiatt JR, Ko CY, Cryer HM (2007) Negative appendectomy in pregnant women is associated with a substantial risk of fetal loss. J Am Coll Surg 205:534–540
Oto A, Srinivasan PN, Ernst RD et al (2006) Revisiting MRI for appendix location during pregnancy. AJR Am J Roentgenol 186:883–887
Parangi S, Levine D, Henry A, Isakovich N, Pories S (2007) Surgical gastrointestinal disorders during pregnancy. Am J Surg 193:223–232
Paulson EK, Coursey CA (2009) CT protocols for acute appendicitis: time for change. AJR Am J Roentgenol 193: 1268–1271
Paulson EK, Harris JP, Jaffe TA, Haugan PA, Nelson RC (2005) Acute appendicitis: added diagnostic value of coronal reformations from isotropic voxels at multi-detector row CT. Radiology 235:879–885
Pedrosa I, Levine D, Eyvazzadeh AD, Siewert B, Ngo L, Rofsky NM (2006) MR imaging evaluation of acute appendicitis in pregnancy. Radiology 238:891–899
Pedrosa I, Lafornara M, Pandharipande PV, Goldsmith JD, Rofsky NM (2009) Pregnant patients suspected of having acute appendicitis: effect of MR imaging on negative laparotomy rate and appendiceal perforation rate. Radiology 250:749–757
Shetty MK, Garrett NM, Carpenter WS, Shah YP, Roberts C (2010) Abdominal computed tomography during pregnancy for suspected appendicitis: a 5-year experience at a maternity hospital. Semin Ultrasound CT MR 31:8–13
Singh A, Danrad R, Hahn PF, Blake MA, Mueller PR, Novelline RA (2007) MR imaging of the acute abdomen and pelvis: acute appendicitis and beyond. Radiographics 27:1419–1431
Valentin J (2000) Pregnancy and medical radiation, ICRP Publication 84. Ann ICRP 30:39
Vu L, Ambrose D, Vos P, Tiwari P, Rosengarten M, Wiseman S (2009) Evaluation of MRI for the diagnosis of appendicitis during pregnancy when ultrasound is inconclusive. J Surg Res 156:145–149
Wall BF, Meara JR, Muirhead CR (Health Protection Agency) (2009) Protection of pregnant patients during diagnostic medical exposures to ionising radiation. http://www.hpa.org.uk/web/HPAwebFile/HPAweb_C/1238230848746
Wieseler KM, Bhargava P, Kanal KM, Vaidya S, Stewart BK, Dighe MK (2010) Imaging in pregnant patients: examination appropriateness. Radiographics 30:1215–1229 Discussion 1230–1213
Woodfield CA, Lazarus E, Chen KC, Mayo-Smith WW (2010) Abdominal pain in pregnancy: diagnoses and imaging unique to pregnancy–review. AJR Am J Roentgenol 194:WS14–WS30

Part IV

Imaging of Acute Appendicitis in Children

Imaging of Acute Appendicitis in Children: Radiography

Daniel N. Vinocur and Edward Y. Lee

Contents

D. N. Vinocur (✉) · E. Y. Lee
Department of Radiology,
Children's Hospital Boston and Harvard Medical School,
300 Longwood Ave, Boston, MA 02115, USA
e-mail: Daniel.Vinocur@childrens.harvard.edu

Abstract

Acute appendicitis is the most common cause for emergent abdominal surgery in pediatric patients. Although most children with acute appendicitis typically present with clinical signs and symptoms that suggest acute appendicitis, approximately one-third of children with acute appendicitis have uncertain and non-specific clinical signs and symptoms. In these pediatric patients, further evaluation with imaging studies is often necessary for proper patient management. The overarching goal of this chapter is to review the plain radiographic evaluation of acute appendicitis in children including current imaging technique, characteristic primary and secondary imaging findings, and interpretation of plain radiographs of acute appendicitis in pediatric population.

1 Introduction

Acute appendicitis is the most common cause for emergent abdominal surgery in pediatric patients (Sivit and Applegate 2003; Kwok et al. 2004; Puig et al. 2008). It accounts for approximately 1–8% of children who present with abdominal pain to the emergency department (Kwok et al. 2004; Rothrock and Pagane 2000). The incidence of acute appendicitis is estimated to be approximately in every 1000 children (Vasavada 2004; Sivit et al. 2001; Sivit 2004). Although most children with acute appendicitis typically present with clinical signs and symptoms that suggest acute appendicitis, approximately one-third of children with acute appendicitis have

C. Keyzer and P. A. Gevenois (eds.), *Imaging of Acute Appendicitis in Adults and Children*, Medical Radiology. Diagnostic Imaging, DOI: 10.1007/174_2011_224, © Springer-Verlag Berlin Heidelberg 2011

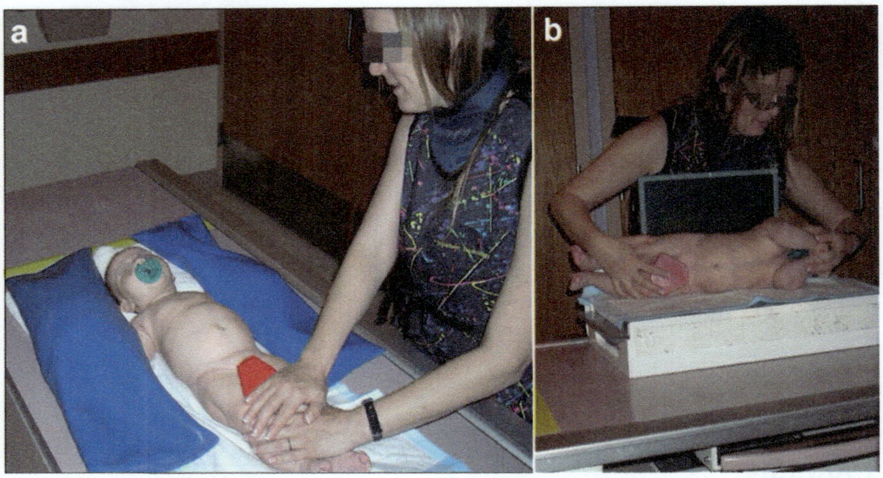

Fig. 1 Eleven-week-old infant. Immobilization for proper patient positioning for AP (**a**) and left lateral decubitus (**b**) views of abdominal radiographs can be achieved by combining sandbags and manual holding of the patient

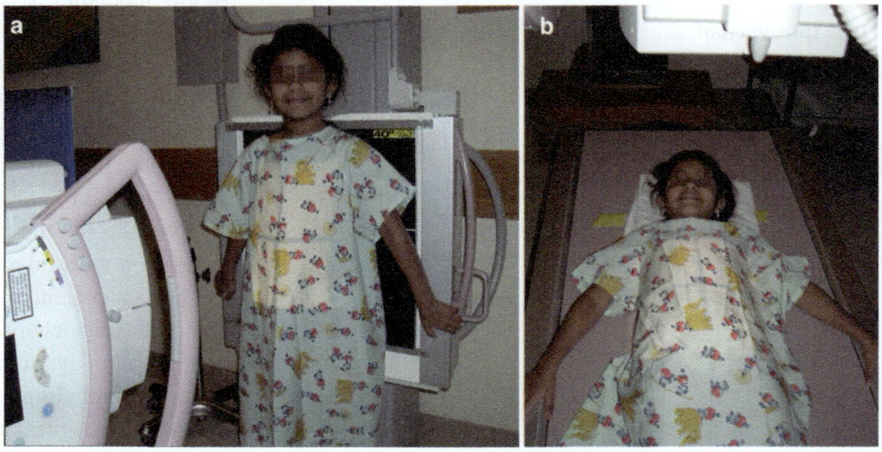

Fig. 2 Seven-year-old girl. School age children are typically cooperative for supine (**a**) and upright (**b**) views of abdominal radiographs

uncertain and non-specific clinical signs and symptoms (Smink et al. 2004; Kaneko and Tsuda 2004). In these pediatric patients, further evaluation with imaging studies is often necessary for proper patient management. In this chapter, we review the plain radiographic evaluation of acute appendicitis in children. Current imaging technique, findings, and interpretation of acute appendicitis on plain radiographs in children are highlighted.

2 Plain Radiographic Evaluation

Traditionally, plain abdominal radiographs have been regarded as a useful initial imaging study in evaluating children with suspected appendicitis (Rothrock and Pagane 2000). Although there is extensive literature regarding the plain radiographic findings of appendicitis, sufficient scientific evidence of sensitivity and specificity for detecting appendicitis based on plain radiographs in children is currently lacking (Leonidas et al. 1975). Furthermore, most of the previously published studies consist of a relatively small number of patients and were published many years ago, prior to the widespread utilization of ultrasound and computed tomography for diagnosing appendicitis in children. Currently, the diagnostic imaging approach and the choice of imaging study for evaluating appendicitis in children are widely varied and depend on each institutional practice guidelines.

At our practice, almost all the imaging evaluation for acute appendicitis is initiated from the emergency department. The selection of the initial and subsequent imaging modality is usually at the discretion of the emergency department physician and consulting surgeon. In most instances, an ultrasound would

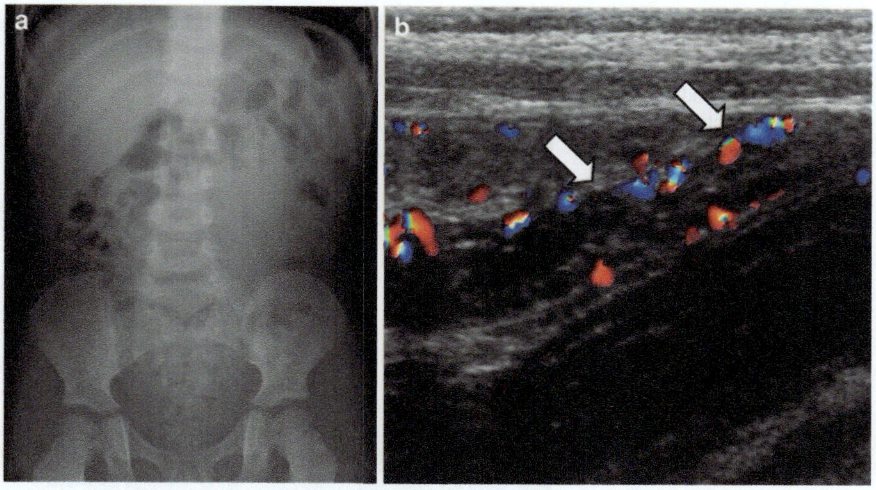

Fig. 3 Three-year-old boy with fever, elevated white blood cell count, and right lower quadrant pain for two days. Supine abdominal radiograph **a** shows normal bowel gas pattern. Subsequently obtained transverse oblique view **b** of ultrasound demonstrates a hyperemic and thickened wall of the enlarged appendix (*arrows*) in the right lower quadrant consistent with acute appendicitis. The patient underwent surgery which confirmed acute appendicitis without perforation

be requested first, with or without a complementary plain abdominal radiograph. When plain abdominal radiographs are requested, the number of views is usually left to the discretion of the referring physician, but typically a supine anteroposterior (AP) radiograph is the routine view, which may be complemented with either an upright or a decubitus view, depending on the age of the patient. At our practice, all the plain radiographs for the emergency department are obtained in a dedicated radiography suite located within the emergency department, which decreases patient transport and delays.

Table 1 Plain radiographic imaging findings of acute appendicitis in children

Appendicolith
Air–fluid levels in the expected location of the terminal ileum and cecum
Loss of the obturator internus and properitoneal fat planes
Displacement of the cecum from the properitoneal fat line
Secondary scoliosis
Free intraperitoneal air
Small bowel obstruction
Colon cut-off sign
Disproportionate jejunal dilatation

2.1 Patient Preparation

Patient motion during imaging evaluation is always problematic in children. The goal of pediatric imaging is to obtain motion-free diagnostic quality images while minimizing the number of re-takes and radiation dose. Dedicated pediatric technologists, specially trained in utilization of helpful techniques to decrease patient motion including distraction and immobilization devices, are essential for obtaining optimal diagnostic quality images. In general, the decision for patient preparation is guided by the age of the child as discussed in the following paragraphs in this section.

2.1.1 Newborns and Infants (<12 months old)

For newborns and infants, swaddling with blankets during imaging, usually sooths the patients and reduces motion. It is important to remove their diapers to avoid potentially confusing artifacts on plain abdominal radiographs (Godderidge 1995). Infants are especially frightened when separated from their parents while obtaining imaging studies. In this age group, having a parent in the examination room assisting with holding his or her child, usually reassures the patient, which in turn, can greatly reduces motion. Alternatively, immobilization while obtaining abdominal radiographs can be achieved with a combination of linens, tapes, Velcro belts, and sandbags in addition to manual holding of patient (Fig. 1).

2.1.2 Toddlers (1–3 years)

Toddlers are perhaps the most challenging group of patients because they are often uncooperative for

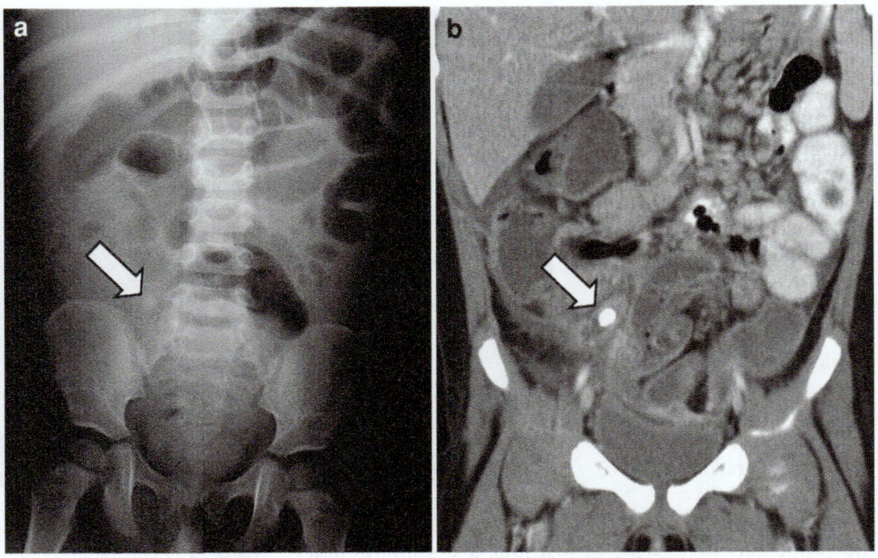

Fig. 4 Two-year-old girl with abdominal pain. Supine abdominal radiograph **a** shows a round radiopaque density consistent with an appendicolith (*arrow*) in the right lower quadrant. Subsequently obtained post-contrast coronal CT image demonstrates **b** an inflamed and enlarged appendix with an appendicolith (*arrow*). Surgery confirmed the presence of acute appendicitis with an appendicolith

imaging studies. Although a great deal of calmness may eventually prove to be successful, we have often found that allowing toddlers to hold on to their favorite toys during imaging studies helps decreasing motion.

2.1.3 Pre-School Children (3–6 years)

Preschool children are usually cooperative particularly when they are invited to actively participate in imaging studies. At our practice, we typically reward these young pre-school children with cartoon stickers or small toys at the successful completion of the imaging studies. We found that this also facilitates future imaging studies.

2.1.4 School Age Children (6–12 years)

School age children usually have a great deal of understanding of the situation. A friendly explanation prior to imaging studies is usually all that is necessary for obtaining successful studies (Fig. 2).

2.1.5 Adolescent Patients (>12 years)

Adolescent patients usually have a complete understanding of the situation. Therefore, we found that these patients are typically cooperative for imaging studies without difficulty.

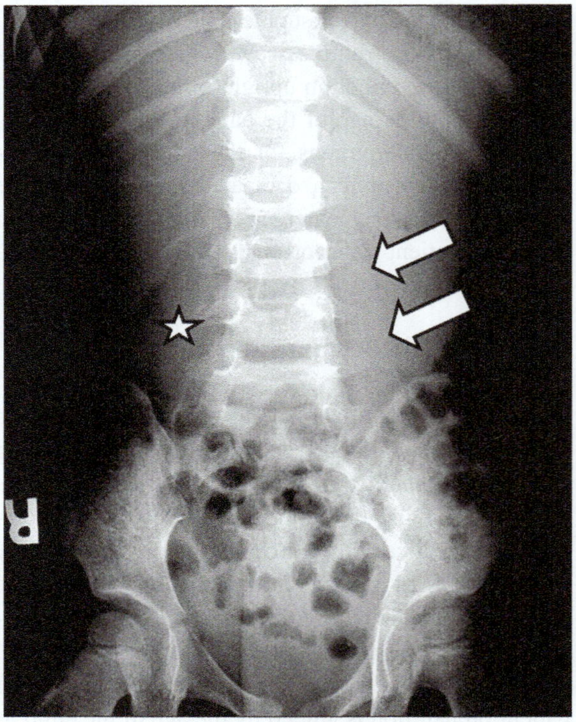

Fig. 5 Three-year-old girl with appendicitis. Upright abdominal radiograph demonstrates loss of the right psoas muscle contour (*star*). The normal appearing left psoas margin (*arrows*) is seen

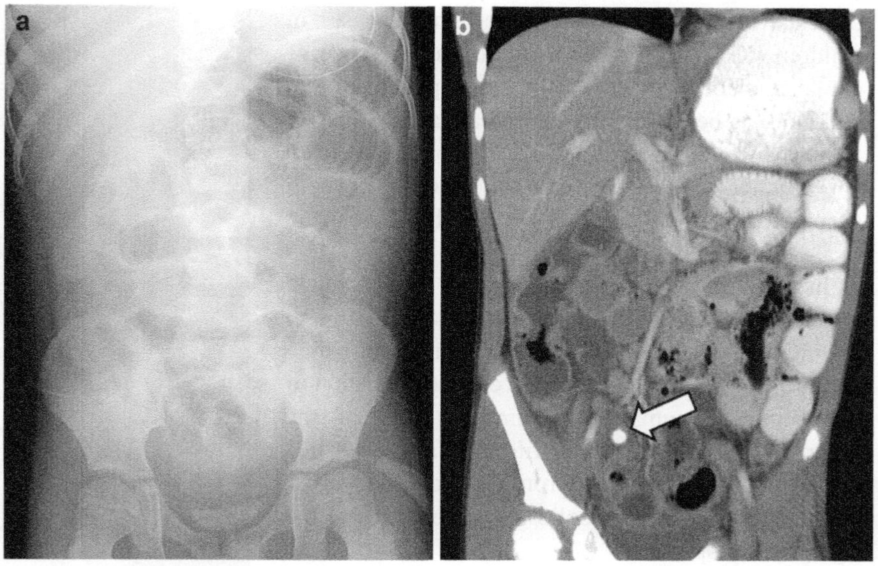

Fig. 6 Eight-year-old boy with perforated appendicitis. Supine abdominal radiograph **a** shows multiple dilated loops of small bowel. Post-contrast coronal CT image **b** demonstrates appendicitis with an appendicolith (*arrow*). Also noted are multiple dilated loops of small bowel along with lack of oral contrast opacification of distal small bowel loops, concerning for at least partial small bowel obstruction

2.2 Plain Radiography Technique

At our practice, AP abdominal radiographs are obtained utilizing commercial digital radiograph equipment (Phillips of North America), standard 40 inches distance from focal zone to cassette and a grid. The mAs and kVp are age adjusted in order to reduce radiation dose, following the ALARA principle ("as low as reasonably achievable"). Typical mAs and kVp are as follows: For a newborn, 65 kVp and 2 mAs; 3–12 month infant, 70 kVp and 2.8 mAs; 1–3 year child, 75 kVp and 4 mAs; 3–6 year child, 75 kVp and 4 mAs; 6–9 year child, 75 kVp and 5 mAs; 10–15 year child, 80 kVp and 6.5 mAs; older than 15 years, 85 kVp and 6.5 mAs. These parameters are general guidelines and the technologists are instructed to adjust them based on the patients' size and in the presence of unusual situations (i.e., marked body deformities). The proper anatomic coverage of the plain abdominal radiographs should capture the entire abdomen from the diaphragms to the pubic symphysis.

2.3 Plain Radiographic Imaging Findings and Interpretation of Acute Appendicitis in Children

Numerous published studies suggest that most plain radiographic imaging findings associated with appendicitis may be non-specific and insensitive (Rothrock and Pagane 2000; Leonidas et al. 1975; Godderidge 1995; Cobb et al. 1993; Isdale 1978). Furthermore, it is well-established in clinical practice and literature that plain abdominal radiographs can be normal in the setting of acute appendicitis (Steinert et al. 1943) (Fig. 3). Therefore, appendicitis should not be excluded from the differential diagnostic considerations on the basis of a normal plain abdominal radiograph alone in children. On the other hand, there are several characteristic plain radiographic imaging appearances of appendicitis (Table 1). Although plain radiographic imaging findings of acute appendicitis depend on many factors, they can be grouped into two categories: imaging findings in non-perforated appendicitis and imaging findings in perforated appendicitis.

2.3.1 Non-Perforated Appendicitis

The most widely recognized finding of acute appendicitis on radiographs is the presence of a radiopaque appendicolith. This finding can be seen in up to 14–22% of positive cases in children (Leonidas et al. 1975; Isdale 1978). It is reported to be the most specific radiographic finding of acute appendicitis in children (Leonidas et al. 1975; Cobb et al. 1993) (Fig. 4). When present, the appendicolith is typically located in the right lower quadrant and may have a laminated configuration (Shimkin 1978). It has been reported that right posterior oblique views of the abdomen and pelvis may be of help in confirming the presence of appendicoliths in questionable cases in children (Kirks 1998). Furthermore, the presence of an appendicolith in the setting of appendicitis in children has been reported to indicate approximately 50% chance of having a complication from acute appendicitis such as perforation, abscess, or both (Leonidas et al. 1975; Hatten et al. 1973; Johnson et al. 1988).

In pediatric patients with acute appendicitis, abdominal radiographs may demonstrate indirect findings of right lower quadrant inflammation which include: (1) air–fluid levels in the expected location of the terminal ileum and cecum; (2) loss of the obturator internus and properitoneal fat planes; (3) displacement of the cecum from the properitoneal fat line; and (4) secondary scoliosis (i.e., concave to the right) due to splinting.

The presence of air–fluid levels in the expected location of the ileum and cecum is a controversial plain abdominal radiographic sign in children. While some investigators found this imaging finding to be helpful for evaluating suspected acute appendicitis (Isdale 1978), other investigators have not found this imaging finding to be useful (Cobb et al. 1993). Loss of the obturator internus and properitoneal fat planes have shown to be suggestive of the diagnosis of acute appendicitis (Isdale 1978) (Fig. 5). However, some investigators disregard this imaging finding as nonspecific because it may be seen with the same prevalence on normal patients (Leonidas et al. 1975) and it cannot be identified with certainty in many instances (Rothrock and Pagane 2000). Rightward secondary scoliosis on plain radiographs of the abdomen in patients with acute appendicitis has been historically considered a useful imaging finding of acute appendicitis. It is presumed to be secondary to antalgic posture ("splinting"). Several previously published reports support its diagnostic value in assessing acute appendicitis in the pediatric population (Rothrock and Pagane 2000; Leonidas et al. 1975; Isdale 1978). Lastly, Bakha et al. reported the disturbance of the normal intestinal bowel gas pattern such as localized ileus, generalized ileus, or obstructive pattern as the most useful plain radiographic imaging findings of acute appendicitis in pediatric patients (Leonidas et al. 1975).

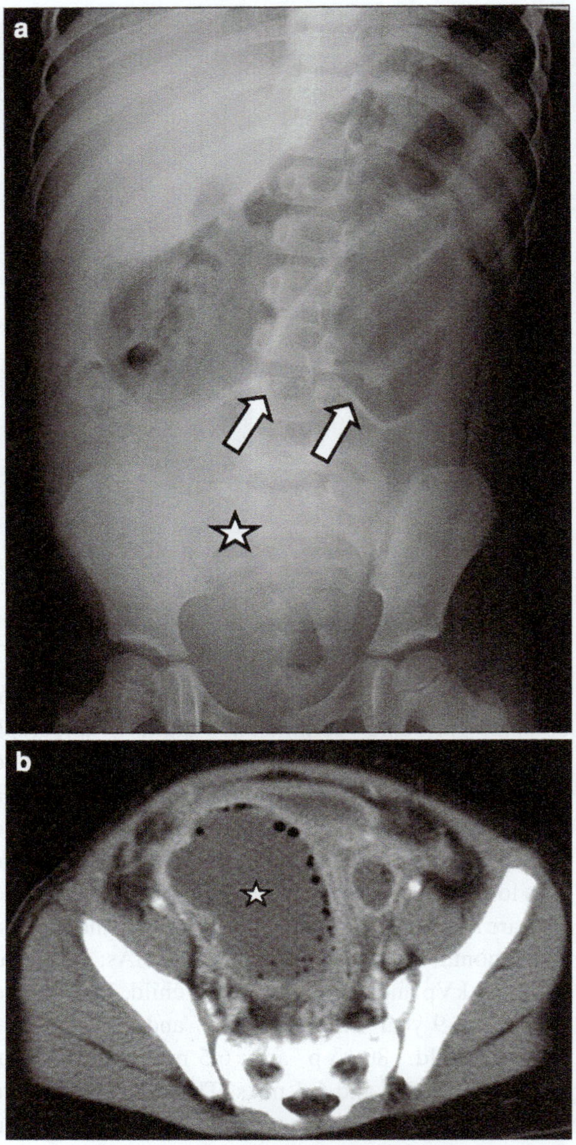

Fig. 7 Three-year-old girl with periappendiceal abscess due to perforated appendicitis. Supine abdominal radiograph **a** shows faint soft tissue density (*star*) in the right lower quadrant with subtle mass-effect (*arrows*) over the loops of small bowel. Post-contrast axial CT image **b** shows a large abscess formation (*star*) in the right lower quadrant with surrounding inflammatory changes

2.3.2 Perforated Appendicitis

In cases of perforated appendicitis, other plain radiographic imaging findings may be seen in addition to

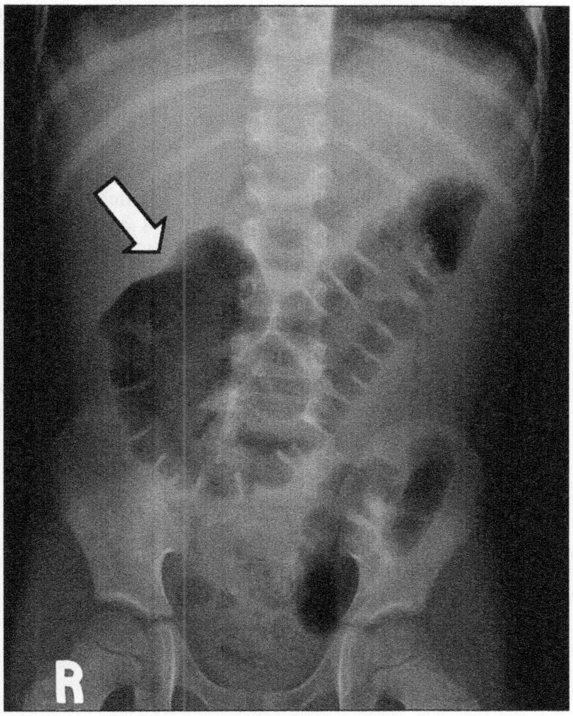

Fig. 8 Five-year-old boy with acute appendicitis. Supine abdominal radiograph demonstrates distended transverse colon and empty ascending colon with a sharp demarcation (*arrow*) of these two segments

the previously listed plain radiographic imaging findings of non-perforated appendicitis. Small foci of extraluminal gas may be present on plain radiographs, although they are usually difficult to detect. The presence of a large amount of free intraperitoneal gas on plain abdominal radiographs is uncommon in pediatric patients with perforated appendicitis.

Small bowel obstruction may be a result of complicated perforated appendicitis (Rothrock and Pagane 2000; Johnson et al. 1988) (Fig. 6). In fact, it has been reported that acute small bowel obstruction is the most common imaging findings of appendiceal perforation in children on plain radiographs (Johnson et al. 1988). This is speculated to be secondary to inflammatory adhesions resulting in small bowel obstruction in the vicinity of the perforated appendix. In this situation, multiple dilated small bowel loops are typically seen on plain radiographs of abdomen. If a well-defined abscess forms as a result of perforated appendicitis, it may produce a soft tissue mass-like opacity with or without an air–fluid level on plain radiographs (Fig. 7).

Furthermore, the colon cutoff sign may be present, which is characterized by the constellations of absence of gas and feces in the cecum and right colon, reflex dilatation of the transverse colon, and amputation of colonic gas at the hepatic flexure (Swischuk and Hayden 1980) (Fig. 8). Finally, disproportionate jejunal dilation in cases of perforated appendicitis in children on plain radiographs has also been reported in the past (Riggs and Parvey 1976).

3 Conclusion

Plain abdominal radiographs are often obtained in the initial evaluation of children with suspected appendicitis. Despite their lack of high sensitivity and specificity, plain abdominal radiographs play an important role in assessing appendicitis in children by providing imaging findings suggestive of underlying acute appendicitis, excluding alternatively diagnosis, and guiding the next appropriate step in both imaging and clinical management. Understanding plain radiographic imaging findings of appendicitis in children enables an early and accurate diagnosis, which in turn, can optimize proper pediatric patient care.

References

Cobb LM, Lelli JL (1993) Appendicitis. In: Reisdorf EJ, Roberts MR, Wiegenstein JG (eds) Pediatric emergency medicine. WB Saunders, Philadelphia, PA 314–321

Godderidge C (1995) Pediatric Imaging. Saunders Company, Philadelphia, PA

Hatten LE, Miller RC, Hester CL Jr, Moynihan PC (1973) Appendicitis and the abdominal roentgenogram in children. South Med J 66:803–806

Isdale JM (1978) The radiological signs of acute appendicitis in infancy and childhood. S Afr Med J 53:363–364

Johnson JF, Coughlin WF, Stark P (1988) The sensitivity of plain films for detecting perforation in children with appendicitis. Rofo 149:619–623

Kaneko K, Tsuda M (2004) Ultrasound-based decision making in the treatment of acute appendicitis in children. J Pediatr Surg 39:1316–1320

Kirks DR (1998) Practical pediatric imaging, diagnostic radiology of infants and children. Lippincott-Raven, Philadelphia, PA

Kwok MY, Kim MK, Gorelick MH (2004) Evidence-based approach to the diagnosis of appendicitis in children. Pediatr Emerg Care 20:690–698 (quiz 699–701)

Leonidas JC, Harris DJ, Amoury RA (1975) How accurate is the roentgen diagnosis of acute appendicitis in children. Ann Radiol (Paris) 18:479–487

Puig S, Staudenherz A, Felder-Puig R, Paya K (2008) Imaging of appendicitis in children and adolescents: useful or useless? A comparison of imaging techniques and a critical review of the current literature. Semin Roentgenol 43:22–28

Riggs W Jr, Parvey LS (1976) Perforated appendix presenting with disproportionate jejunal distention. Pediatr Radiol 5:47–49

Rothrock SG, Pagane J (2000) Acute appendicitis in children: emergency department diagnosis and management. Ann Emerg Med 36:39–51

Shimkin PM (1978) Radiology of acute appendicitis. AJR Am J Roentgenol 130:1001–1004

Sivit CJ (2004) Imaging the child with right lower quadrant pain and suspected appendicitis: current concepts. Pediatr Radiol 34:447–453

Sivit CJ, Applegate KE (2003) Imaging of acute appendicitis in children. Semin Ultrasound CT MR 24:74–82

Sivit CJ, Siegel MJ, Applegate KE, Newman KD (2001) When appendicitis is suspected in children. Radiographics 21:247–262 (questionnaire 288–294)

Smink DS, Finkelstein JA, Garcia Pena BM, Shannon MW, Taylor GA, Fishman SJ (2004) Diagnosis of acute appendicitis in children using a clinical practice guideline. J Pediatr Surg 39:458–463 (discussion 458–463)

Steinert R, Hareide I, Christiansen T (1943) Roentgenolic examination of acute appendicitis. Acta Radiol 24:13–27

Swischuk LE, Hayden CK Jr (1980) Appendicitis with perforation: the dilated transverse colon sign. AJR Am J Roentgenol 135:687–689

Vasavada P (2004) Ultrasound evaluation of acute abdominal emergencies in infants and children. Radiol Clin North Am 42:445–456

Imaging of Acute Appendicitis in Children: Ultrasonography

Herma C. Holscher

Contents

Abstract

This chapter describes the normal and abnormal findings in ultrasound when imaging the appendiceal region in a child. Next to practical tips in imaging the appendix, potential pitfalls in diagnosing appendicitis are highlighted. The criteria for diagnosing appendicitis are summarized and clear guidelines are pointed out to handle equivocal cases. A wide range of illustrations make this chapter a very practical approach to imaging appendicitis in childhood.

1 Introduction

In the literature there is debate about the preferred imaging modality in appendicitis but, for children, ultrasonography is the most advocated modality, especially in Europe (Holscher and Heij 2009). It can result in changes in the proposed management in more than 25% of cases (Puylaert et al. 1987). Nowadays most authors agree on the fact that ultrasound and CT are complementary rather than opposites (Strouse 2010). The advantages of ultrasound are agreed upon: no radiation dose, easy accessibility for the radiologist and less frightening for the child. Furthermore, the radiologist can correlate the clinical findings during the sonography (where does it hurt?) with the imaging findings. Ultrasound scanning may, however, have suboptimal accuracy in obese children with a low likelihood of appendicitis (Schuh et al. 2010).

H. C. Holscher (✉)
HAGA Teaching Hospital, Juliana Children's Hospital, Sportlaan, 600, 2566 MJ Den Haag, The Netherlands
e-mail: h.holscher@hagaziekenhuis.nl

C. Keyzer and P. A. Gevenois (eds.), *Imaging of Acute Appendicitis in Adults and Children*,
Medical Radiology. Diagnostic Imaging, DOI: 10.1007/174_2011_225, © Springer-Verlag Berlin Heidelberg 2011

2 Imaging Technique, Tips and Tricks

Imaging children with clinical signs of appendicitis starts with the routine ultrasound examination of the whole abdomen. The gel is preferably warmed to near-body temperature before being applied to the skin of the child. It is important to examine the diaphragmatic area in order to look for pleural effusion and/or pulmonary consolidation as children with pneumonia can present with symptoms mimicking appendicitis (Jona and Belin 1976). Coincidental findings or other findings that may explain the physical condition of the patients are important to notice before concentrating on the right lower quadrant. Furthermore the child can get used to the ultrasound, before the more painful part of the body is examined.

2.1 Equipment

For the survey a convex array low frequency probe (3–7 MHZ) can be used.

For right lower quadrant, specific examination is done with a high-frequency linear probe transducer (7–12 MHz), which has limited penetration but high image quality.

2.2 Graded Compression

Graded compression sonography, first described by Puylaert (1986), consists of anterior forced compression used to reduce the abdominal cavity between the pathologic process and the high-frequency transducer with a short focus (Fig. 1a).

A more recent amendment to this technique is a modified bimanual compression technique (Lee et al. 2001). If the appendix is not visualized after completion of the graded compression scans, posterior manual compression techniques can improve visualization of the appendix. This technique is an adjuvant to graded compression sonography and is composed of forced extrinsic compression of the opposite side of the right lower quadrant abdomen in the anterior or anteromedial direction using the palms or the four fingers of the left hand' thereby allowing compression of the posterior aspects of the cecum or pericecal space with or without anteromedial displacement of the right lower quadrant bowel structures onto the psoas muscle (Fig. 1b).

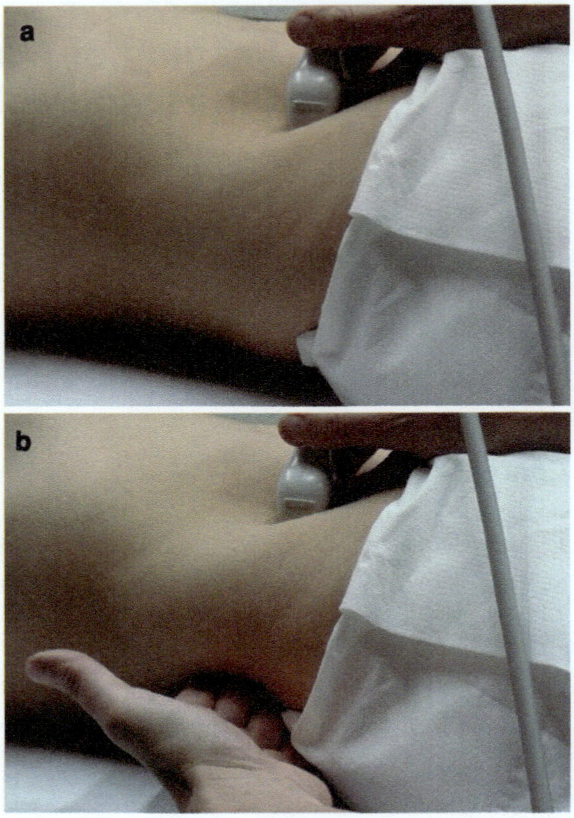

Fig. 1 Graded compression techniques. **a** Original graded compression with the transducer by using the hand on the transducer, gradually increasing the force of compression. **b** Modified bimanual technique. With the other hand compression is applied from the back, thereby diminishing the distance from the psoas to the transducer

In some cases a full bladder may push the appendix into a higher position, thereby concealing it behind bowel loops and making it non-visible. After voiding the appendix has more space to unfold and repeated ultrasound after voiding may be helpful.

In some cases a left oblique lateral decubitus change of body position allows better visualization of the appendix (Lee et al. 2005).

If necessary the US examination can be repeated if clinical management allows.

3 The Normal Appendix

With the improvement of ultrasound machines, it is possible to image the normal appendix in children. The normal appendix can be visualized in about 80% of

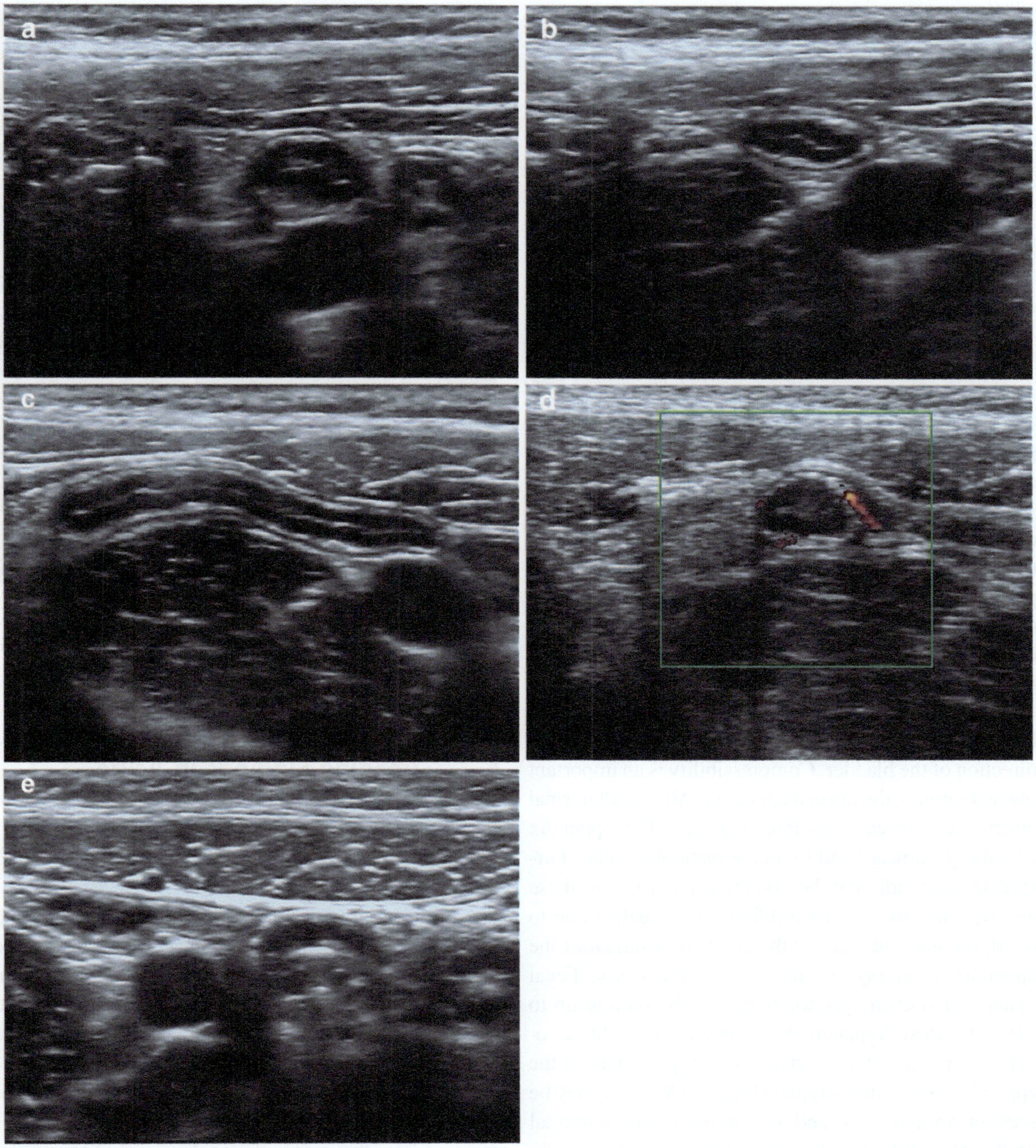

Fig. 2 Normal appendix. **a** Axial, non-compressed image. A small round structure with a concentric layered wall is visualized. **c** After compression a slight indentation of the anterior wall is seen. The axial diameter of the appendix is decreased compared to the non-compressed image. **b** Longitudinal image. Four layers of the appendiceal wall can be identified. **e** Color Doppler. Very sparse flow in appendiceal wall and surrounding tissue. **d** Bright central reflection in the appendix representing gas in the normal appendix

normal asymptomatic children (Wiersma et al. 2005). It is seen as a blind-ending lamellated structure, without peristalsis (Fig. 2a, b). The five concentric layers of the wall are alternatingly echo lucent and hyperechoic, just like the layers in the wall in other parts of the gastrointestinal tract. From outside to inside this

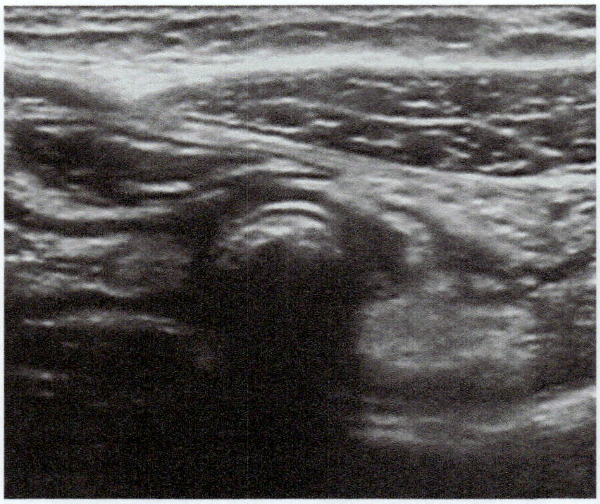

Fig. 3 Appendicolith. Large echogenic focus within the appendix with acoustic shadowing in a patient with early appendicitis

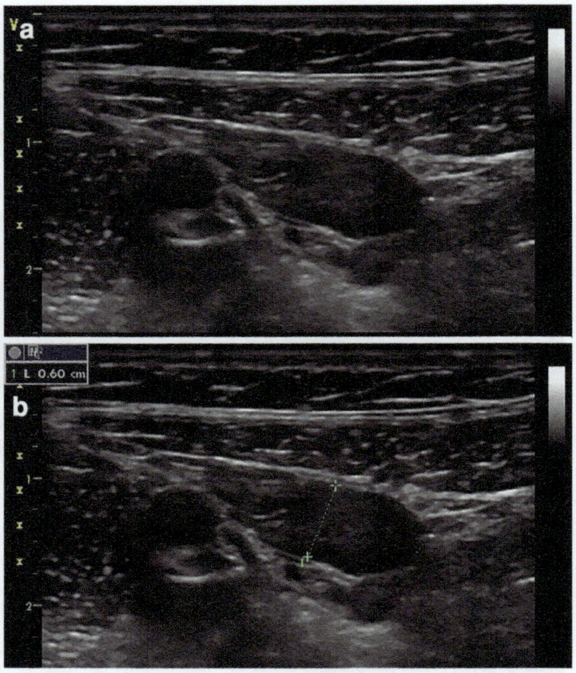

Fig. 4 Normal lymphnode. **a** Small almond-like hypoechoic lymph node with tiny echogenic hilum. **b** The axial diameter is 6 mm

consist of the serosa (hyperechoic), the muscularis (hypoechoic), the submucosa (hyperechoic), lamina propia (hypoechoic) and central the mucosal surface (hyperechoic) (Kimmey et al. 1989). On ultrasound the hyperechoic serosa is often not seen due to the surrounding tissue (Fig. 2b).

The classical position is coming out of the cecum lying caudally above the iliac vessels pointing in the direction of the bladder. Compressibility is an important phenomenon in the normal appendix. Almost all normal appendices are compressible (Fig. 2c). The appendix can also go upward and lie in the paracolic gutter. Further, the appendix can be completely retrocecal, these are the ones that are more difficult to visualize due to overlying gas and feces in the colon. The lumen of the appendix is empty in majority of the cases. Fecal material and even appendicoliths can be seen in up to 25% of cases. Appendicoliths appear as bright echogenic foci with acoustic shadowing (Fig. 3). Gas in the appendix, appearing as typical bright reflections, may be seen in around 15% and is considered as a normal finding (Fig. 2d). The diameter of the normal appendix may vary in healthy children (mean 4 mm) but is generally less than 6 mm in AP diameter. The left to right diameter may be higher, up to 8 mm due to compression. The diameter of the appendix does not correlate significantly with age (Simonovský 2002). With color Doppler the normal appendix does not show flow or occasionally very sparse flow (Fig. 2e). In the surrounding area small lymph nodes (<8 mm AP diameter) can be considered a normal finding (Fig. 4).

4 Imaging Findings in Acute Appendicitis

4.1 The Appendix in Appendicitis

The ultrasonographic findings in appendicitis depend on the stage of disease. In the early phase of disease the lumen of the appendix distends due to obstruction of the lumen. The appendiceal wall gets swollen and the diameter of the appendix increases. In appearance it is like a concentrically layered sausage-like structure (Fig. 5). The diameter of the appendix is one of the most important hallmarks of the disease and is measured in the axial plane. An axial diameter of more than 8 mm is generally believed to be abnormal. A diameter below 6 mm is generally normal (Jeffrey et al. 1988). Some difficulty may be found when the diameter is between 6 and 8 mm. More caution is needed and the radiologist needs to focus on additional signs.

Non-compressibility is an important sign of appendicitis. Due to swelling of the appendix it cannot be compressed as normal appendices.

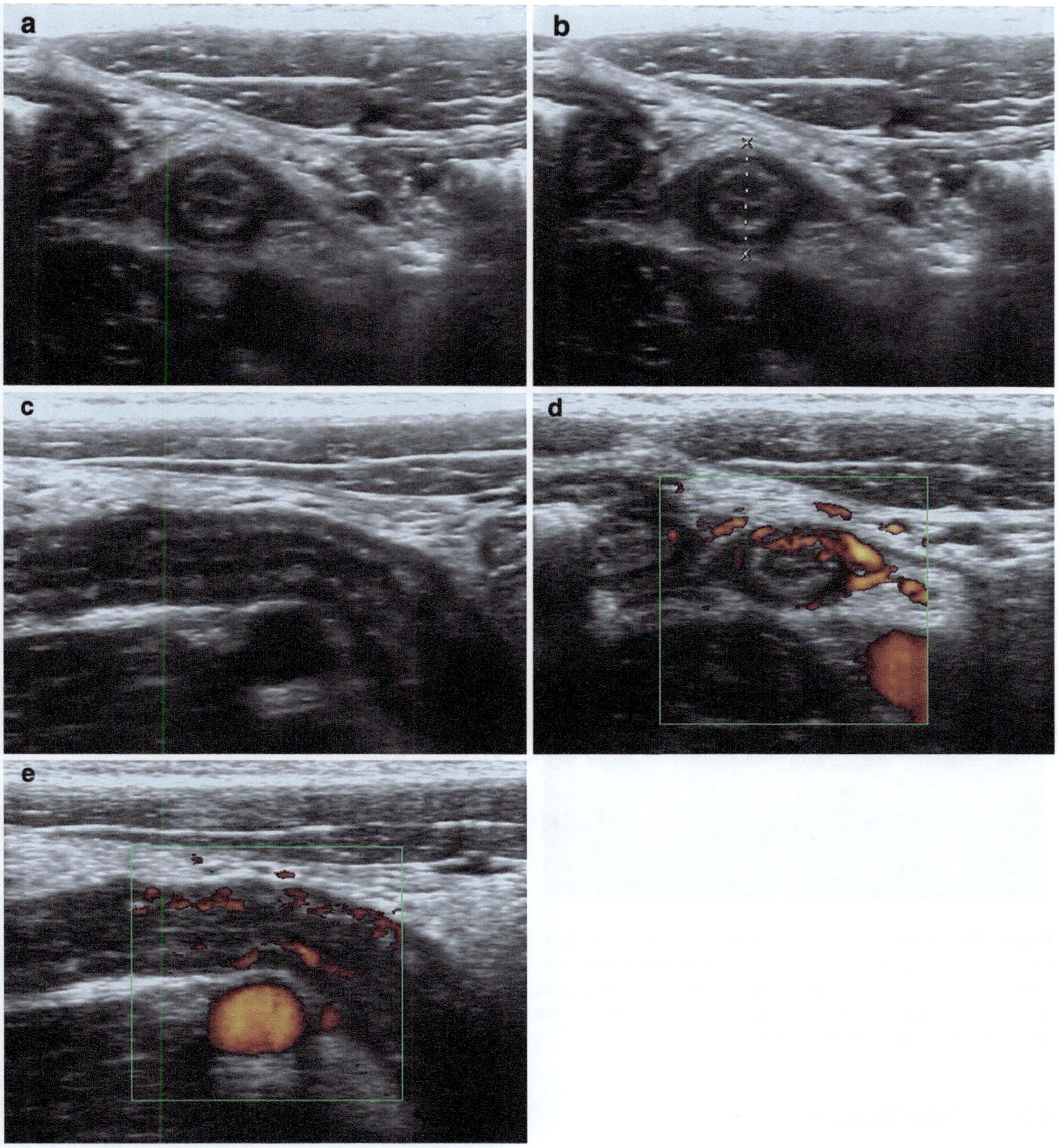

Fig. 5 Early appendicitis. **a** Axial image shows slight dilation of the non-compressible appendix, with mild swelling of the wall. Some minor echogenic changes in the surrounding fat. **b** Axial measurement shows an appendiceal diameter of 7.7 mm. **c** Corresponding longitudinal image, inflamed appendix lying in the classical position. **d** On Color Doppler imaging some increase in flow in the wall. **e** Corresponding longitudinal image

Appendicoliths may be or may not be present, but is not a differentiating finding in appendicitis (Fig. 6). It is, however, an important feature to describe in the radiologic report, as an appendicolith of an inflamed appendix, if not surgically removed may stay in the peritoneal cavity and may give rise to postoperative abscess formation. This can occur up to a month after operation.

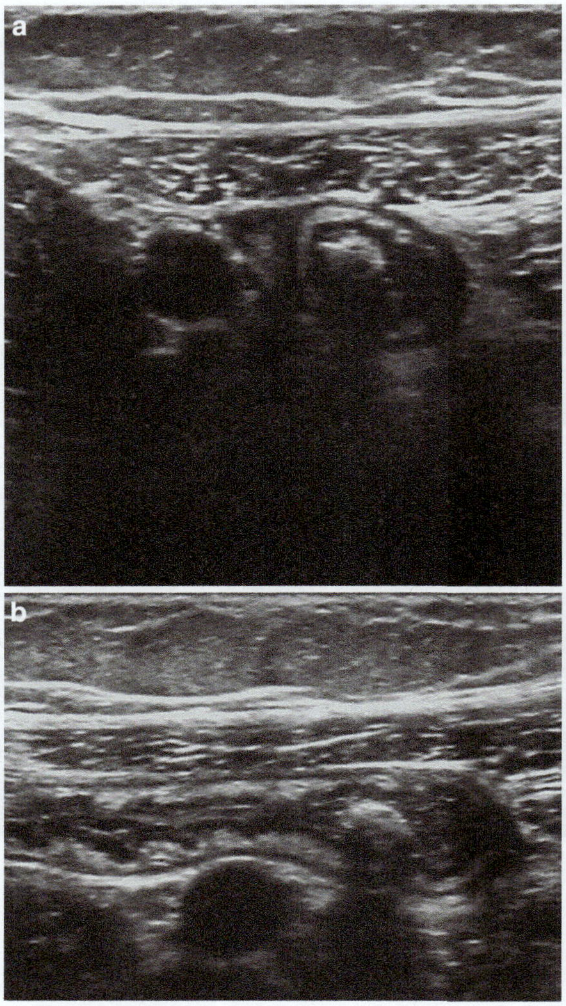

Fig. 6 Appendicitis with appendicolith. **a** Axial image showing slightly enlarged non-compressible appendix with appendicolith. Some echogenic infiltration of the surrounding fat, indicative of appendicitis. **b** Longitudinal image shows the appendicolith in the tip of the appendix

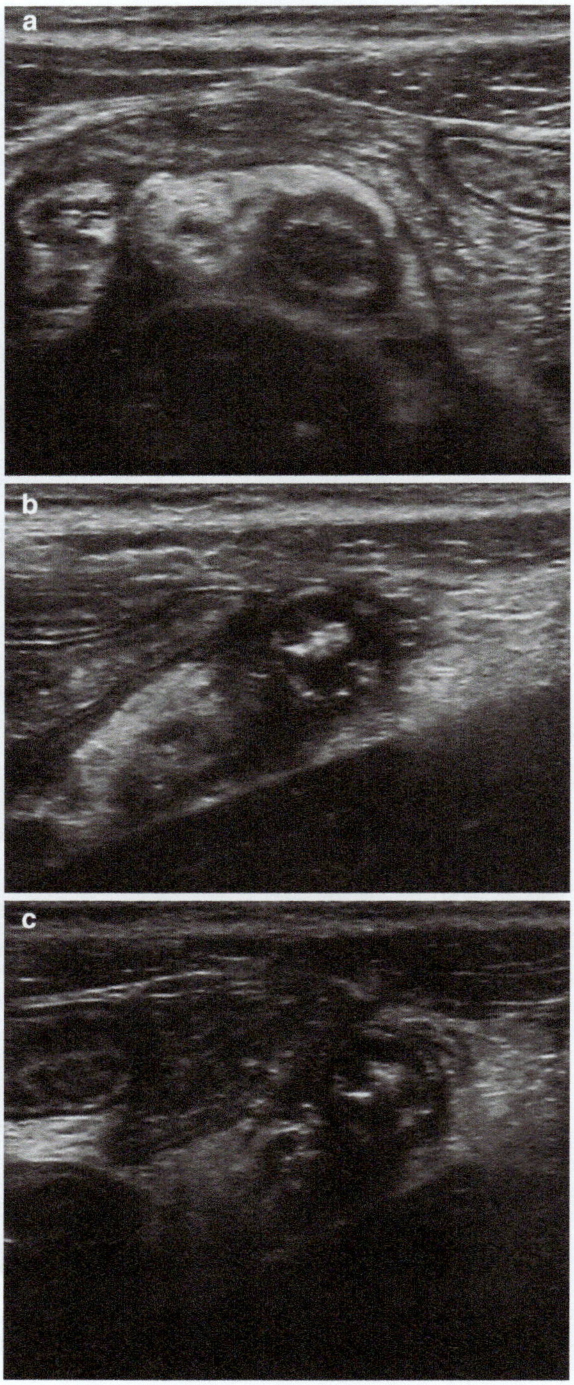

Fig. 7 Appendicitis with phlegmon. **a** Axial image shows enlarged non-compressible appendix and echogenic mesentery. **b** Some fecal material is seen in the lumen. **c** Local distortion of the wall of the appendix indicates that perforation is imminent

4.2 Color Doppler

The rate of vascularization of the appendix is related to the stage of the disease. A normal appendix shows virtually no wall-enhancement. When the appendix becomes hypervascularized due to inflammation the flow in the wall will increase in the phlegmonous stage of the disease (Fig. 5c, d). When the appendix reaches the gangrenous stage of the disease the vascularization is diminished again due to necrosis, thereby no flow with color Doppler is visualized in this phase, and the wall of the appendix is sometimes disintegrated. The absence of flow in perforated appendicitis is less well understood, but might be

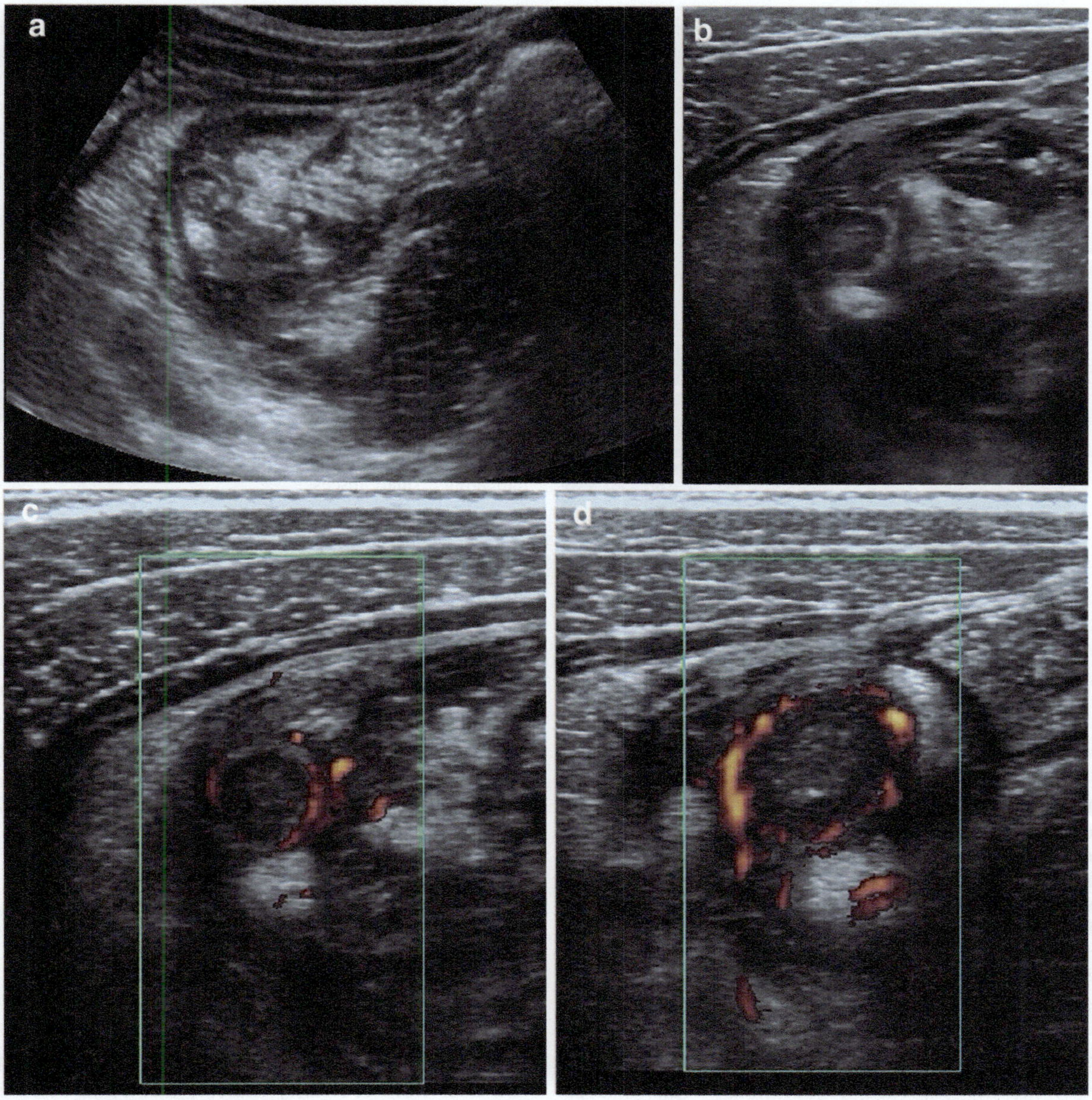

Fig. 8 Appendicitis of paracolic appendix. **a** Overview: In the paracolic gutter the distended appendix is already visualized in an area with mixed hyper- and hypoechogeneity. **b** Detailed view of enlarged appendix with surrounding phlegmon. **c**, **d** On color Doppler increased flow in the non-necrotic appendiceal wall

either due to early inflammation with early perforation, or due to necrosis (Quillin and Siegel 1995).

4.3 Secondary Signs

Around the appendix inflammation of the mesenteric fat causes increased echogenicity and non-compressibility of this mesenteric tissue adjacent to the appendix (Figs. 7 and 8). Some reactive fluid may develop and after perforation local abscess formation might be seen. Local peritonitis causes focal dilatation of the small bowel without peristalsis. In some cases just a kind of "messy" image is seen, indicating peri-appendicular phlegmon (Fig. 9). These secondary signs are very indicative of appendicitis, even without visualizing the appendix itself (Wiersma et al. 2009).

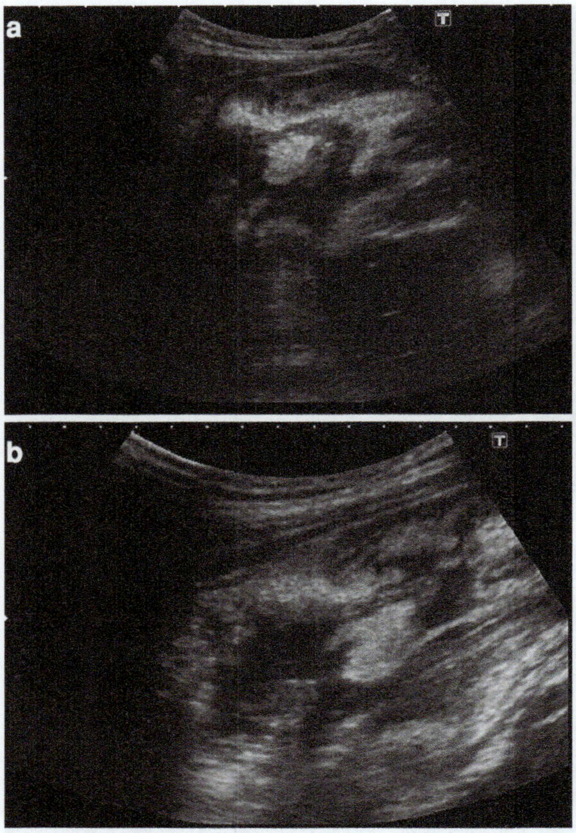

Fig. 9 Secondary signs. **a** Overview of the right lower quadrant. "Messy" appearance with hyper- and hypoechogenicity, indicating infiltrated mesenteric and omental fat and local fluid. **b** The appendix could not be found. These secondary signs are sufficient to diagnose appendicitis with high accuracy

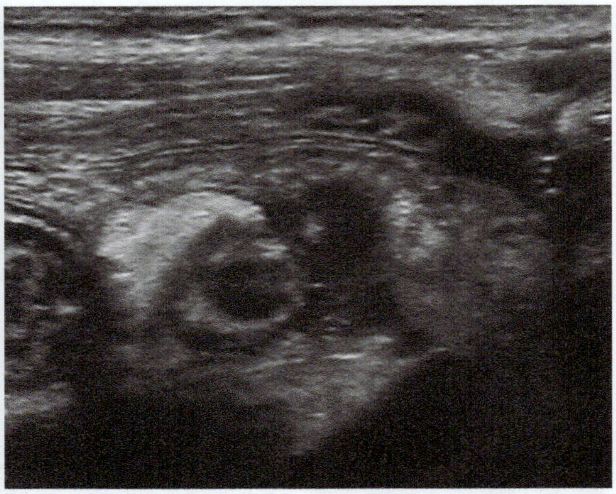

Fig. 10 Small fluid collection adjacent to the appendix indicating a small abscess

Non-visualization of the appendix without these secondary signs, safely rules out appendicitis, whereas the presence of secondary signs without depiction of the appendix itself is a strong indicator of acute appendicitis.

4.4 Abscess Formation

Irregular masses with reduced echogenicity may indicate the formation of an abscess. Usually it lies in close contact with the inflamed appendix (Fig. 10). The appendix can also be seen lying in the cavity itself. If perforation results in peritoneal spread of pus throughout the whole peritoneal cavity abscess formation can be seen distant from the appendix, usually in the pouch of Douglas, the pouch of Morrisson or subphrenic (Fig. 11).

In adults percutaneous drainage of abscesses is much advocated and is successful in many cases, in children this technique is not widely used. In general in children small collections will spontaneously resolve, while for larger abscesses surgical intervention is usually necessary. This is due to the fact that the children will require general anesthesia anyway. In older cooperative children though, percutaneous drainage might be considered.

4.5 Coincidental Findings

Increased echogenicity of the renal cortex in children with acute abdominal illness is a non-specific finding and does not necessarily indicate true renal disease. Increased echogenicity of the renal cortex is a transient phenomenon in this clinical setting. Hyperechogenicity of the renal cortex in children with acute abdominal illness should alert the radiologist to search the abdomen more thoroughly for a cause of the acute abdominal illness, such as appendicitis (Wiersma et al. 2008). Mild to severe hydronephrosis of the right kidney may be seen in a case of appendicitis when the distal ureter is obstructed by peri-apppendicular infiltrate or abscess formation (Fig. 12).

In children who present with acute abdominal symptoms, no matter the course, strong periportal reflections may be noticed (Fig. 13). In this setting

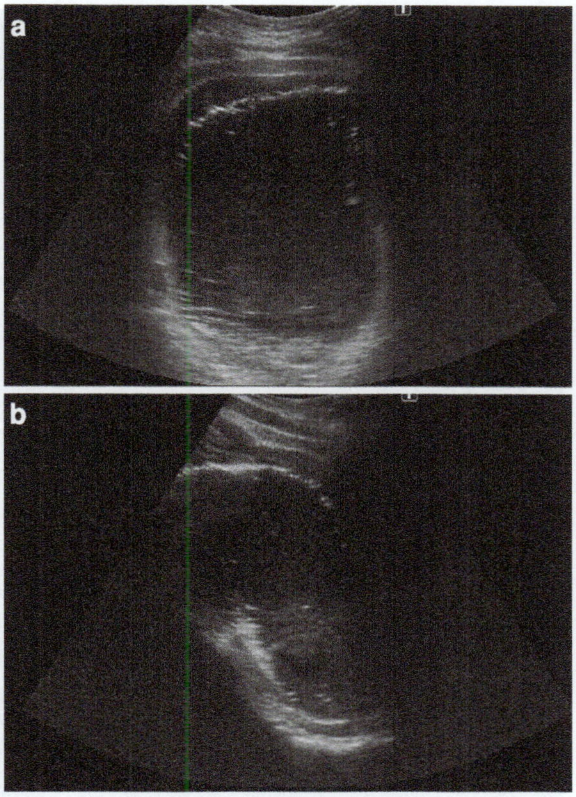

Fig. 11 Abscess in Pouch of Douglas. **a** Axial image shows large fluid collection with some reflections, due to pus. **b** Longitudinal image. The abscess follows the contours of the Pouch of Douglas

this is a coincidental and transient finding and should not be confused with hepatic disease.

4.6 Abortive and Recurrent Appendicitis

Though there are controversies in the literature about this entity, ultrasonography is the imaging method which shows the findings in spontaneous resolving appendicitis. The incidence of the phenomenon in the total group of patients with appendicitis is not known, but is estimated for at least 8% (Cobben et al. 2000). The findings are those of an enlarged non-compressible appendix with a diameter of more than 6 mm at US, and rapidly subsiding symptoms. There are no US or clinical signs of an peri-appendiceal spread or abscess. Spontaneous resolvement resulting in normalization of the appendix occurs within days. The decision on whether or not to operate on these children depends on the clinician who may decide to observe a patient who has relatively mild symptoms. The incidence of recurrence in the patients with spontaneous resolving appendicitis is around 38%, with the majority of cases recurring within 1 year (Cobben et al. 2000). Spontaneously resolving and chronic appendicitis will be extensively discussed by L Cobben in chapter “Spontaneously Resolving and Chronic Appendicitis”.

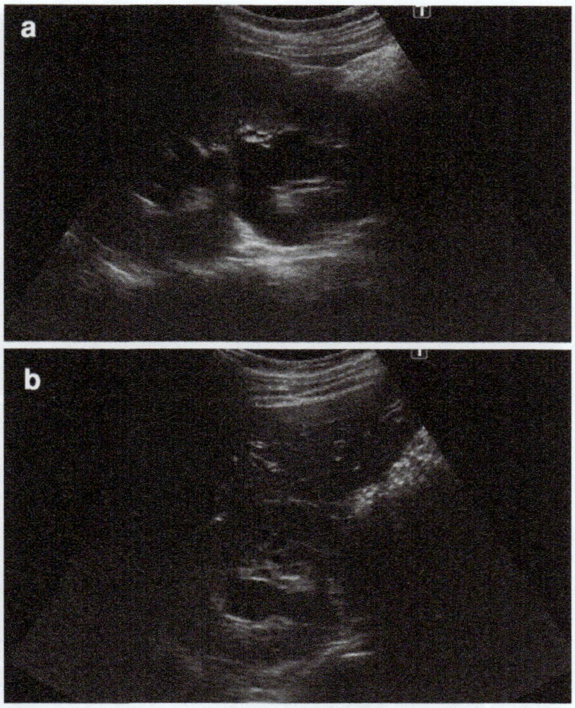

Fig. 12 Renal coincidental finding in patient with periappendicular abscess. **a** Longitudinal image. Marked hydronephrosis of the right kidney. **b** Axial image. The renal cortex is somewhat more echogenic than the liver

5 Pitfalls

There are several conditions that may cause ultrasonographic features resembling appendicitis.

5.1 Cystic Fibrosis

The appendiceal diameter on US scans in asymptomatic children with cystic fibrosis (CF) is significantly larger than in the normal population (mean diameter 8.3 mm) (Lardenoye et al. 2004). Often the appendix in these patients is non-compressible

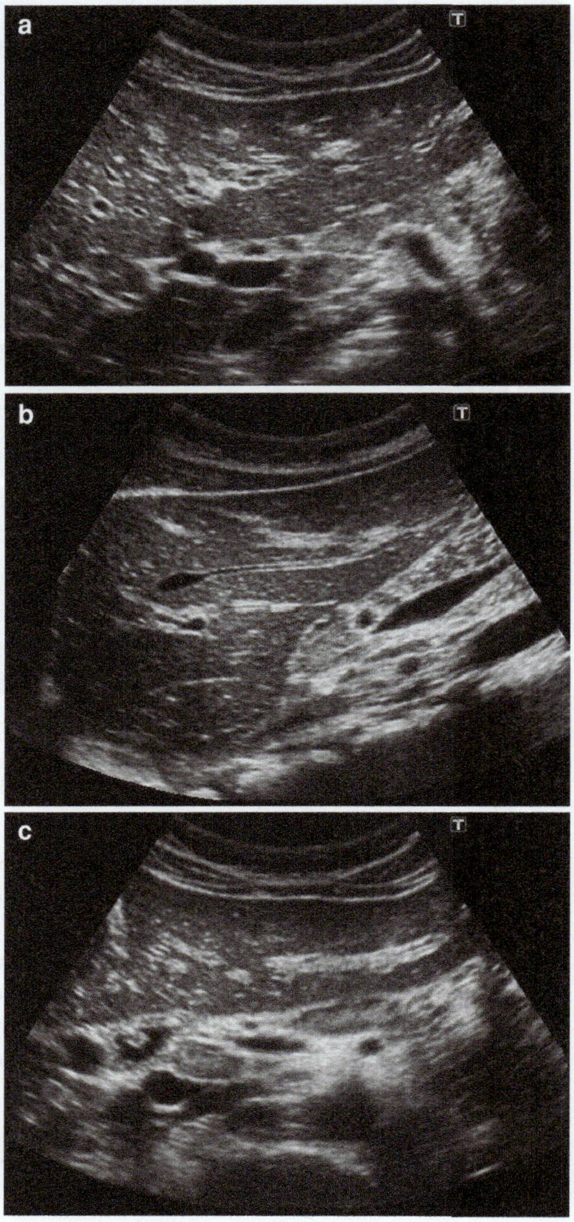

Fig. 13 **a**, **b**, **c** Three images of strong periportal reflections in a patient with appendicitis

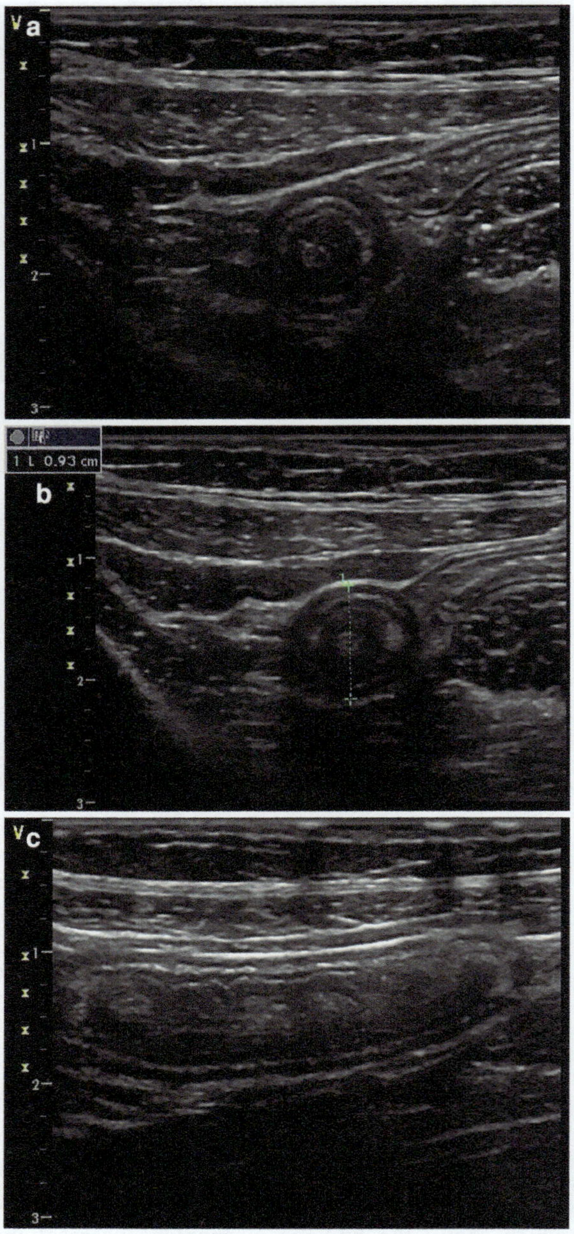

Fig. 14 Normal appendix in cystic fibrosis. **a** Axial image. Non-compressible appendix with mucous impaction in the lumen. **b** Appendiceal diameter 9 mm. **c** Longitudinal view. No signs of inflammation

(Fig. 14). This is due to mucoid impaction in the appendix. As lower abdominal pain is a relatively common complaint in patients with CF, the appendiceal diameter and non-compressibility cannot be used as a criteria for diagnosing appendicitis. The diagnosis of acute appendicitis in patients with CF should, therefore be based on other signs of inflammation, including the correspondence of the point of maximal tenderness to the appendix itself, pain during compression of the appendix, distortion of the concentric layers of the appendiceal wall and/or infiltration of neighboring omental or mesenteric fat.

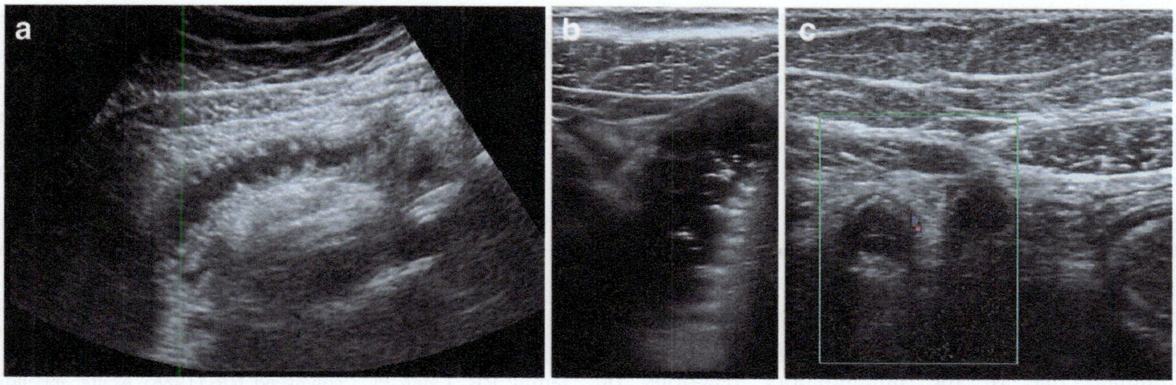

Fig. 15 Primary peritoneal peritonitis. **a** Aperistalsis of a small bowel loop and hyperechoic surrounding area. **b** Dilatation of small bowel indicating peritonitis. **c** A normal appendix was visualized, thereby excluding appendicitis

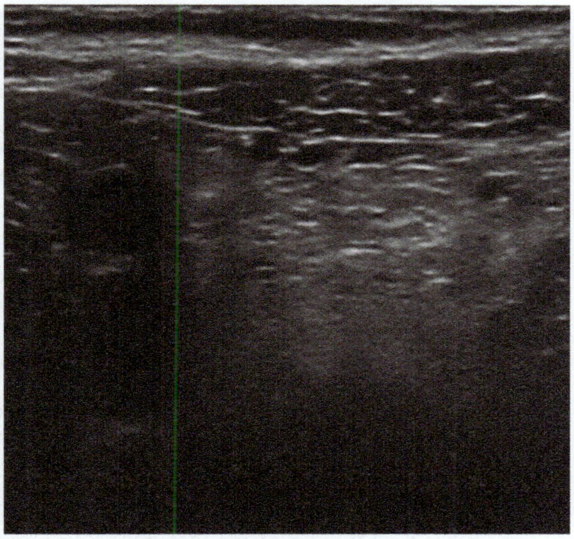

Fig. 16 Non-specific hyperechogeneity in the right lower quadrant. Extra care has to be taken to find the appendix; differentiation with appendagitis epiploica or omental infarction can be difficult

Table 1 Four potential outcomes of US

US Findings	Diagnosis
Appendix seen, normal	No appendicitis
Appendix not seen, but no secondary signs, and/or alternative diagnosis	
Appendix seen, appendicitis	Appendicitis
Appendix not seen, secondary signs of appendicitis	

5.2 Primary Bacterial Peritonitis

Primary bacterial peritonitis in children is a spontaneously acute bacterial infection of the peritoneal fluid. In general the source of the infecting agent is not easily identifiable. Children with nephrotic syndrome have a higher risk of developing spontaneous bacterial peritonitis (Uncu et al. 2010). Clinical symptoms may mimic appendicitis and with ultrasound signs of focal peritonitis may be seen, which are undistinguishable from the secondary signs in appendicitis. If a normal appendix is visualized, the diagnosis of primary bacterial peritonitis can be suggested, but if the appendix is not seen, the findings may lead to a false positive diagnosis of appendicitis (Fig. 15).

5.3 Omental Infarction and Appendagitis Epiploica

Though relatively infrequent in children these entities may present with symptoms similar to appendicitis. Although its pathogenesis is still unknown, omental infarction has been shown to occur with or without torsion. Some predisposing factors have been reported, such as a bifid omentum, a tongue like portion of omentum and obesity (Vertuno et al. 1980). On ultrasound a hyperechoic mass containing poorly defined nodular or linear hypoechoic areas with few vessels within the mass and hyperemia in the peripheral area are seen (Baldisserotto et al. 2005).

Appendagitis epiploica is an inflammatory or ischemic process involving an appendix epiploica of the colon. At the site of maximum tenderness, a non-compressible hyperechoic small ovoid or round solid mass of adipose tissue is seen between the colon and the abdominal wall in the anterior or anterolateral compartment of the abdomen (van Breda Vriesman and Puylaert 1999).

Both of these entities are self-limiting and do not need surgical intervention. It is possible that the echogenic aspect of the infiltrated mesentery might simulate one of the inflammatory reactions of appendicitis (Fig. 16) (van Breda Vriesman and Puylaert 2002, 2006). These conditions may lead to a false positive diagnosis of appendicitis in cases where the appendix itself is not seen.

6 Radiology Report

Clear communication of the radiologic information is of substantial importance. Terms 'no evidence of appendicitis' or 'probably appendicitis' should be avoided. The radiological report should contain all the clinical relevant information, of the survey and the local findings in right lower quadrant. In the conclusion there are four possibilities (see Table 1).

Using this classification specificity, sensitivity and accuracy may rise to 97–99% (Wiersma et al. 2009).

It must be kept in mind that no matter which imaging technique is used, there still may be equivocal cases, even in experienced hands. In those children who are not critically ill repeated ultrasound is optional, without being concerned about radiation issues.

7 Conclusion

Ultrasonography is the first imaging modality in children with clinical signs of appendicitis. If attention is paid to finding the appendix and the secondary signs of appendicitis, sensitivity and specificity are comparable with CT. Visualization of a normal appendix rules out appendicitis. Due to the lack of radiation repeated ultrasound can be done easily. With special skill, care and knowledge of the pitfalls ultrasound remains the hallmark in the diagnosis of appendicitis.

References

Baldisserotto M, Maffazzoni DR, Dora MD (2005) Omental infarction in children: Color Doppler sonography correlated with surgery and pathology findings. Am J Roentgenol 184:156–162

Cobben LP, van Otterloo AM, Puylaert JBCM (2000) Spontaneously resolving appendicitis: Frequency and natural history in 60 patients. Radiology 215:349–352

Holscher HC, Heij HA (2009) Imaging of acute appendicitis in children EU versus U.S. …or US versus CT? a European perspective. Pediatr Radiol 39:497–499

Jeffrey RB, Laing FC, Townsend RR (1988) Acute appendicitis: Sonographic criteria based on 250 cases. Radiology 167:327–329

Jona JZ, Belin RP (1976) Basilar pneumonia simulating acute appendicitis in children. Arch Surg 111:552–553

Kimmey MB, Martin RW, Haggit RC, Wang KY, Franklin DW, Silverstein FE (1989) Histological correlates of gastrointestinal ultrasound images. Gastroenterology 96: 433–441

Lardenoye SW, Puylaert JBCM, Smit MJ, Holscher HC (2004) Appendix in children with cystic fibrosis: US features. Radiology 232:187–189

Lee JH, Jeong YK, Hwang JC, Ham SY, Yang SO (2001) Graded compression sonography with adjuvant use of a posterior manual compression technique in the sonographic diagnosis of acute appendicitis. Am J Roentgenol 178:863–868

Lee JH, Jeong YK, Park KB, Park JK, Jeong AK, Hwnag JC (2005) Operator-dependent techniques for graded compression sonography to detect the appendix and the diagnose acute appendicitis. Am J Roentgenol 184:91–97

Puylaert JBCM (1986) Acute appendicitis: US evaluation using graded compression. Radiology 158:355–360

Puylaert JBCM, Rutgers PH, Lalisang RI (1987) A prospective study of ultrasonography in the diagnosis of appendicitis. N Engl J Med 317:666–669

Quillin SP, Siegel MJ (1995) Diagnosis of appendiceal abscess in children with acute appendicitis: Value of color Doppler sonography. Am J Roentgenol 164:1251–1254

Schuh S, Man C, Cheng A, Murphy A, Mohanta A, Moineddin R, Tomlinson G, Langer JC, Doria AS (2010) Predictors of non-diagnostic ultrasound scanning in children with suspected appendicitis. J Pediatr 158:123–129

Simonovský V (2002) Normal appendix: is there any significant difference in the maximal mural thickness at US between pediatric and adult populations? Radiology 224:333–337

Strouse PJ (2010) Pediatric appendicitis: an argument for US. Radiology 255:8–13

Uncu N, Bülbül M, Yildiz N, Noyan A, Koşan C, Kavukçu S, Calişkan S, Gündüz Z, Beşbaş N, Gür Güven A (2010) Primary peritonitis in children with nephrotic syndrome: Results of a 5 year multicenter study. Eur J Pediatr 169:73–76

van Breda Vriesman AC, Puylaert JBCM (1999) Old and new infarction of an epiploic appendage: Ultrasound mimicry of appendicitis. Abdom Imaging 24:129–131

van Breda Vriesman AC, Puylaert JBCM (2002) Epiploic appendagitis and omental infarction: Pitfalls and look-alikes. Abdom Imaging 27:20–28 van Breda Vriesman AC, Puylaert JBCM (2006) Mimics of appendicitis: Alternative nonsurgical diagnoses with sonography and CT. Am J Roentgenol 186:1103–1112

Vertuno LL, Dan JR, Wood W (1980) Segmental infarction of the omentum: a cause of the semi-acute abdomen. Am J Gastroenterol 74:443–446

Wiersma F, Šrámek A, Holscher HC (2005) Ultrasonographic features of the normal appendix and surrounding area in children. Radiology 235:1018–1022

Wiersma F, Toorenvliet BR, Ruige M, Holscher HC (2008) Increased echogenicity of renal cortex: a transient feature in acutely ill children. Am J Roentgenol 190:240–243

Wiersma F, Toorenvliet BR, Bloem JL, Allema JH, Holscher HC (2009) US examination of the appendix in children with suspected appendicitis: the additional value of secondary signs. Eur Radiol 19:455–461

Imaging of Acute Appendicitis in Children: Computed Tomography Including Radiation Issues

Andrew J. Spencer, Megan R. Saettele, and Lisa H. Lowe

Contents

A. J. Spencer (✉) · M. R. Saettele · L. H. Lowe
School of Medicine, University of Missouri-Kansas City, Red 1, 2411 Holmes Street, Kansas City, MO 64108, USA
e-mail: ajszq7@mail.umkc.edu

M. R. Saettele
Department of Radiology, St. Luke's Hospital, University of Missouri-Kansas City, 4401 Wornall Road, Kansas City, MO 64111, USA

L. H. Lowe
Department of Radiology, Children's Mercy Hospitals and Clinics, University of Missouri-Kansas City, 2401 Gillham Road, Kansas City, MO 64108, USA

Abstract

Clinical presentation, along with careful diagnostic imaging, should be employed when appendicitis is suspected in a child. Because computed tomography (CT) is becoming increasingly utilized for the diagnosis of acute appendicitis in children, radiologists must carefully and responsibly consider the issue of radiation exposure.

Abbreviations

CT	Computed tomography
ALARA	As low as reasonably achievable

1 Radiation Issues

1.1 Introduction

Computed tomography (CT) scans expose patients to low-dose radiation, which carries a statistically significant increased risk of cancer over a lifetime (Brenner et al. 2001). The excess risk is outlined in the Life Span Study cohort of atomic bomb survivors and tracked by the Radiation Effects Research Foundation. Compiling data over a half century, results indicate that children exposed to the atomic bombings of Hiroshima and Nagasaki had the highest excessive relative risk of solid organ cancer, and individuals exposed in childhood had the highest cancer mortality rates. Children are inherently more sensitive to radiation than adults because they are growing (their cells are dividing) and they have a longer life span during

Medical Radiology. Diagnostic Imaging, DOI: 10.1007/174_2011_226,

which time they may express radiation-induced cell damage (Charles 2003). For comparison, a one-year-old infant is ten to fifteen times more likely to develop a malignancy than an adult when exposed to the same dose of radiation (Mountford and Temperton 1992). Further, the risk of malignancy increases in a linear fashion from a dose range of 0–120 mSv (Charles 2003).

Studies have found that radiation exposure to a child from a CT scan carries a significantly elevated lifetime risk of mortality from cancer. According to Brenner et al. (2001), up to 1 in 550 (0.18%) infants exposed to radiation from a single abdominal CT scan will die from cancer induced by the associated radiation. In a fifteen-year-old, the radiation-induced malignancy rate falls to 0.11% (Brenner et al. 2001, 2002). Females are twice as susceptible to carcinogenesis as males when exposed to radiation (Brenner et al. 2001).

Developing tissues and organs of children are more sensitive to the effects of radiation than those of adults (Charles 2003; Hall 2002). Several factors contribute to organ radiation dose, including the number of scans, tube current, patient size, axial scan range, scan pitch, maximum tube voltage, and specific scanner design (Cody 2002). Organ dose and risk of radiation-induced malignancy are greater for children than for adults when exposed to an equivalent dose of radiation, and a single acute dose of radiation is more threatening than an identical dose given in fractions over time (Hall 2002). A child's large organ to overall body size ratio, lack of protective tissue (adipose tissue), and smaller cross-sectional area compared to that of an adult results in higher effective radiation organ doses in children (Brenner et al. 2002; Huda et al. 1997).

A rapid increase in the rate of pediatric CT imaging can be largely attributed to the development of fast helical CT technique, which allows for less sedation and superior image quality (Frush and Donnelly 1998). Approximately 80 million CT scans are performed annually in the United States, a dramatic increase compared to three million in 1980. This marks an annual increase of approximately 10% per year and a greater than 20-fold increase in the number of scans since 1980 (IMV 2006; Brenner et al. 2003; Mettler et al. 2009). Presently, 11% of CT scans are performed in children, which accounts for more than 8 million studies per year in the United States (Frush and Applegate 2004; Mettler et al. 2000). More recently though, there is convincing data that CTs ordered in children have not been increasing as a percentage of cross-sectional imaging studies since 2003. Townsend et al. have shown a trend in decreased CT utilization in pediatric institutions in North America over the last 7 years (Townsend et al. 2010). However, radiation dose from medical imaging has increased more than 6-fold, and the average radiation dose an individual is exposed to has doubled over the last 30 years (Mettler et al. 2009; Brenner and Hall 2007). Medical imaging is now responsible for 50% of the overall radiation dose to the United States population, compared to 15% in 1980 (Mettler et al. 2009). CT represents only 17% of all radiologic and nuclear medicine examinations in the world (excluding dental radiographic examinations), but it accounts for almost 50% of the collective effective radiation dose (Mettler et al. 2009).

Although individual risk may be small, the number of CT scans is in the tens of millions causing exposure to CT radiation to be a public health concern. To decrease this risk, collective dose reduction can be accomplished most easily by decreasing the number of CT scans performed annually. In addition, it is essential to employ the as low as reasonably achievable (ALARA) concept when using CT. This implies reducing the amount of radiation used per scan, the number of radiation-producing tests performed, and scanning only the indicated region with a single phase study whenever possible (Voss et al. 2009; Goske et al. 2008). Initiated by the Society for Pediatric Radiology, the Image Gently campaign emphasizes the importance of radiation safety in children (Goske et al. 2009). Universal protocols to lower CT dose based on age and/or weight can be found at Image-Gently.org (Arch and Frush 2008; Thomas and Wang 2008). Moreover, many authors advocate the importance of establishing standard radiation doses for pediatric patients by modifying CT parameters such as tube current, filtration, pitch, collimation, and peak tube voltage. These can be individually adjusted to reduce dose on a case by case basis, while preserving image quality (McCollough et al. 2006; Strauss et al. 2010). Optimization of MDCT parameters in abdominal imaging is reviewed in "Radiation Dose from MDCT Examinations for Suspected Acute Appendicitis" by Tack. To help minimize radiation exposure to the pediatric population, CT vendors have developed automated exposure control methods (McCollough et al. 2006; Kalra et al. 2004; Aldrich et al. 2006). Automated exposure control can decrease radiation dose by altering the tube current in response to the pathway length of the X-rays through the patient's body, creating an image of equivalent quality and quantum mottle (Strauss et al. 2010). With the successful use of automated exposure control, image noise does not interfere with scan interpretation. Manufacturers continue to introduce new techniques to lower radiation dose, such as noise reduction software which will further reduce radiation exposure. Radiologists must be vigilant in reducing radiation exposure to children, and in doing so, change their practice patterns by reducing tube current settings and radiation dose for CT scans.

There is wide agreement that potential benefits of a single CT scan frequently far outweigh the individual risks. However, to put the radiation exposure in perspective, one must keep in mind that the effective dose of an abdominal CT is equal to 500 chest radiographs, which is also equivalent to the average background radiation received over more than a 3-year period (Hall 2002). As mentioned above, extensive data from atomic bomb survivors indicate a small but significant risk of developing radiation-induced malignancy from a single abdominal CT examination (Charles 2003). Pediatric clinicians must be aware that the radiation-induced cancer risk from a single abdominal CT scan is not insignificant, and thus incorporate the ALARA and Image Gently campaign concepts when imaging for suspected acute appendicitis. When scanning children for suspected acute appendicitis, CT imaging should be used judiciously and preferably after failure to make an obvious clinical or ultrasound diagnosis (Johansson et al. 2007; Doria et al. 2006; Teo et al. 2000).

2 Acute Appendicitis

2.1 Introduction

Abdominal pain is a frequent complaint among children presenting to the emergency department and appendicitis is the most common cause of acute abdominal pain requiring surgical intervention (Brown 1991). Pediatric patients may present with an extensive array of clinical manifestations, making accurate diagnosis challenging. Timely diagnosis is critical to avoid complications and minimize morbidity.

The objectives when evaluating children with abdominal pain are to correctly identify the pathology causing the pain, and in the case of acute appendicitis, intervene early. Medical history and physical examination are the foundations for a diagnosis. However, in recent years clinicians have relied much more heavily on CT scanning to make a diagnosis of appendicitis, as evidenced by the impressive increase in the number of annual CT scans performed (Frei et al. 2008; Martin et al. 2004). Indeed, CT is a fast, effective, and accurate method for the evaluation and diagnosis of acute appendicitis (Taylor et al. 2006; Kaiser et al. 2004; Kaiser et al. 2002; Stephen et al. 2003; Sivit et al. 2000).

Historically it has been acceptable to have a 15–20% false positive appendectomy rate in order to minimize risks of diagnostic delay, which are associated with higher morbidity due to a greater incidence of perforated appendicitis (Flum and Koepsell 2002). However, several studies have shown that CT scanning can reduce the rate of unnecessary appendectomies in children without leading to significantly higher perforation rates (Kaiser et al. 2002; Applegate et al. 2001; Pena et al. 2000). One study revealed that the negative appendectomy rate sequentially decreased as the use of diagnostic CT imaging increased. The negative appendectomy rate in 2000 was 17%, with CT utilization in 52% of cases (Jones et al. 2004); in 2001 and 2002, this changed to 5 and 74% and 2 and 86%, respectively ($P = 0.001$) (Jones et al. 2004). Rao et al. (1999) investigated the influence of CT imaging on the negative appendectomy rate in children between 5 and 18 years of ages by comparing the negative appendectomy rates before and after the availability of CT at their institution. They found the negative appendectomy rates decreased from 10% to 5% in boys and 18% to 12% in girls. They also found a decrease in the rate of perforated appendicitis from 22% to 14% concluding that increased utilization of CT resulted in decreased negative appendectomy and perforation rates.

2.2 Imaging

Imaging methods are employed to avoid a misdiagnosis and decrease morbidity (Doria et al. 2006), while improving diagnostic accuracy (van Randen et al. 2008).

Use of pre-operative CT imaging has led to improved clinical outcomes and lower false positive appendicitis diagnosis rates (Raman et al. 2008). Menes et al. (2006) found that the accuracy and efficiency of CT imaging improved over the years studied and that there was a shorter time to surgery with increased CT use.

Many authors advocate the use of ultrasound as the initial study of choice in order to avoid unnecessary radiation. Ultrasound is unfortunately highly operator-dependent, is not always readily available, and requires significant sonographic skill to diagnose appendicitis that is gained from experience. These same authors suggest using CT as the study of choice for patients with inconclusive sonograms and obese children with a body habitus that prevents performance of adequate sonography (Kaiser et al. 2004; Lameris et al. 2009; Birnbaum and Wilson 2000; Puylaert et al. 1997; Gaitini et al. 2008). This approach works well in centers with skilled sonographers.

2.3 Technique

2.3.1 Computed Tomography

A multitude of techniques have been utilized in pediatric appendiceal CT scanning, all of which have been shown to be highly accurate. These techniques include abdominal and/or pelvic CT ranging from no contrast what so ever to every imaginable combination of intravenous, oral and rectal contrast materials. The choice of which technique to use varies widely despite little change in accuracy rates.

Administration of rectal contrast material may require sedation in many children under the age of five years (Acosta et al. 2005). Acosta et al. found that the appendix could be visualized more than 80% of the time when rectal contrast extended into the ileum, and that when appendiceal visualization was accomplished, CT imaging with rectal contrast achieved 100% sensitivity, 97.7% specificity, and 98% accuracy (Acosta et al. 2005). The amount of contrast material used varies from 500 mL in small children to 1000 mL in adolescents, based on patient size and degree of tolerated discomfort (Acosta et al. 2005).

A study by Kharbanda et al. (2007) compared CT scanning with rectal and intravenous contrast to CT with only intravenous contrast and demonstrated accuracies of 89 and 92%, respectively. For children under five years of age, collimation of 5 mm is suggested. In older children, 5–8 mm collimation may be used depending on patient size (Rosendahl et al. 2004). Thin collimation technique of 5 mm may increase sensitivity and the ability to better identify individual features of acute appendicitis (Weltman et al. 2000).

Advantages of CT imaging include lack of operator dependence, greater examination reproducibility, easier visualization of retrocecal appendices, the ability to utilize multi-planar data reconstruction, and at many institutions rapid, consistent availability (Frush and Donnelly 1998; Sivit and Applegate 2003; Sivit 2004; Sivit et al. 2001). CT also has the advantages of allowing detailed evaluation of complications (such as abscess formation), frequent detection of an alternative diagnosis, and can be used to plan radiological interventions (Sivit and Applegate 2003). One key advantage of CT is a very low false-negative rate, being 0% in some studies, and the resultant improvement in accuracy of 97% compared to sonography 91% (Vermeulen et al. 1999; Lowe et al. 2001a). Multi-detector helical CT can be performed so rapidly that sedation is usually unnecessary (Garcia Pena et al. 1999). It is able to demonstrate a wide, sequential field of view, which allows reconstruction of images for visualization of the appendix in various planes (Hernanz-Schulman 2010). Further, extremes of body habitus do not limit interpretation (Lowe et al. 2001a). A study prospectively comparing the ability of residents versus pediatric radiologists ability to diagnose appendicitis on unenhanced CT showed no statistically significant difference in accuracy (Lowe et al. 2001b).

Disadvantages of CT imaging are not to be taken lightly and include radiation exposure, cost, and risk of contrast reaction, when intravenous contrast is used (Frei et al. 2008).

2.4 Findings

Imaging criteria for a normal appendix on CT include transverse diameter less than 6 mm and no evidence of surrounding inflammation (Figs. 1 and 2). The normal appendix may or may not contain intraluminal gas. When intraluminal gas is present, it should not be included in the transverse measurement of the appendix (Birnbaum and Wilson 2000; Rettenbacher et al. 2000). Occasionally, the normal appendix

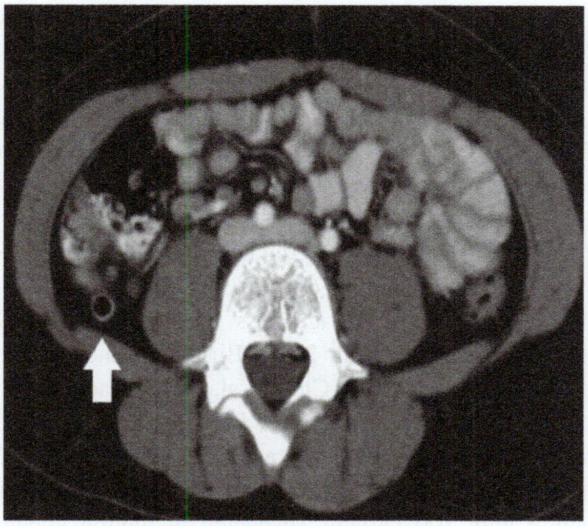

Fig. 1 Normal appendix in a 9-year-old-female. Axial contrast-enhanced CT image shows the normal appendix with intraluminal air (*arrow*). Recall that when measuring the appendix, the air containing lumen is not included. Note the lack of appendiceal enlargement and periappendiceal inflammation

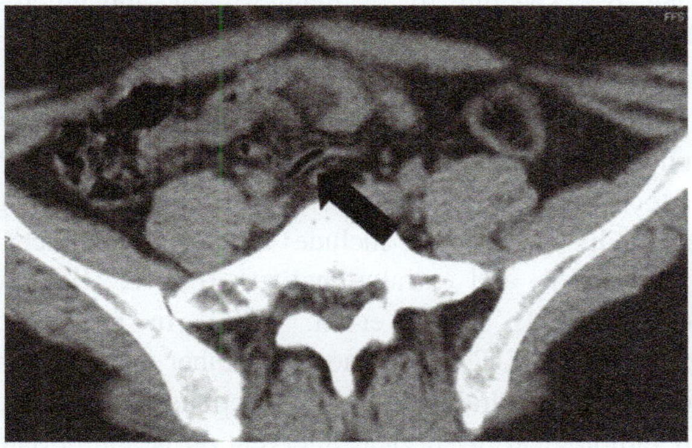

Fig. 2 Normal appendix in a 14-year-old-female. Axial contrast-enhanced CT identifies the normal appendix (*arrow*). Note presence of intraluminal air without appendiceal thickening or periappendiceal inflammation

contains a tiny fecolith (<3 mm) or other nonspecific uncalcified radiodense material such as barium or pepto bismol (Lowe et al. 2000). The most frequent CT finding in false negative studies is a calcified appendicolith (Taylor et al. 2006). This can be understood when one compares older literature investigating the significance of fecoliths seen on abdominal radiographs to recent descriptions of fecolith significance seen on CT. It is well established that fecoliths seen on plain abdominal radiographs are 100% specific for a diagnosis of appendicitis (Figs. 3 and 4) (Siegel 1992).

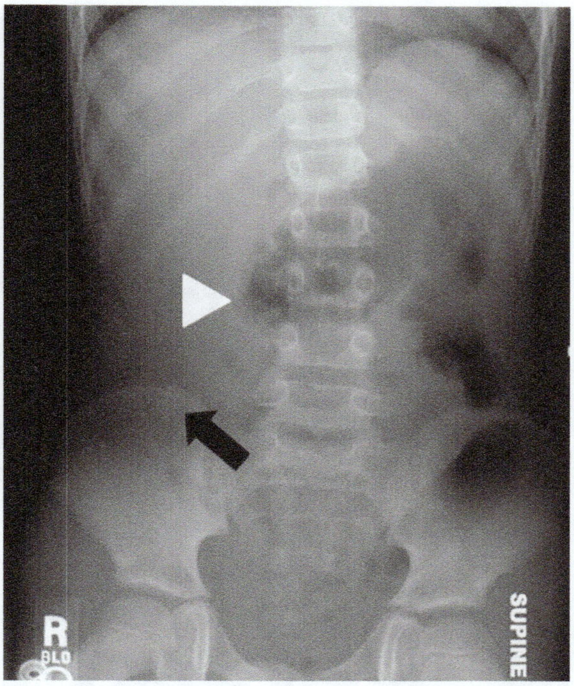

Fig. 3 Appendicitis with an appendicolith in a 14-year-old-female with abdominal pain. Frontal radiograph shows a large appendicolith (*arrow*) projecting over the right iliac crest. In addition, the colon cut-off sign (*triangle*) is shown with abrupt non-visualization of the colon due to surrounding appendiceal inflammatory changes

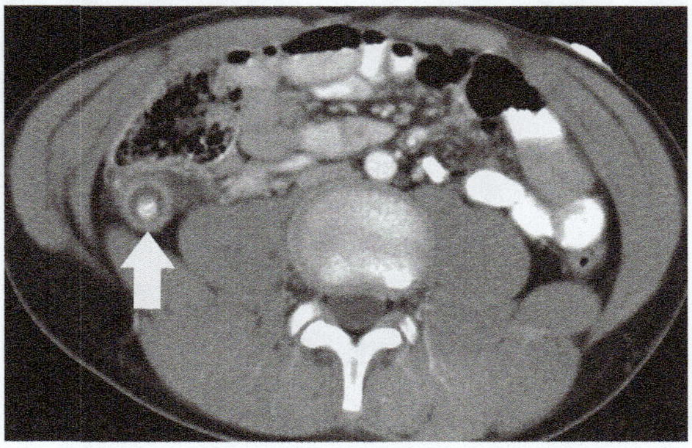

Fig. 4 Appendicitis with large appendicolith on CT in a 12-year-old-male with abdominal pain. Axial contrast-enhanced CT reveals enlarged, enhancing fluid filled appendix containing a large central fecolith (*arrow*). Periappendiceal inflammation is also noted

However, the same cannot be said of fecoliths seen on modern helical CT, which are often detected when they are much smaller in size. In a study by Penney et al. 3% of children imaged due to trauma

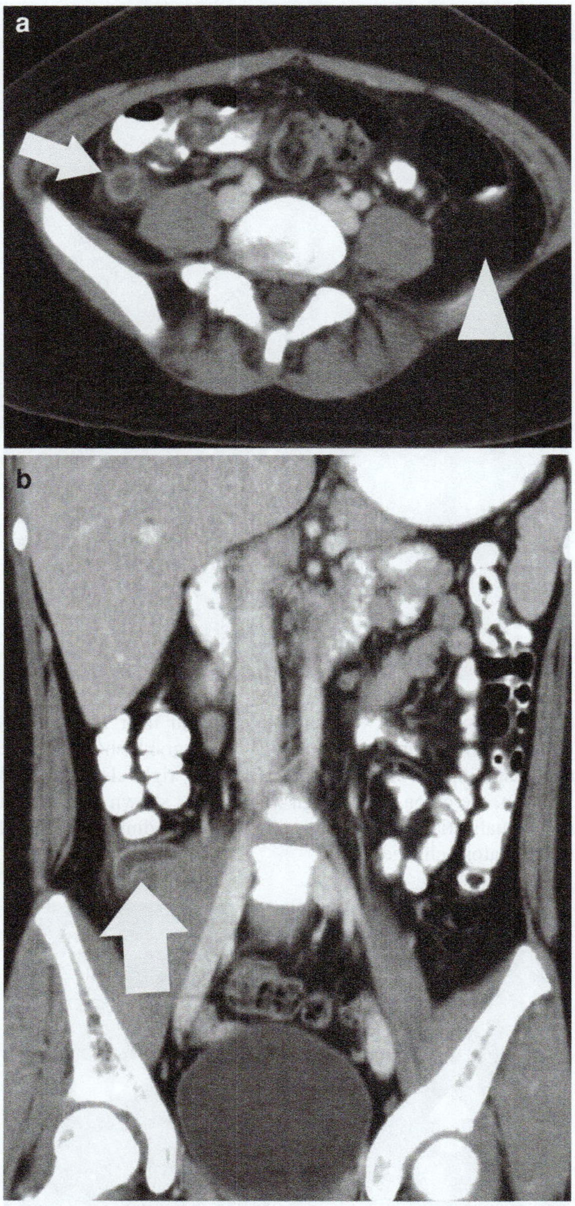

Fig. 5 Appendicitis in a 10-year-old-female with abdominal pain. **a** Axial contrast-enhanced CT demonstrates an enlarged (>6 mm), enhancing appendix with surrounding periappendiceal inflammatory fat stranding (*arrow*) posterior to the cecum. Note normal fat in the left flank (*triangle*). **b** Coronal reconstructed image confirms an enlarged appendix with periappendiceal fat stranding (*arrow*)

were found to have a tiny fecolith (<3 mm). None of these children had acute appendicitis and none developed appendicitis on follow up (Lowe et al. 2000).

CT diagnostic criteria for appendicitis include identification of an enlarged appendix (transverse diameter >6 mm) and/or evidence of periappendiceal inflammation (Fig. 5). Periappendiceal fat stranding (100%), an appendix greater than 6 mm in diameter (93%), and focal cecal thickening (69%) are the most sensitive signs of appendicitis on CT (Rao et al. 1997). Enhancement and thickening of the appendix wall, intraluminal appendix fluid, free fluid, phlegmon, and/or abscess are less sensitive secondary signs (Applegate et al. 2001; Birnbaum and Wilson 2000; Rao et al. 1997; Choi et al. 2003; Macari et al. 2002; Rodriguez et al. 2006; Puig et al. 2008). Rao et al. (1997) found the CT arrowhead sign was 30% sensitive and 100% specific for appendicitis in a study with 100 patients suspected of having appendicitis (Fig. 6). The arrowhead sign is formed by the gradual thickening of inflammation extending from the appendix to the cecum, causing contrast to form an arrowhead pointing away from the base of the appendix. Fecoliths seen on CT are 65% sensitive and 6% specific for a diagnosis of appendicitis yielding a positive predictive value of 75% (Lowe et al. 2000). Perforated appendicitis with abscess formation occurs four times more often in children under five years of age compared to older children (Rodriguez et al. 2006). CT criteria suggesting appendix perforation include abscess, appendiceal wall deficit, and extraluminal gas (Fig. 7) (Horrow et al. 2003; Yeung et al. 2004). In perforated appendicitis, CT can define the number and location of potentially drainable fluid collections to determine if radiological or surgical intervention is appropriate (Fig. 8) (Sivit 2004).

2.5 Alternative Diagnoses

The primary presentation of appendicitis is often mimicked by other common childhood disorders, which may lead to false negative imaging or a delay in diagnosis (Rodriguez et al. 2006). Some of the more common alternative diagnoses include mesenteric adenitis, Meckel diverticulum, Crohn's disease, ileocecal intussusception, urolithiasis, omental infarction, carcinoid tumor of the small intestine, hemorrhagic ovarian cyst, ovarian torsion, ovarian dermoid, and pelvic inflammatory disease. Clinical presentation and imaging evaluation may be unclear in many of the

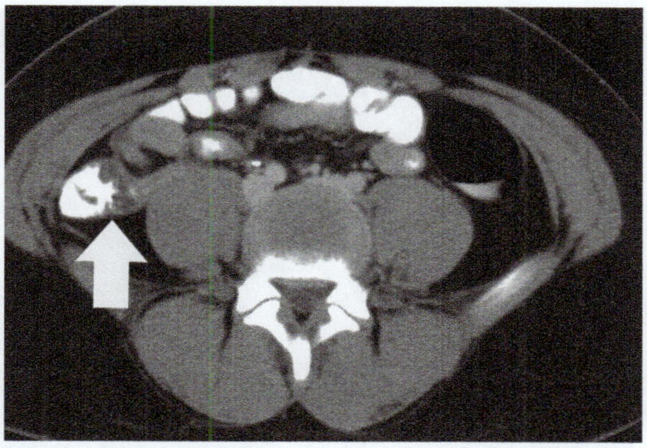

Fig. 6 Appendicitis in a 12-year-old-male with abdominal pain. Axial contrast-enhanced CT shows the arrowhead sign formed by inflammation at the base of the appendicitis. Note that the *arrowhead* points to the base of the appendix

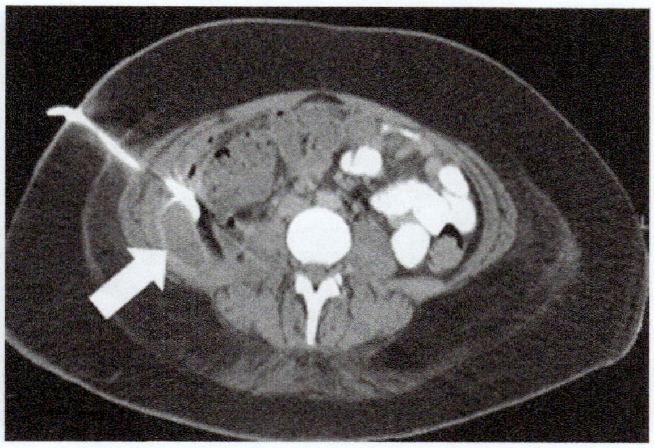

Fig. 8 Abscess with drain in place in a 14-year-old-female who presented with abdominal pain. Axial contrast-enhanced CT reveals a drain in place within an abscess (*arrow*) from a ruptured appendix. The appendix could not be identified

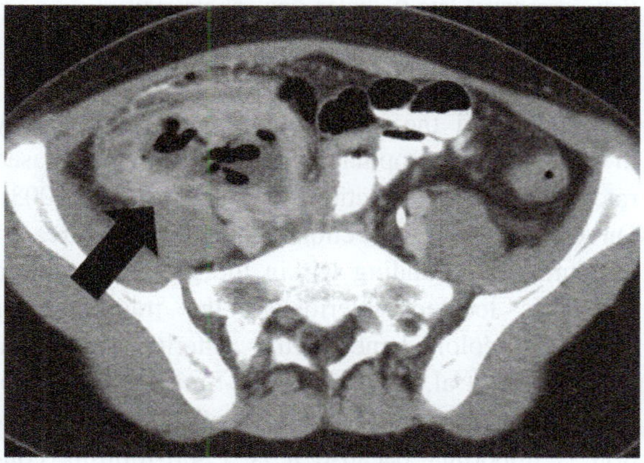

Fig. 7 Abscess due to appendicitis in an 11-year-old-female with right lower quadrant pain. Axial contrast-enhanced CT image identifies a right lower quadrant fluid collection with a thick, lobular-enhancing wall and several foci of internal air (*arrow*). No appendix could be seen with CT

aforementioned disorders, especially in a teen-aged female (Rodriguez et al. 2006).

2.5.1 Gastrointestinal

2.5.1.1 Mesenteric Adenitis

Mesenteric adenitis is reported to be the second most common cause of right lower quadrant pain in children, as well as the most common alternative pathological diagnosis to appendicitis (Sivit et al. 2001; Macari et al. 2002; Callahan et al. 2002). It is an inflammatory process affecting the mesenteric lymph nodes in the right lower quadrant resulting in abdominal pain, fever, and elevated white blood cell count often mimicking appendicitis symptoms (Lowe et al. 2001c). It occurs most often in teenagers (Macari et al. 2002; Yu et al. 2005). CT imaging demonstrates clusters of enlarged lymph nodes (<5 mm) in the lower right quadrant and mild thickening of the terminal ileum in conjunction with a normal appendix (Macari et al. 2002).

2.5.1.2 Inflammatory Bowel Disease

Inflammatory bowel disease is the second most common alternative diagnosis. Accurate identification of this disorder can be difficult when a child presents with a first occurrence of right lower quadrant pain, fever, and elevated white blood cell count mimicking appendicitis (Ruess et al. 2000). Moreover, CT diagnosis is complicated by the fact that inflammatory changes in the terminal ileum frequently involve the cecum, appendix, and periappendiceal fat (Callahan et al. 2002). Children with inflammatory bowel disease may be initially misdiagnosed in up to one-third of patients with ileocecal Crohn's disease (Yu et al. 2005a; Sturm et al. 2004). CT imaging shows bowel wall thickening and luminal narrowing of terminal ileum with regional mesenteric fat stranding (Fig. 9). Terminal ileal thickening, circumferential mural thickening of the cecum, skip lesions, and a focal region of inflammation away from the appendix are chief characteristics that distinguish inflammatory bowel disease from appendicitis. Uncomplicated

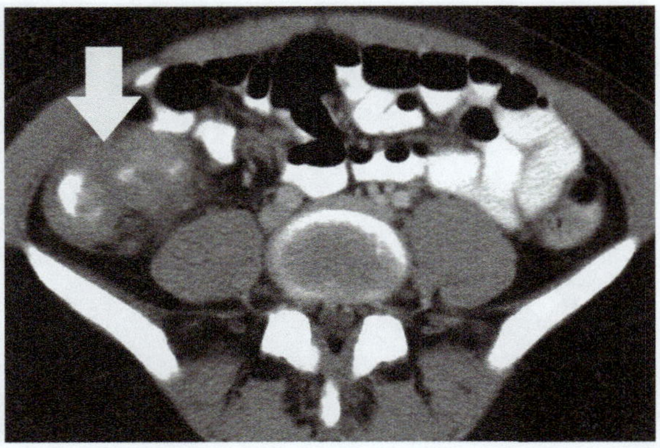

Fig. 9 Inflammatory bowel disease in a 14-year-old-female with abdominal pain for two weeks. Axial contrast-enhanced CT image demonstrates extensive thickening and enhancement of the ileocecal region (*arrow*). The appendix, likely included in the phlegmon, could not be visualized

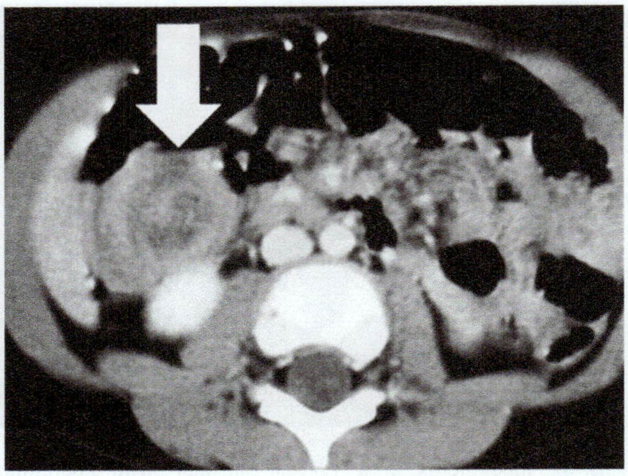

Fig. 10 Intussusception in a 2-year-old-female with abdominal pain. Axial contrast-enhanced CT image shows a right lower quadrant mass forming a target appearance with alternating layers of bowel wall and mesenteric fat (*arrow*). The target appearance is due to the infolding of the small bowel (intussusceptum) into the colon (intussuscipiens)

Crohn's disease can be treated first with anti-inflammatory drugs. Unfortunately, due to the overlap of clinical presentations and imaging findings, surgical exploration may be required to distinguish between acute appendicitis and inflammatory bowel disease in many children (Lowe et al. 2001c).

2.5.1.3 Ileocecal Intussusception

Ileocecal intussusception primarily occurs in infants and children. The usual history is a child under 3 years of age with episodic acute right lower quadrant pain (Koumanidou et al. 2002). Lymphoid hyperplasia in the distal ileum can act as a lead point for intussusception. Other potential lead points may include inflammation of Peyer patches, Meckel diverticulum, gastrointestinal duplication cysts, polyps, and lymphoma (Carty 2002; van Breda Vriesman and Puylaert 2006). CT imaging of intussusception shows circumferential layers of thickened bowel wall surrounding lymph nodes and mesenteric fat. The appearance of intussusception on CT is that of a target with layers of bowel wall thickening alternating with intussuscepted mesenteric nodes and fat (Fig. 10). Treatment includes image guided pneumatic or hydrostatic reduction in most cases, and if unsuccessful, surgery is required.

2.5.1.4 Omental Infarction

Omental infarction may present with findings suggestive of appendicitis (Helmrath et al. 2001; Nagar et al. 2003). Obesity is a risk factor for omental infarction, and the increasing incidence of obesity in the pediatric population may lead to increased rates of omental infarction (Varjavandi et al. 2003). On CT, omental infarction shows a focal area of inflammatory stranding within the greater omentum which is located anterior to the transverse or ascending colon beneath the anterior abdominal wall (Lowe et al. 2001c; Grattan-Smith et al. 2002). For the radiologist, recognition of omental infarction is important because it is a self-limiting condition not requiring surgery. Rarely, omental infarction may require laparoscopic removal of the infarcted tissue to avoid possible abscess or adhesions (Varjavandi et al. 2003; Grattan-Smith et al. 2002).

2.5.2 Gynecological

2.5.2.1 Pelvic Inflammatory Disease

Pelvic inflammatory disease may present with acute right lower quadrant pain. Imaging findings may include adnexal prominence and free pelvic fluid in the cul-de-sac. Confusion can arise due to overlapping imaging features of hydrosalpinx and a dilated appendix found in the right lower quadrant (Yu et al. 2005a). Identification of adnexal tenderness on physical examination may be the most practical way to distinguish between pelvic inflammatory disease

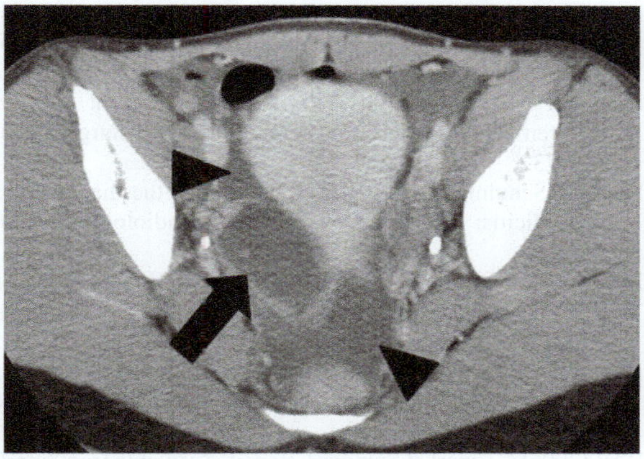

Fig. 11 Hemorrhagic ovarian cyst in a 16-year-old-female with acute right lower abdominal pain. Axial contrast-enhanced CT reveals a cystic structure in the right adnexa (*arrow*) with wall thickening and enhancement. In addition, a moderate amount of free pelvic fluid (*triangles*) is present indicating rupture of the hemorrhagic ovarian cyst

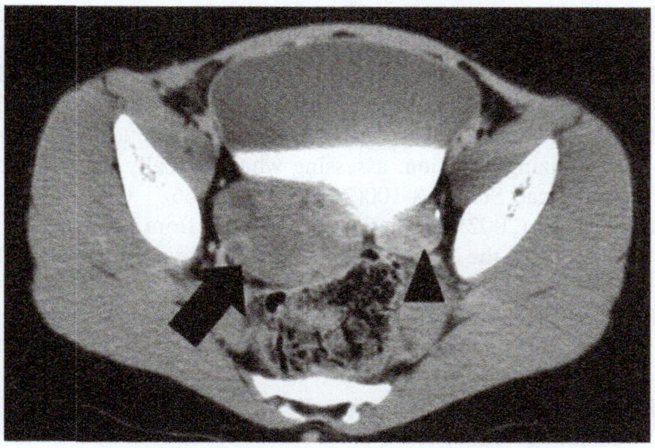

Fig. 12 Ovarian torsion in a 13-year-old-female with right pelvic pain. Axial contrast-enhanced CT image shows a well-defined enlarged ovary with multiple peripherally enhancing subcapsular cysts (*arrow*) located posterior to the contrast filled bladder. Note the normal ovary on the left side (*triangle*)

and appendicitis. Treatment of pelvic inflammatory disease usually involves antibiotics (Yu et al. 2005a).

2.5.2.2 Hemorrhagic Ovarian Cyst

The most common gynecologic condition mimicking appendicitis is a hemorrhagic ovarian cyst (Yu et al. 2005a). Helical CT findings include a well-defined cystic adnexal mass containing internal high attenuation material (Fig. 11). Rupture of a hemorrhagic ovarian cyst releasing free pelvic fluid and causing fat stranding can lead to a false-positive diagnosis of acute appendicitis (Yu et al. 2005a). Identification of an ovarian cyst and a normal appendix are helpful to determine a correct diagnosis.

2.5.2.3 Ovarian Torsion

Ovarian torsion is a surgical emergency that involves twisting of the ovary resulting in vascular compromise. Adolescents have increased mobility of the adnexa, which can lead to an increased risk of torsion (Bennett et al. 2002). Key non-contrast CT findings of ovarian torsion include ovarian enlargement and tubal thickening due to vascular congestion (Moore et al. 2009; Yu et al. 2005b). Contrast-enhanced CT demonstrating an enlarged ovary with multiple subcapsular foci of low attenuation is 93% specific for a diagnosis of ovarian torsion (Fig. 12). Right lower quadrant fat stranding may extend to the appendix erroneously suggesting a diagnosis of appendicitis.

2.5.3 Genitourinary

2.5.3.1 Urolithiasis

Ureteral obstruction may present with right lower quadrant pain when the obstruction is caused by an obstructing stone. Presenting symptoms in children are more unpredictable than adults (Fisher and Reeves 2004). Dilation of the right renal collecting system and urine extravasation from the ureter may occur, extending into the right lower quadrant, rarely causing fat standing mimicking acute appendicitis (Yu et al. 2005a).

References

Acosta R, Crain EF, Goldman HS (2005) CT can reduce hospitalization for observation in children with suspected appendicitis. Pediatr Radiol 35(5):495–500

Aldrich JE et al (2006) Radiation dose in abdominal computed tomography: the role of patient size and the selection of tube current. Can Assoc Radiol J 57(3):152–158

Applegate KE et al (2001) Effect of cross-sectional imaging on negative appendectomy and perforation rates in children. Radiology 220(1):103–107

Arch ME, Frush DP (2008) Pediatric body MDCT: a 5-year follow-up survey of scanning parameters used by pediatric radiologists. AJR Am J Roentgenol 191(2):611–617

Bennett GL, Slywotzky CM, Giovanniello G (2002) Gynecologic causes of acute pelvic pain: spectrum of CT findings. Radiographics 22(4):785–801

Birnbaum BA, Wilson SR (2000) Appendicitis at the millennium. Radiology 215(2):337–348
Brenner D et al (2001) Estimated risks of radiation-induced fatal cancer from pediatric CT. AJR Am J Roentgenol 176(2):289–296
Brenner DJ et al (2003) Cancer risks attributable to low doses of ionizing radiation: assessing what we really know. Proc Natl Acad Sci USA 100(24):13761–13766
Brenner DJ (2002) Estimating cancer risks from pediatric CT: going from the qualitative to the quantitative. Pediatr Radiol 32(4):228–231 (discussion 242–244)
Brenner DJ, Hall EJ (2007) Computed tomography—an increasing source of radiation exposure. N Engl J Med 357(22):2277–2284
Brown JJ (1991) Acute appendicitis: the radiologist's role. Radiology 180(1):13–14
Callahan MJ, Rodriguez DP, Taylor GA (2002) CT of appendicitis in children. Radiology 224(2):325–332
Carty HM (2002) Paediatric emergencies: non-traumatic abdominal emergencies. Eur Radiol 12(12):2835–2848
Charles MW (2003) Studies of mortality of atomic bomb survivors. Report 13: solid cancer and noncancer disease mortality: 1950–1997. J Radiol Prot 23(4):457–459
Choi D et al (2003) The most useful findings for diagnosing acute appendicitis on contrast-enhanced helical CT. Acta Radiol 44(6):574–582
Cody DD (2002) AAPM/RSNA physics tutorial for residents: topics in CT. Image processing in CT. Radiographics 22(5): 1255–1268
Doria AS et al (2006) US or CT for diagnosis of appendicitis in children and adults? a meta-analysis. Radiology 241(1):83–94
Fisher JD, Reeves JJ (2004) Presentation variability of acute urolithiasis in school-aged children. Am J Emerg Med 22(2):108–110
Flum DR, Koepsell T (2002) The clinical and economic correlates of misdiagnosed appendicitis: nationwide analysis. Arch Surg 137(7):799–804 (discussion 804)
Frei SP et al (2008) Appendicitis outcomes with increasing computed tomographic scanning. Am J Emerg Med 26(1):39–44
Frush DP, Applegate K (2004) Computed tomography and radiation: understanding the issues. J Am Coll Radiol 1(2):113–119
Frush DP, Donnelly LF (1998) Helical CT in children: technical considerations and body applications. Radiology 209(1):37–48
Gaitini D et al (2008) Diagnosing acute appendicitis in adults: accuracy of color doppler sonography and MDCT compared with surgery and clinical follow-up. AJR Am J Roentgenol 190(5):1300–1306
Garcia Pena BM et al (1999) Ultrasonography and limited computed tomography in the diagnosis and management of appendicitis in children. JAMA 282(11):1041–1046
Goske MJ et al (2008) The Image Gently campaign: working together to change practice. AJR Am J Roentgenol 190(2): 273–274
Goske MJ, Frush DP, Schauer DA (2009) Image Gently campaign promotes radiation protection for children. Radiat Prot Dosimetry 135(4):276
Grattan-Smith JD, Blews DE, Brand T (2002) Omental infarction in pediatric patients: sonographic and CT findings. AJR Am J Roentgenol 178(6):1537–1539
Hall EJ (2002) Lessons we have learned from our children: cancer risks from diagnostic radiology. Pediatr Radiol 32(10):700–706
Helmrath MA et al (2001) Right lower quadrant pain in children caused by omental infarction. Am J Surg 182(6): 729–732
Hernanz-Schulman M (2010) CT and US in the diagnosis of appendicitis: an argument for CT. Radiology 255(1): 3–7
Horrow MM, White DS, Horrow JC (2003) Differentiation of perforated from nonperforated appendicitis at CT. Radiology 227(1):46–51
Huda W et al (1997) An approach for the estimation of effective radiation dose at CT in pediatric patients. Radiology 203(2):417–422
IMV (2006) CT market Summary Report. Available from http://www.imvinfo.com/user/documents/content_documents/nws_rad/MS_CT_DSandTOC.pdf. Cited 12 July 2010
Johansson EP, Rydh A, Riklund KA (2007) Ultrasound computed tomography, and laboratory findings in the diagnosis of appendicitis. Acta Radiologica 48(3):267–273
Jones K et al (2004) Are negative appendectomies still acceptable? Am J Surg 188(6):748–754
Kaiser S et al (2004) Impact of radiologic imaging on the surgical decision-making process in suspected appendicitis in children. Acad Radiol 11(9):971–979
Kaiser S, Frenckner B, Jorulf HK (2002) Suspected appendicitis in children: US and CT—a prospective randomized study. Radiology 223(3):633–638
Kalra MK et al (2004) Techniques and applications of automatic tube current modulation for CT. Radiology 233(3):649–657
Kharbanda AB, Taylor GA, Bachur RG (2007) Suspected appendicitis in children: rectal and intravenous contrast-enhanced versus intravenous contrast-enhanced CT. Radiology 243(2):520–526
Koumanidou C et al (2002) Sonographic detection of lymph nodes in the intussusception of infants and young children: clinical evaluation and hydrostatic reduction. AJR Am J Roentgenol 178(2):445–450
Lameris W et al (2009) Imaging strategies for detection of urgent conditions in patients with acute abdominal pain: diagnostic accuracy study. BMJ 338:b2431
Lowe LH et al (2000) Appendicolith revealed on CT in children with suspected appendicitis: how specific is it in the diagnosis of appendicitis? AJR Am J Roentgenol 175(4): 981–984
Lowe LH et al (2001a) Unenhanced limited CT of the abdomen in the diagnosis of appendicitis in children: comparison with sonography. AJR Am J Roentgenol 176(1):31–35
Lowe LH et al (2001b) Nonenhanced limited CT in children suspected of having appendicitis: prospective comparison of attending and resident interpretations. Radiology 221(3): 755–759
Lowe LH et al (2001c) Appendicitis and alternate diagnoses in children: findings on unenhanced limited helical CT. Pediatr Radiol 31(8):569–577
Macari M et al (2002) Mesenteric adenitis: CT diagnosis of primary versus secondary causes, incidence, and clinical significance in pediatric and adult patients. AJR Am J Roentgenol 178(4):853–858

Martin AE et al (2004) CT scans may not reduce the negative appendectomy rate in children. J Pediatr Surg 39(6) 886–890 (discussion 886–890)
McCollough CH, Bruesewitz MR, Kofler JM Jr (2006) CT dose reduction and dose management tools: overview of available options. Radiographics 26(2):503–512
Menes TS et al (2005) Increased use of computed tomography does not harm patients with acute appendicitis. Am Surg 72(4):326–329
Mettler FA Jr et al (2000) CT scanning: patterns of use and dose. J Radiol Prot 20(4):353–359
Mettler FA Jr et al (2009) Radiologic and nuclear medicine studies in the United States and worldwide: frequency, radiation dose, and comparison with other radiation sources—1950–2007. Radiology 253(2):520–531
Moore C et al (2009) Prevalence of abnormal CT findings in patients with proven ovarian torsion and a proposed triage schema. Emerg Radiol 16(2):115–120
Mountford PJ, Temperton DH (1992) Recommendations of the international commission on radiological protection (ICRP) 1990. Eur J Nuc Med 19(2):77–79
Nagar H et al (2003) Omental infarction: an unusual cause of acute abdomen in children. Pediatr Surg Int 19(9–10):677–679
Pena BM et al (2000) Costs and effectiveness of ultrasonography and limited computed tomography for diagnosing appendicitis in children. Pediatrics 106(4):672–676
Puig S et al (2008) Imaging of appendicitis in children and adolescents: useful or useless? A comparison of imaging techniques and a critical review of the current literature. Semin Roentgenol 43(1):22–28
Puylaert JB, van der Zant FM, Rijke AM (1997) Sonography and the acute abdomen: practical considerations. AJR Am J Roentgenol 168(1):179–186
Raman SS et al (2008) Effect of CT on false positive diagnosis of appendicitis and perforation. N Engl J Med 358(9): 972–973
Rao PM et al (1997) Appendicitis: use of arrowhead sign for diagnosis at CT. Radiology 202(2):363–366
Rao PM et al (1999) Introduction of appendiceal CT: impact on negative appendectomy and appendiceal perforation rates. Ann Surg 229(3):344–349
Rao PM, Rhea JT, Novelline RA (1997) Sensitivity and specificity of the individual CT signs of appendicitis: experience with 200 helical appendiceal CT examinations. J Comput Assist Tomogr 21(5):686–692
Rettenbacher T et al (2000) Presence or absence of gas in the appendix: additional criteria to rule out or confirm acute appendicitis–evaluation with US. Radiology 214(1):183–187
Rodriguez DP et al (2006) Appendicitis in young children: imaging experience and clinical outcomes. AJR Am J Roentgenol 186(4):1158–1164
Rosendahl K, Aukland SM, Fosse K (2004) Imaging strategies in children with suspected appendicitis. Eur Radiol 14(Suppl 4):L138–L145
Ruess L et al (2000) Inflammatory bowel disease in children and young adults: correlation of sonographic and clinical parameters during treatment. AJR Am J Roentgenol 175(1): 79–84
Siegel MJ (1992) Acute appendicitis in childhood: the role of US. Radiology 185(2):341–342
Sivit CJ et al (2000) Imaging evaluation of suspected appendicitis in a pediatric population: effectiveness of sonography versus CT. AJR Am J Roentgenol 175(4):977–980
Sivit CJ (2004) Imaging the child with right lower quadrant pain and suspected appendicitis: current concepts. Pediatr Radiol 34(6):447–453
Sivit CJ, Applegate KE (2003) Imaging of acute appendicitis in children. Semin Ultrasound CT MR 24(2):74–82
Sivit CJ et al (2001) When appendicitis is suspected in children. Radiographics 21(1):247–262 (questionnaire 288–294)
Stephen AE et al (2003) The diagnosis of acute appendicitis in a pediatric population: to CT or not to CT. J Pediatr Surg 38(3):367–371 (discsussion 367–371)
Strauss KJ et al (2010) Image gently: Ten steps you can take to optimize image quality and lower CT dose for pediatric patients. AJR Am J Roentgenol 194(4):868–873
Sturm EJ et al (2004) Detection of ileocecal Crohn's disease using ultrasound as the primary imaging modality. Eur Radiol 14(5):778–782
Taylor GA et al (2006) CT for suspected appendicitis in children: an analysis of diagnostic errors. Pediatr Radiol 36(4):331–337
Teo EL et al (2000) Ultrasonography and computed tomography in a clinical algorithm for the evaluation of suspected acute appendicitis in children. Singapore Med J 41(8): 387–392
Thomas KE, Wang B (2008) Age-specific effective doses for pediatric MSCT examinations at a large children's hospital using DLP conversion coefficients: a simple estimation method. Pediatr Radiol 38(6):645–656
Townsend BA, Callahan MJ, Zuralowski D, Taylor GA (2010) Has the use of pediatric CT at children's hospitals reached its peak? Am J Roentgenol 194:1194–31196
van Breda Vriesman AC, Puylaert JB (2006) Mimics of appendicitis: alternative nonsurgical diagnoses with sonography and CT. AJR Am J Roentgenol 186(4):1103–1112
van Randen A et al (2008) Acute appendicitis: meta-analysis of diagnostic performance of CT and graded compression US related to prevalence of disease. Radiology 249(1): 97–106
Varjavandi V et al (2003) Omental infarction: risk factors in children. J Pediatr Surg 38(2):233–235
Vermeulen B et al (1999) Acute appendicitis: influence of early pain relief on the accuracy of clinical and US findings in the decision to operate—a randomized trial. Radiology 210(3): 639–643
Voss SD et al (2009) The ALARA concept in pediatric oncology. Pediatr Radiol 39(11):1142–1146
Weltman DI et al (2000) Diagnosis of acute appendicitis: comparison of 5- and 10-mm CT sections in the same patient. Radiology 216(1):172–177
Yeung KW, Chang MS, Hsiao CP (2004) Evaluation of perforated and nonperforated appendicitis with CT. Clin Imaging 28(6):422–427
Yu J et al (2005a) Helical CT evaluation of acute right lower quadrant pain: part I, common mimics of appendicitis. AJR Am J Roentgenol 184(4):1136–1142
Yu J et al (2005b) Helical CT evaluation of acute right lower quadrant pain: part II, uncommon mimics of appendicitis. AJR Am J Roentgenol 184(4):1143–1149

US Versus CT: Evidence-Based Medicine and Cost-Effectiveness in Imaging Acute Appendicitis in Children

Shyama Kamat, Barbara M. Garcia Peña, Craig Blackmore, and L. Santiago Medina

Contents

Abstract

Despite the high incidence of acute appendicitis in children, its diagnosis remains difficult. This chapter will discuss the usefulness of ultrasound vs computed tomography in diagnosing pediatric appendicitis and the cost-effectiveness of imaging these patients based on recently published studies. The cost-effectiveness and financial impact of imaging in patients with acute appendicitis should be taken into account by clinicians who seek accurate diagnosis. Clinicians must aim to avoid radiation exposure in children whenever possible, but should also seek to minimize costs in an increasingly expensive health care system.

1 Introduction

Acute appendicitis is the most common reason for abdominal surgery in children (Sivit and Applegate 2003; Kwok et al. 2004; Puig et al. 2008) and is diagnosed in 1–8% of children presenting with abdominal pain to the emergency room (ER) (Kwok et al. 2004; Rothrock and Pagane 2000). There are approximately 70,000–90,000 pediatric cases of acute appendicitis yearly in the United States (Brennan 2006, Agency for Healthcare Research and Quality (AHRQ) 2000). The estimated incidence ranges from 75 to 233 per 100,000 pediatric patients per year, with boys affected more commonly than girls at a rate of 1.4/1.0 (Puig et al. 2008). Acute appendicitis is more common in 10–19-year-old patients, although it can present even under 1 year of age (Sivit and Applegate 2003; Puig et al. 2008). The rate of perforation in pediatric patients

S. Kamat · B. M. Garcia Peña (✉) · C. Blackmore · L. Santiago Medina
Division of Emergency Medicine,
Miami Children Hospital, 3100 SW 62nd Avenue,
Miami, FL 33155, USA
e-mail: barbpena@gmail.com

C. Keyzer and P. A. Gevenois (eds.), *Imaging of Acute Appendicitis in Adults and Children*,
Medical Radiology. Diagnostic Imaging, DOI: 10.1007/174_2011_236,

ranges from 23 to 73% in various series and is higher in young children (Sivit and Applegate 2003; Kwok et al. 2004; Rothrock and Pagane 2000; Garcia Pena et al. 1999a). This may be related to the fact that clinical diagnosis is often difficult in these patients. In general, it is more difficult to obtain a clear history and physical examination in children than in adults. Many laboratory tests such as the white blood cell count are non-specific and can be elevated in many non-surgical conditions. Therefore, there is an ongoing interest in identifying an imaging test that could help in diagnosing acute appendicitis.

Acute appendicitis in children is a very common reason for hospitalization and incurs costs in terms of health care resources. In the United States, 238 appendectomies are, on average, performed daily in children (Agency for Healthcare Research and Quality (AHRQ) 2000). Annually, acute appendicitis accounts for approximately 87,000 pediatric hospital stays, representing 4% of all hospital stays for pediatric illness (Agency for Healthcare Research and Quality (AHRQ) 2000). Appendicitis is the second-most common reason for hospitalization for children and adolescents 6–17 years old. The aggregate total charges related to care of pediatric patients with acute appendicitis sum up to over $800,000,000 annually (Agency for Healthcare Research and Quality (AHRQ) 2000). At an institutional level, a retrospective chart review by our group showed that 308 pediatric patients who were observed for possible acute appendicitis collectively accumulated 487 inpatient observation days, with a per patient cost of $5,831 (Garcia Pena et al. 1999a).

The goals of imaging in suspected acute appendicitis are (1) to provide an earlier diagnosis, and (2) to identify complications, such as perforation or abscess, which may change the surgical management. It is also imperative to perform imaging in a cost-effective manner as well as in a way where the patient will have a beneficial outcome with improved care by both the pediatrician and surgeon.

2 Accuracy of Imaging for Acute Appendicitis (Ultrasound vs. Computed Tomography)

Extensive review reveals that there are evidence-based studies investigating this particular topic. First described in 1981, ultrasound (US) was the diagnostic procedure of choice for appendicitis. In 1998, Rao et al. (1998) advocated computed tomography (CT) scans for improved patient care in the diagnosis of acute appendicitis. Since then there have been numerous studies investigating the accuracy of diagnosis with ultrasound and CT with regard to acute appendicitis.

A recent meta-analysis by Doria et al. (2006) found 26 prospective and retrospective studies of graded compression US and/or CT in pediatric patients (mean age range, 7–12 years) with suspected acute appendicitis. These studies included results from US only, CT only, or combined US and CT in 6,850, 598, and 1,908 patients, respectively. The mean sample prevalence of acute appendicitis in these studies was 0.31 for both US and CT articles (range, 0.15–0.75). The weighted perforation rate in positive appendicitis cases was 26.5%.

This meta-analysis identified eight studies of CT in pediatric patients, which demonstrated a pooled sensitivity of 94% (95% confidence interval (CI), 92–97%), a combined specificity of 95% (95% CI, 94–97%), and a summary diagnostic odds ratio of 239 (95% CI, 118–487). For the extracted data, the positive and negative likelihood ratios were 18.8 and 0.06, respectively (Puig et al. 2008). When these test specifications were applied to a population with the mean prevalence of appendicitis found in the trials examined by Doria et al. (31%), the positive predictive value was 89%, and the negative predictive value was 97%.

There were 23 studies of graded compression US that met inclusion criteria in this meta-analysis. With one outlier removed, the pooled sensitivity of US in the pediatric population was 88% (95% CI, 86–90%), the pooled specificity was 94% (95% CI, 92–95%), and the summary diagnostic odds ratio was 202 (95% CI, 159–258). The positive and negative likelihood ratios were 14.7 and 0.13, respectively (Puig et al. 2008). The positive predictive value of graded compression US was 87%, and the negative predictive value was 95% using the mean prevalence of 31% for calculations.

Thus, in children with suspected acute appendicitis in whom further evaluation with imaging is desired, the meta-analysis by Doria et al., demonstrated that there is a significant difference in the weighted pooled sensitivities in favor of CT, with no significant difference in specificity of CT compared to US. However, as the authors noted, pediatric patients in general demonstrate greater sensitivity to ionizing radiation, which is produced with CT scanning. This radiation risk linked to CT use should be balanced by the risk of additional false negative cases with US.

Several limitations were identified in the examined studies, including potential verification and selection biases, which could result in falsely inflated sensitivity and specificity estimates. The degree of differential verification bias is probably similar between CT and US since patients with negative imaging results were likely to be managed nonoperatively regardless of modality. Additional difficulties in analysis included lack of randomization of patients to imaging groups. It may be difficult to generalize these results worldwide since CT was more commonly used in North America whereas US was more prevalently used in Europe and Asia. In addition, relatively few children under the age of 5 years were included in many of the studies, so that their results may not hold true for infants and preschool age children.

Reviewing the literature published after the article by Doria et al., only one single prospective study examining CT in pediatric patients with suspected acute appendicitis was identified (Acosta et al. 2005). This study, published in 2005, included 94 patients aged from 6 to17 years admitted to the hospital for possible acute appendicitis, and reported that CT with rectal contrast had a sensitivity of 100%, specificity of 98%, positive predictive value of 90%, and negative predictive value of 100% for the 53 patients in whom the appendix was visualized. It is important to notice that these investigators considered the CT examinations in which the radiologist could not identify the appendix as positive for possible appendicitis. Given the relatively small sample size, these results are consistent with the results of the meta-analysis by Doria et al., although the absence of data in the many individuals in whom the appendix was not seen limits the conclusions.

An additional consideration in deciding on the use of US vs. CT is the patient body habitus. A high body mass index (BMI) can limit the visualization of the appendix at US: the appendix is indeed not detectable in 79% of overweight children compared to 33% in normal weight and 25% in underweight children (Puig et al. 2008). Importantly, the vast majority of studies evaluating diagnostic imaging do not report any information on patient's weight or BMI, and it is thus difficult to propose any cutoff at which a particular child with a given weight would benefit more from CT than US. A retrospective study by Grayson et al. found that increased intraperitoneal fat was correlated with a significantly increased likelihood of visualizing a normal appendix on CT in pediatric patients (Grayson et al. 2001).

3 US and CT Protocols: An Effort to Minimize Radiation Risk

In the emergency department (ED), a significant amount of radiation exposure is due to CT scans performed for the diagnosis of appendicitis (Ramarajan et al. 2009). Children are at increased risk of developing cancer from low-dose radiation and it is therefore desirable to utilize CT only when appropriate (Ramarajan et al. 2009). US eliminates radiation but has a lower sensitivity than CT. There has been recent interest in an interdisciplinary initiative to use a staged US and CT pathway to maximize diagnostic accuracy while minimizing radiation exposure in children.

Ideally, an imaging protocol would combine the sensitivity of CT with the lack of ionizing radiation afforded by US in order to maximize diagnostic accuracy while minimizing patient risk. In our literature search, two prospective studies were identified which examined the combination of graded compression US as the initial imaging, followed by CT study if the appendix was not visualized at US or if US was inconclusive (Teo et al. 2000; Garcia Pena et al. 1999b). These studies enrolled a total of 585 patients with a prevalence of appendicitis ranging from 23 to 43% with a pooled prevalence of 39%. The sensitivity varied from 77 to 97% with a pooled sensitivity of 95% (95% CI, 83–100%). The range of specificity was 89–99%, with a pooled result of 93% (95% CI, 97–97%). As expected, these series demonstrated a greater sensitivity and lower specificity when the combined US followed by CT results were considered than when the US data were considered alone. Another randomized trial of 600 patients compared results of CT and US versus US alone in a pediatric population (Kaiser et al. 2002). This study demonstrated similar results to the two aforementioned series, with the combined CT and US protocol demonstrating a sensitivity of 99% and specificity of 89% while ultrasound alone showed a sensitivity of 86% and specificity of 95%.

Another recent study published in 2009 by Ramarajan et al. emphasized similar findings regarding a protocol of US followed by CT in the diagnosis of pediatric appendicitis (Ramarajan et al. 2009). This study was a retrospective outcomes analysis of patients presenting for suspected appendicitis at an academic children's hospital ED over a 6-year period. The pathway established US as the initial imaging modality. CT was recommended only if US was equivocal. Clinical and pathologic outcomes from ED diagnosis and disposition, histopathology, and return visits were correlated with the US and CT. ED diagnosis and disposition, pathology, and return visits were used to determine outcome.

A total of 680 patients met the study criteria. A total of 407 patients (60%) followed the pathway. Two hundred of these (49%) were managed definitively without CT. A total of 106 patients (26%) had a positive US for appendicitis; 94 (23%) had a negative US. A total of 207 patients had equivocal US with follow-up CT. A total of 144 patients went to the operating room; 10 patients (7%) had negative appendectomies. One case of appendicitis was missed (<0.5%). The sensitivity, specificity, negative predictive value, and positive predictive values of this staged US-CT pathway were 99, 91, 99, and 85%, respectively. A total of 228 of 680 patients (34%) had an equivocal US with no follow-up CT. Of these patients, 10 (4%) went to the operating room with one negative appendectomy. A total of 218 patients (32%) were observed clinically without complications. This study had a negative appendectomy rate of 7% and a missed appendicitis rate less than 0.5%, both relatively acceptable.

It therefore can be concluded that there is moderate evidence-based medicine that supports the idea that acute appendicitis can be diagnosed in children with a protocol that emphasizes minimizing radiation risks without losing diagnostic accuracy. Further prospective studies are needed in regard to the use of the pathway coupled with patient demographics, clinical characteristics, and laboratory values that can help in the diagnosis of acute appendicitis.

4 Cost-Effectiveness and Financial Impact of Imaging in Acute Appendicitis

The data examining the cost impact of imaging in pediatric patients with suspected acute appendicitis are limited. Since patients with equivocal appendicitis have traditionally been admitted for observation, it has been postulated that use of imaging could decrease costs by allowing for more patients to be definitely diagnosed as negative in terms of appendicitis and sent home. However, no formal cost-effectiveness analyses are available.

A prospective cohort study of 94 pediatric patients to be admitted for observation for possible acute appendicitis found that if all of the patients who had a normal appendix clearly visualized on CT had been discharged home, the admission rate would have decreased by 41.8% with no missed diagnosis given the high accuracy of CT (Acosta et al. 2005). This could have theoretically resulted in considerable savings, as the mean length of hospital stay was 2.0 days.

In contrast, a retrospective review of 197 consecutive children who underwent appendectomy found no significant improvement in diagnostic accuracy or outcome in imaged compared to non-imaged groups, with a delay in surgical treatment (12.1 h in imaged group versus 5.4 h in non-imaged group, $P < .001$), and a 26% increase in hospital charges, from $11,791 (imaged) compared to $9,360 (non-imaged, $P = .001$) (York et al. 2005). However, significant selection bias between the non-imaged versus the imaged groups is likely, with the non-imaged group representing more typical cases which could be taken directly to the operating room. In addition, this study did not include the potential cost impact from avoiding surgery or observation on subjects without appendicitis who had negative imaging.

A study by Garcia Peña et al. used a decision analytic model to examine a retrospective consecutive cohort of children admitted to the hospital for observation for suspected appendicitis (Garcia Pena et al. 1999b). Three proposed strategies for patient management were evaluated using empirical data from this cohort, which demonstrated sensitivity and specificity of CT for appendicitis of 97 and 97% in imaged patients. All three of the protocols involved getting CT scans on children whom under the practice of the time would have simply been admitted for observation without CT imaging. Costs for average charges from 1997 were applied to each situation and were calculated using the average hospital charge data. The total cost per patient using the traditional practice strategy was $5,831, compared to $3,813 if CT examinations were obtained in all patients and those with negative examinations sent home. This second strategy would have resulted in the same number of projected missed acute appendicitis cases and a decrease in the negative appendectomy rate. Two additional strategies involved admitting and getting CT examinations in all and getting CT examinations only in patients with elevated white blood cells count. These strategies resulted in projected costs per patient of $5,277 and $5,140, respectively. It was found that all three proposed CT strategies would have reduced the number of observation days, surgical procedures, negative laparotomies, and cost per patient compared to traditional practice. The analysis was also repeated for a range of sensitivities from 80 to 100%, which no change in the relative ordering of the strategies. These modeling data have not been validated in actual clinical practice.

Garcia Peña et al. also completed a prospective cohort study of 139 children with equivocal clinical findings of acute appendicitis (Garcia Pena et al. 2000). Subjects were evaluated with US, and those with negative or unequivocal US findings then had CT with rectal contrast. Surgical management plans were recorded before imaging, following US, and following CT, and total hospital direct and indirect costs incurred or saved were determined at each point. The imaging protocol resulted in a total cost savings of $565 per patient, in this cohort with a 36% prevalence of acute appendicitis.

These limited data suggest that there could be cost savings associated with imaging pediatric patients with suspected acute appendicitis, but the exact effects are unclear particularly given our present inconclusive knowledge of the effects of imaging on the negative appendectomy rate and clinical decision making.

A recent article by Wan et al. used a Markov decision analytic model to investigate the cost-effectiveness of US vs. CT in pediatric acute appendicitis (Wan et al. 2009). This decision model was constructed by using costs, utilities, and probabilities from the literature. As the base-case scenario, the study selected a 5-year-old child clinically suspected of having acute appendicitis at presentation. The age of 5 years was chosen because the risk of radiation-induced malignancy is highest and most relevant for young patients. The model simulated the course of events, starting from the initial diagnostic imaging test at the age of 5 years, and ending when the patient died or reached 100 years of age.

The risk of radiation-induced cancer was modeled by using the Biological Effects of Ionizing Radiation VII report, which is based primarily on data from atomic bomb survivors (Committee to Assess Health Risks from Exposure to Low Levels of Ionizing Radiation - National Research Council 2006). The three imaging strategies were US, CT, and US followed by CT if the initial US study was negative. The model simulated the short-term and long-term outcomes of the patients, calculating the average quality-adjusted life span and health care costs.

The results showed that for a single abdominal CT study in a 5-year-old child, the lifetime risk of radiation-induced cancer would be 26.1 per 100,000 in girls and 20.4 per 100,000 in boys. In the base-case analysis, US followed by CT was the most costly and most effective strategy, CT was the second-most costly and second-most effective strategy, and US was the least costly and least effective strategy. The incremental cost-effectiveness ratios (ICERs) of CT to US and of US followed by CT to US were both well below the societal willingness-to-pay threshold of $50,000. The ICER of US followed by CT to CT was less than $10,000 in both boys and girls.

This study incorporated the health care costs and loss of life associated with radiation-induced cancer in association with the cost-effectiveness of radiological imaging. The principal limitation was that there is still an extreme degree of uncertainty associated with current estimates of radiation-induced cancer, especially at very low doses (Wan et al. 2009).

The decision of how to image suspected appendicitis in children depends on many factors including cost and side effects. In this study, when the incidence of acute appendicitis in patients referred for imaging was very low (< 5%), US was the most effective and least costly imaging strategy; conversely, if the incidence was greater than 21%, the strategy of US followed by CT was most effective.

This study concluded that in a Markov-based decision model of pediatric acute appendicitis, the most cost-effective method of imaging was to start with a US study and follow each negative US study with a CT examination (Wan et al. 2009). The cost-effectiveness and financial impact of imaging in patients with acute appendicitis should be taken into account by clinicians who seek accurate diagnosis. Clinicians must aim to avoid radiation exposure in children whenever possible, but should also seek to minimize costs in an increasingly expensive health care system.

References

Acosta R, Crain E, Goldman HS (2005) CT can reduce hospitalization for observation in children with suspected appendicitis. Pediatr Radiol 35:495–500

Agency for Healthcare Research and Quality (AHRQ) (2000) Care of Children and Adolescents in U.S. Hospitals: HCUP Fact Book No. 4. Available from: http://www.ahrq.gov/data/hcup/factbk4/factbk4.htm#why

Brennan GD (2006) Pediatric appendicitis: pathophysiology and appropriate use of diagnostic imaging. CJEM 8:425–432

Committee to Assess Health Risks from Exposure to Low Levels of Ionizing Radiation – National Research Council (2006) Health risks from exposure to low levels of ionizing radiation: BEIR VII Phase 2. National Research Council, Washington, DC

Doria AS, Moineddin R, Kellenberger C, Epelmen M, Beyene J, Schuh S, Babyn PS, Dick PT (2006) US or CT for diagnosis of appendicitis in children and adults? A meta-analysis. Radiology 241:83–94

Garcia Pena BM, Taylor GA, Lund DP, Mandl KD (1999a) Costs and effectiveness of ultrasonography and limited computed tomography for diagnosing appendicitis in children. Pediatrics 104:440–446

Garcia Pena BM, Mandl KD, Kraus SJ, Fischer AC, Fleisher GR, Lund DP, Taylor GA (1999b) Ultrasonography and limited computed tomography in the diagnosis and management of appendicitis in children. JAMA 282: 1041–1046

Garcia Pena BM, Taylor GA, Fishman SJ, Mandl KD (2000) Costs and effectiveness of ultrasonography and limited computed tomography for diagnosing appendicitis in children. Pediatrics 106:672–676

Grayson DE, Wettlaufer JR, Dalrymple NC, Keesling CA (2001) Appendiceal CT in pediatric patients: relationship of visualization to amount of peritoneal fat. AJR Am J Roentgenol 176:497–500

Kaiser S, Frenckner B, Jorulf HK (2002) Suspected appendicitis in children: US and CT–a prospective randomized study. Radiology 223:633–638

Kwok MY, Kim MK, Gorelick MH (2004) Evidence-based approach to the diagnosis of appendicitis in children. Pediatr Emerg Care 20:690–698

Puig S, Staudenherz A, Felder-Puig R, Paya K (2008) Imaging of appendicitis in children and adolescents: useful or useless? A comparison of imaging techniques and a critical review of the current literature. Semin Roentgenol 43: 22–28

Ramarajan N, Krishnamoorthi R, Barth R, Ghanouni P, Mueller C, Dannenburg B, Wang NE (2009) An interdisciplinary initiative to reduce radiation exposure: evaluation of appendicitis in a pediatric emergency department with clinical assessment supported by a staged ultrasound and computed tomography pathway. Acad Emerg Med 16: 1258–1265

Rao PM, Rhea JT, Novelline RA, Mostafavi AA, McCabe CJ (1998) Effect of CT of the appendix on treatment of patients and use of hospital resources. N Engl J Med 338: 141–146

Rothrock SG, Pagane J (2000) Acute appendicitis in children: emergency department diagnosis and management. Ann Emerg Med 36:39–51

Sivit CJ, Applegate KE (2003) Imaging of acute appendicitis in children. Semin Ultrasound CT MR 24:74–82

Teo EL, Tan KP, Lam SL, Ong CL, Wong CS (2000) Ultrasonography and computed tomography in a clinical algorithm for the evaluation of suspected acute appendicitis in children. Singapore Med J 41:387–392

Wan M, Krahn M, Ungar W, Caku E, Sung L, Medina LS, Doria A (2009) Acute appendicitis in young children: cost effectiveness of US versus CT in diagnosis—A Markov decision analytic model. Radiology 250:378–386

York D, Smith A, Phillips JD, von Allmen D (2005) The influence of advanced radiographic imaging on the treatment of pediatric appendicitis. J Pediatr Surg 40:1908–1911

Imaging of Acute Appendicitis in Children: MRI

Marcus Hörmann

Contents

M. Hörmann (✉)
Department of Radiology, City Diagnostic Center Bellaria,
Bellariastrasse, 6, 1010 Vienna, Austria
e-mail: marcus.hoermann@citydc.at

Abstract

In children, it is widely recommended to avoid, or at least minimize, ionizing radiations. Ultrasonography and more recently MRI have become more widespread in clinical imaging departments. Even if MRI is sensitive to breathing artefacts that are not easily avoidable in children, ultrafast sequences that reduce them substantially are now widely available. MRI is thus an attractive alternative imaging technique in children suspected of acute appendicitis, with high negative predictive value, and sensitivity and specificity slightly superior to those of CT.

1 Introduction

As a non-ionizing imaging technique, MR is appropriate for imaging children, adolescents, women in childbearing age, and pregnant women. Nevertheless, publications dealing with MR in children suspected of acute appendicitis are rare and mostly based on small number of patients (Hörmann et al. 1998, 2002; Inescu et al. 1997; Doria et al. 2006).

As children are often difficult to explore clinically, they need imaging examinations in order to rule out indication for surgery, to avoid unnecessary surgery, and to reduce the perforation rate in case of acute appendicitis. This has to be done in accordance with the ALARA (as low as reasonably achievable) principle, by minimizing the delivered radiation dose (Brenner et al. 2001).

There are still several reasons why MR imaging is not usually performed in children. First, although the number of MR scanners has increased over years,

C. Keyzer and P. A. Gevenois (eds.), *Imaging of Acute Appendicitis in Adults and Children*,
Medical Radiology. Diagnostic Imaging, DOI: 10.1007/174_2011_237,

their availability in most general hospitals is still limited. Second, sedation may be mandatory to obtain sufficient image quality. Nevertheless, if gently managed children suspected of acute appendicitis–who are mostly at school age–do not require any sedation. Third, most MR units are reserved for neurological patients during night-time and week-ends. However, some hospitals have adopted a policy to not perform appendectomy between 12 PM and 7 AM, unless the patient is very ill (Cobben et al. 2009).

2 Imaging Technique

MR examination in children should be tailored to the patient's size and age. The most useful sequences are T2 or T2*-weighted, and STIR or T2- weighted-fat-saturated (T2 fat sat) sequences that shows best the inflammatory changes in acute appendicitis. T1-weighted images are not usually useful for depicting the normal or detecting the inflamed appendix but it could help in distinguishing tissue composition and in establishing, among multiple differential diagnoses, the definite one. Very recently, diffusion-weighted images were shown to be of value for diagnosing acute appendicitis (Inci et al. 2010).

In an acute setting and in order to act as fast as possible, T2-weighted and STIR/T2 fat sat can be sufficient to rule out acute appendicitis. The MR image should be obtained in coronal and transversal planes. The sagittal plane could give additional and complementary information in pregnant women because their appendix is commonly displaced laterally or cranially to the cecum, but is not recommended in children (Baldisserotto et al. 2008; Nikolaidis et al. 2006). The most appropriate plane depends however on the course of the appendix.

The slice thickness should range from 4 to 6 mm, the intersection gap not more than 2 mm, as the size of normal or inflamed appendix ranges from 3 to 20 mm. The sequence parameters should be chosen according to the used MR scanner as well as to the user's experience. The field of view should be appropriate for patient's size and the MR examination explores from beneath the symphysis pubis to as high as possible in the abdomen in order to rule out differential diagnoses such as hernias and *osteochondritis ischiopubica*. The examination should never be focused on the right lower quadrant of the abdomen

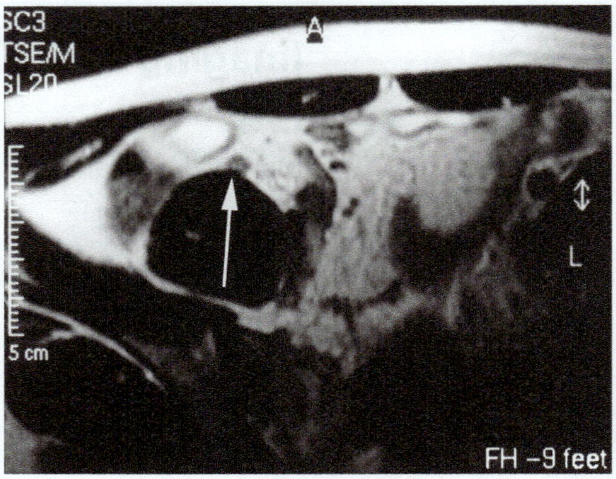

Fig. 1 Axial T2-weighted image showing the normal appendix (*arrow*) coursing on the psoas muscle. The diameter is lower than 6 mm. No inflammatory changes in the surrounding tissue

alone. Especially in girls, the examination should also cover the genital organs as well as the kidneys in both genders. Finally, breathholding after full inspiration (needing patient rehearsal) prevents breathing artefacts and is feasible in children at least in school age (Hörmann et al. 1998; Cobben et al. 2009).

In children, sedation is only seldom necessary as acute appendicitis is not common in children less than 6–7 years of age, the examination time exceeding not approximately 20 min.

Because of the excellent contrast resolution of MR in acute appendicitis, the use of MR contrast agents is not necessary, making this technique an excellent alternative in patients with renal dysfunction.

3 Image Interpretation

The maximal outer diameter of the normal appendix is smaller than 7 mm. The signal of the normal appendix on T1 and T2-weighted images is hypo or hyperintense, depending on the studies (Fig. 1). Its detection rate increases with the amount of intraabdominal fat that yields an intrinsically high contrast (Hörmann et al. 2002).

The inflamed appendix has an outer diameter larger than 6–7 mm and the thickened wall displays a high signal on T2-weighted images (Hörmann et al. 1998, 2002; Inescu et al. 1997; Barger and Nandalur 2010). The appendiceal lumen contains mostly fluid, and appendicolith is detected as a signal void lesion in

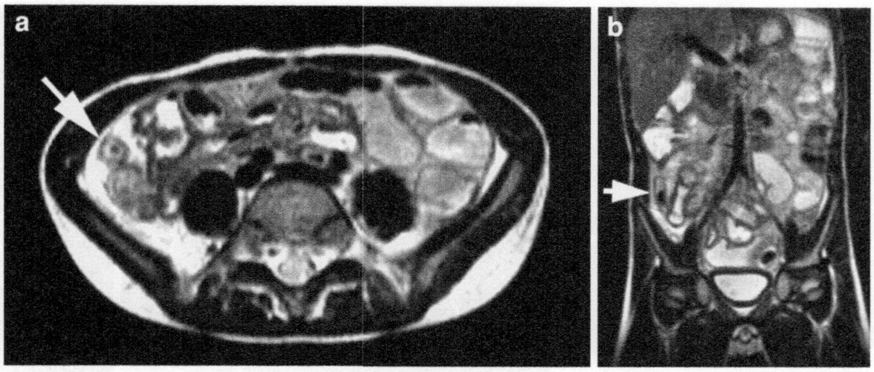

Fig. 2 **a** Axial T2-weighted image showing lateral and ventral to the cecum a target lesion (*arrow*) with a thickened hyperintense wall (outer diameter larger than 7 mm) and periappendiceal fluid collection. **b** Coronal T2-weighted image in the same patient with acute appendicitis. Signal void lesion in the lumen corresponding to an appendicolith. Note extensive ascite

the lumen (Fig. 2). Note that a signal void lesion can also represent gas within the lumen without pathological significance (Hörmann et al. 1998; Barger and Nandalur 2010).

Periappendiceal changes consisting of edematous changes of the periappendiceal fat (i.e., periappendiceal fat stranding) with high signal on T2-weighted images can evolve in fluid collections of various sizes in the cecal region. These changes are important to consider if the appendiceal diameter is not increased. Enlarged lymph nodes can also be seen along the appendiceal artery. Air-fluid levels resulting from local paralysis of the small bowel can be seen in its surrounding loops with sometimes thickened walls. These findings should be interpreted with caution as they could also be seen in inflammatory ileitis with involvement of the appendix, a particular clinical circumstance that should not be operated.

In case of appendiceal perforation, MR findings can be misleading as abscess formation, surrounding inflammatory changes, and reactive thickening of the bowel wall could be misinterpreted as malignancy (Fig. 3).

4 Alternative Diagnoses

As described in the chapters discussing ultrasonography and CT, most of the alternative diagnoses can be detected by these two techniques. However, some alternative diagnoses can be better depicted by MR imaging, especially gynecological disorders and inflammatory bowel disease because of the high soft tissue resolution provided by MR. Ovarian torsion secondary to an ovarian cyst or tumor is one of these diagnoses that should be rapidly detected as it necessitates rapid surgery. *O. ischiopubica*, with edematous changes and thickening of the pubis synchondrosis is another important alternative diagnosis in children at school age that can be easily made at MR. Finally, lymphadenitis mesenterialis is very common in children and is typically seen 2 weeks after a "cold". Lymphadenitis mesenterialis can be diagnosed at MR on the basis of multiple lymph nodes detected in the mesenteric root, predominantly in the region of the belly button and in the area of the right lower quadrant.

List of most common alternative diagnoses in children.

Gastrointestinal
- Any form of inflammatory bowel disease
- Meckel's diverticula
- Hernia
- Intussusception
- Lymphadenitis mesenterialis after viral infection of the tracheobronchial system

Gynecological
- Ovarian torsion (with cyst or tumor)
- Rupture of ovarian cyst
- First menses

Urological
- Ureteropelvic obstruction
- Pyelonephritis
- Obstruction from calculi

Unspecific
- Non-specific abdominal pain (NSAP) with no morphological changes
- Diseases with pain referred to the periumbilical region

Thorax
- Basal pneumonia

Musculoskeletal
- *O. ischiopubica*

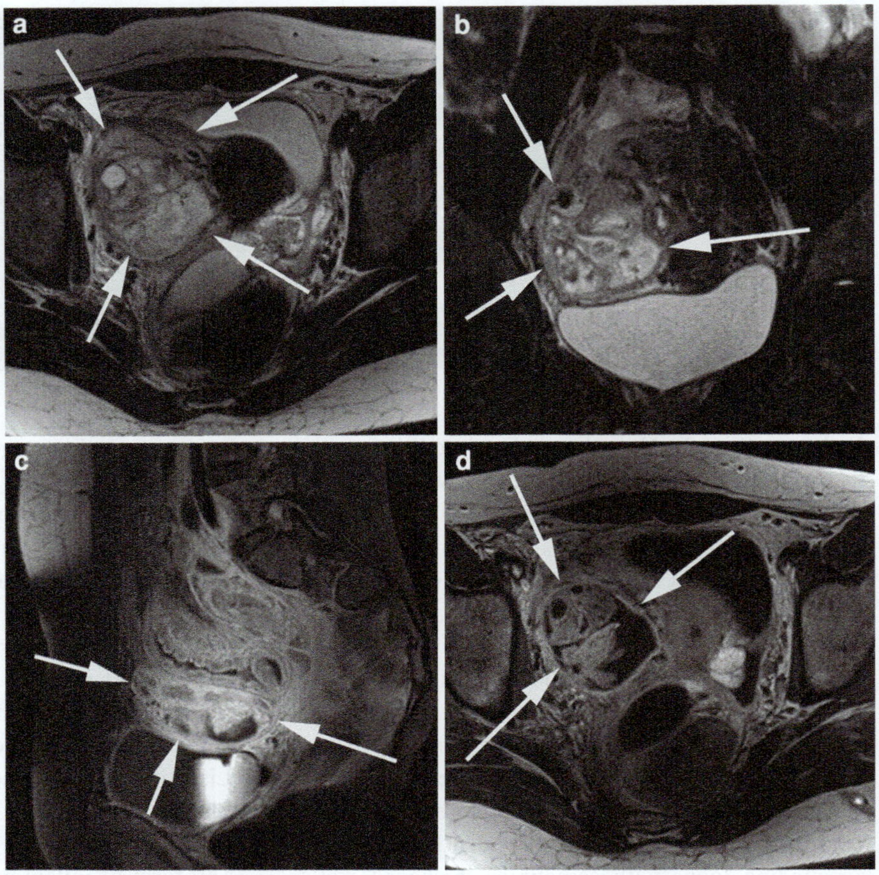

Fig. 3 **a** Axial T2-weighted image in an adolescent girl showing a big mass (*arrows*) in the right lower quadrant with inhomogeneous signal and a pseudo capsule. The adjacent uterus is displaced and there is peritoneal effusion. **b** Coronal T2-weighted image shows in the upper lateral aspect a small signal void lesion. **c** T1-weighted sagittal images after gadolinium IV, showing marked enhancement of the mass, extensive inflammatory changes of the pelvic soft tissues, and inflammatory changes of the adjacent small bowel wall. **d** T1-weighted images without gadolinium, showing a mass of mixed intensities with fluid in the "capsule". Differential diagnosis was: perforated acute appendicitis, tubo ovarian abscess, or tumor. Surgery revealed acute perforated appendicitis

5 Pros and Cons

MR imaging as a complement to ultrasound in case of suspected acute appendicitis is still controversial. There are indeed surgeons who rather rely on their clinical experience than on imaging, whereas others recommend imaging and even further imaging in cases of inconclusive ultrasound. CT is commonly recommended if ultrasound is inconclusive even in children (Doria et al. 2006). However, sensitivity, specificity, positive predictive, and negative predictive values of MR imaging in patient suspected of acute appendicitis are all very high and meta-analyses even reveal sensitivity and specificity (97% each) higher than those of CT (91 and 90%, respectively) (Barger and Nandalur 2010). The preference of CT over MR imaging is probably due to its greater availability as compared to MR on a 24 h basis, and to the fact that CT is believed cheaper than MR. Cobben et al. have evaluated the effect of imaging examinations (Ultrasound, CT, and MR) on the use of hospital resources by calculating the avoided unnecessary appendectomy and avoided observation days. These authors showed significant cost savings resulting from the use of imaging. Furthermore they showed that imaging speeds up the diagnostic process (Cobben et al. 2009). The impact of imaging on negative appendectomy rate, that should be as low as possible, is further discussed in "Impact of Imaging on Negative Appendectomy Rate" by CA Coursey and RD Moreno.

Bearing in mind the radiation burden delivered by CT and the so-called ALARA principle, one should remember that children should be protected from ionizing radiations. We could therefore recommend performing MR imaging in children of any age in case of inconclusive ultrasonography (Hörmann et al. 1998; Inescu et al. 1997; Brenner et al. 2001).

References

Baldisserotto M, Valduga SG, da Cunha CF (2008) MR imaging evaluation of the normal appendix in children and adolescents. Radiology 249:278–284

Barger RL, Nandalur KR (2010) Diagnostic performance of magnetic resonance imaging in the detection of appendicitis in adults: a meta analysis. Acad Radiol 17:1211–1216

Brenner D, Elliston C, Hall E, Berdon W (2001) Estimated risks of radiation-induced fatal cancer from pediatric CT. AJR Am J Roentgenol 176:289–296

Cobben L, Groot I, Kingma L, Coerkamp E, Puylaert J, Blickman J (2009) A simple MRI protocol in patients with clinically suspected appendicitis: results in 138 patients and effect on outcome of appendectomy. Eur Radiol 19:1175–1883

Doria AS, Moineddin R, Kellenberger CJ, Epelman M, Beyene J, Schuh S, Babyn PS, Dick PT (2006) US or CT-Diagnosis of appendicitis in children and adults? A meta-analysis. Radiology 241:83–94

Hörmann M, Paya K, Eibenberger K, Dorffner R, Lang S, Kreuzer S, Metz VM (1998) MR imaging in children with nonperforated acute appendicitis: value of unenhanced MR imaging in sonographically selected cases. AJR Am J Roentgenol 171:467–470

Hörmann M, Puig S, Prokesch SR, Partik B, Helbich TH (2002) MR imaging of the normal appendix in children. Eur Radiol 12:2313–2316

Inci E, Kilicksemez O, Hocaoglu E, Aydin S, Bayramoglu S, Cimilli T. Utility of diffusion-weighted imaging in the diagnosis of acute appendicitis. Eur Radiol 2010, Epub ahead

Inescu L, Coskun A, Selcuk MB, Akan H, Sozubir S, Bernay F (1997) Acute appendicitis: MR imaging and sonographic correlation. AJR Am J Roentgenol 168:669–674

Nikolaidis P, Hammond N, Marko J, Miller FH, Papanicolaou N, Yaghmai V (2006) Incidence of visualization of the normal appendix on different MRI-sequences. Emerg Radiol 12:223–226

Part V

Imaging Findings of Other Appendiceal Diseases, Impact of Imaging on Negative Appendectomy Rate, and Radiation Dose Optimization

Spontaneously Resolving and Chronic Appendicitis

Lodewijk P. J. Cobben and Julien B. C. M. Puijlaert

Contents

Abstract

The term appendicitis covers four pathophysiological concepts: acute appendicitis, chronic appendicitis, recurrent acute appendicitis, and spontaneously resolving appendicitis. Chronic appendicitis is subject to many discussions, and most authors actually conclude that there is no pathological substrate for chronic appendicitis. In contrast, spontaneously resolving appendicitis is well-recognized but management of patients with spontaneously resolving appendicitis is still a matter of debate as conservative treatment could be associated with high rate of recurrence and recurrent episodes sometimes with perforation.

1 Introduction

Appendicitis is the most common abdominal surgical emergency in the Western World. In our hospital about 600 patients are admitted for suspected appendicitis each year, and 200 eventually prove to have it. The term appendicitis covers four pathophysiological entities: acute appendicitis, chronic appendicitis, recurrent acute appendicitis, and spontaneously resolving appendicitis.

The appendix is a blind-ending tube with a narrow lumen, and, as such, prone to obstruction. Obstruction of the appendiceal lumen has been attributed to a number of etiologies including fecaliths, normal stool, viral induced ulcers, lymphoid hyperplasia, and appendicolith. Acute appendicitis is the result of appendiceal obstruction associated with infection, as

L. P. J. Cobben (✉) · J. B. C. M. Puijlaert
Department of Radiology, Medisch Centrum Haaglanden, Lijnbaan 32, 2501 CK Den Haag, The Netherlands
e-mail: coblod@telfort.nl

C. Keyzer and P. A. Gevenois (eds.), *Imaging of Acute Appendicitis in Adults and Children*, Medical Radiology. Diagnostic Imaging, DOI: 10.1007/174_2011_238,

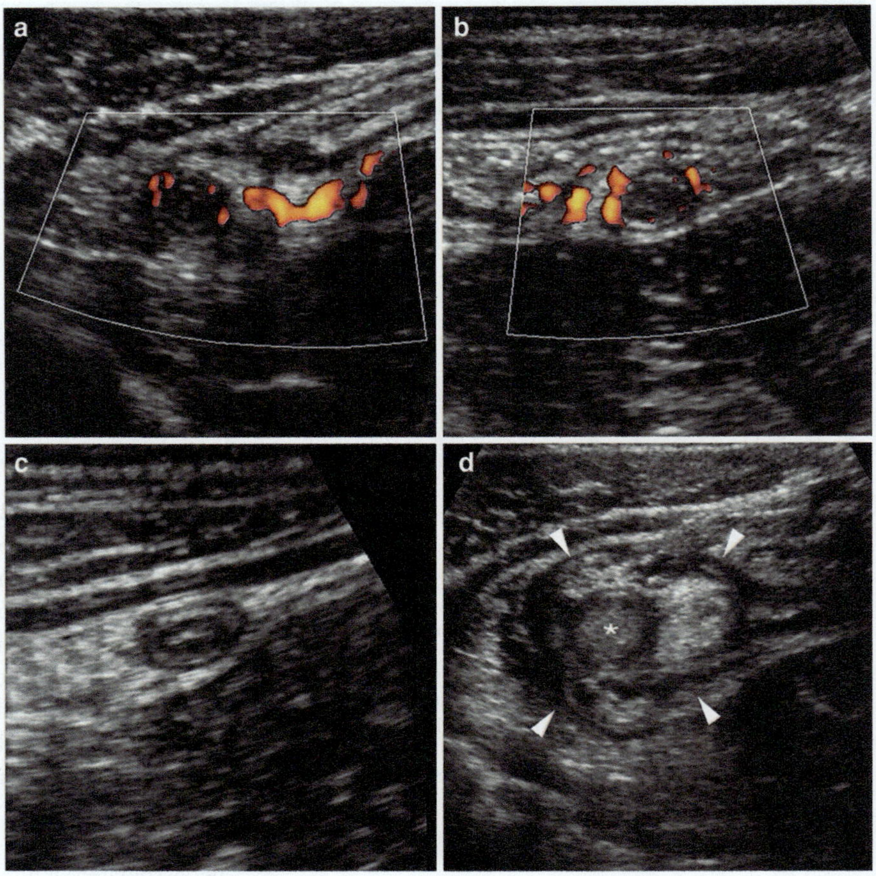

Fig. 1 Spontaneously resolving appendicitis. US studies of a 11 year-old girl suspected of having appendicitis show an enlarged appendix of 7 mm, surrounded by mild periappendicitis (**a**). During the initial examination the clinical symptoms had subsided, and she felt no pain. The surgeons decided not to operate. Close clinical and US follow-up was opted for and the following days she was doing fine, the US studies showed a gradual normalization of the appendix at day 2 (**b**) and 5 (**c**) after the initial examination. Two years later though, she returned with both a clinical and US diagnosed recurrent appendicitis (**d**). A clearly enlarged appendix was seen (*asterisk*) surrounded by periappendicitis (*arrowheads*)

discussed in previous chapters of this volume (Wangensteen and Bowers 1937). If appendectomy is not timely performed, free perforation or the formation of an appendiceal phlegmon or abscess will generally follow. However, in a minority of patients, symptoms of appendicitis spontaneously resolve in an early phase of the disease, usually within 24–48 h after the onset of pain. This phenomenon, which is believed to be caused by relief of obstruction, has been labeled "spontaneously resolving appendicitis" and is firmly documented by US follow-up studies (Cobben et al. 2000; Jeffrey et al. 1988; Puylaert et al. 1987; Rioux 1992; Migraine et al. 1997; Ooms et al. 1991; Puylaert 1986). Chronic appendicitis is subject of many discussions, and most authors now conclude that there is no pathological substrate for chronic appendicitis (Crabbe et al. 1986; Mattei et al. 1994; Rosai 1996).

2 Spontaneously Resolving Appendicitis

The frequent use of US in patients with right lower quadrant pain has learned that it is not unusual to find an unequivocally inflamed appendix, while the patient's symptoms are rapidly subsiding or already have subsided at the time of the examination (Figs. 1, 2, 3). Follow-up US studies usually demonstrate a gradual decrease in appendiceal diameter, until the appendix has reached normal dimensions (Migraine et al. 1997). Also clinical studies endorse the existence of spontaneously resolving appendicitis. From 7 to 25% of patients who undergo appendectomy for acute appendicitis mention a previous episode of similar symptoms (Crabbe et al. 1986; Mattei et al. 1994; Barber et al. 1997; Ferrier 1972; Lewis et al. 1975).

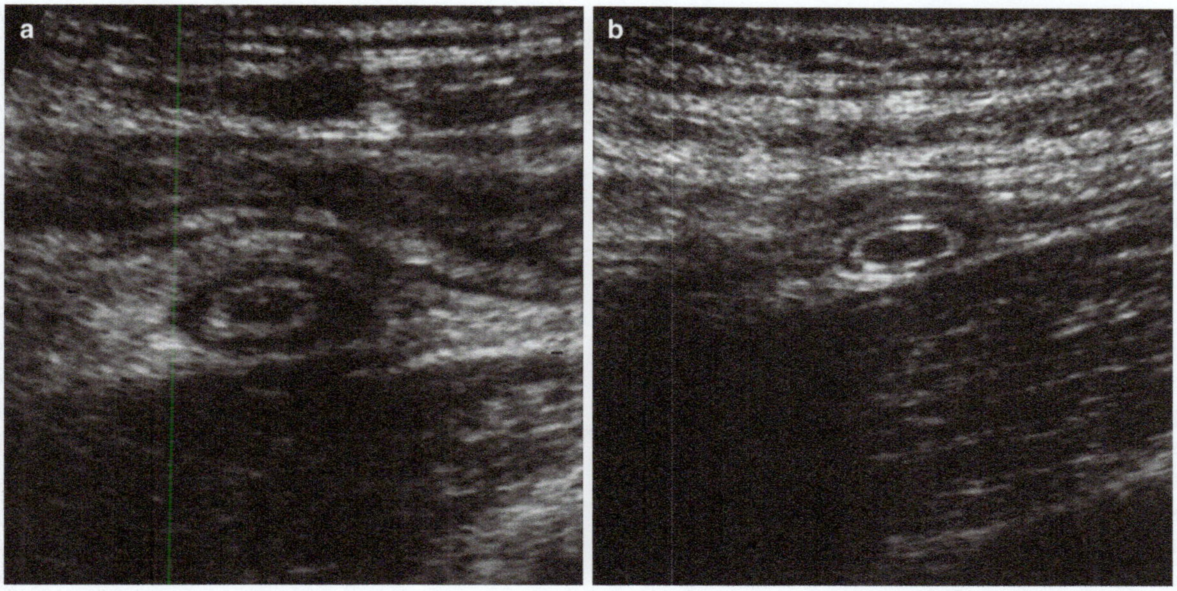

Fig. 2 Spontaneously resolving appendicitis in a 28 year-old man, who had pain in his right lower quadrant for 3 days but at the time of the US examination felt relieved of his symptoms. The initial US study (**a**) showed a mildly inflamed appendix with a diameter of 7 mm surrounded by some inflamed fat. Follow-up US study 3 days later (**b**) showed a completely normal appendix without any sign of inflammation

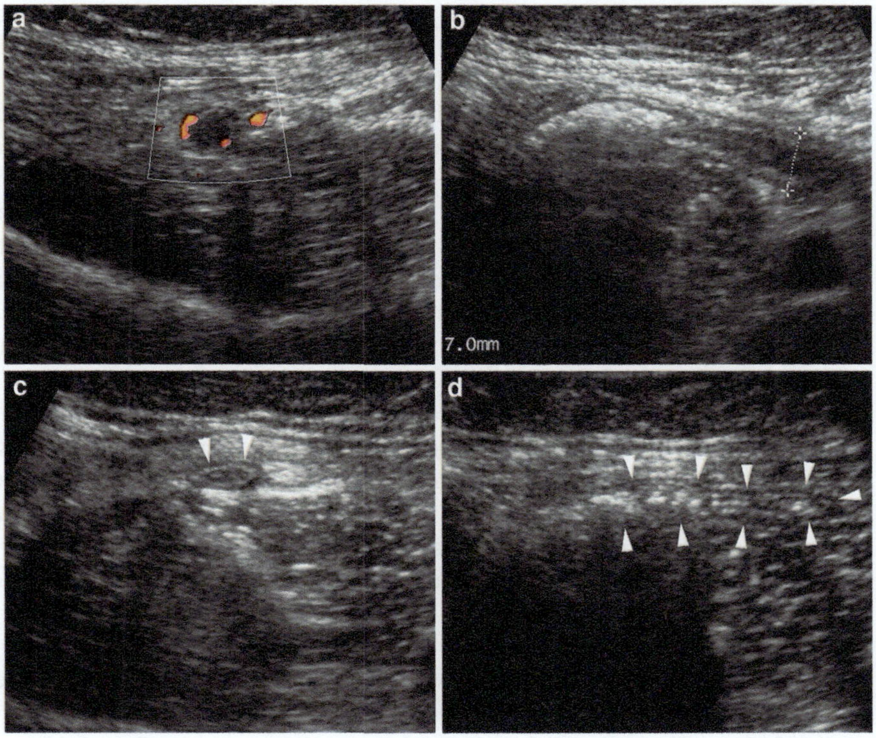

Fig. 3 Spontaneously resolving appendicitis in a 25 year-old woman. On admission US reveals an inflamed appendix (**a, b**) with a diameter of 7 mm, and suggestion of a fecalith at the base of the appendix. Because symptoms were rapidly subsiding the surgeons decided not to operate. Follow-up US 3 days later showed a normal compressible appendix (**c**, **d**) with a diameter of 4 mm (*longitudinal view with arrowheads*)

Spontaneously resolving appendicitis is not a rare phenomenon. In a study of our group (Cobben et al. 2000), we observed this phenomenon in 106 patients during a 10 year period. In the same period, 1,280 appendectomies revealing acute appendicitis were performed. Together with the non-operated spontaneously resolving appendicitis in the same period, the total number of patients with appendicitis was 1,321, so the frequency of spontaneously resolving appendicitis in this study was 8%. This could however be an underestimation of the true frequency of this phenomenon, since some of the patients who were operated upon would have spontaneously been resolved.

Management of patients with spontaneously resolving appendicitis is a controversial issue. Surgeons, who decide to operate despite subsiding symptoms, will find their decision justified by the pathologist confirming acute appendicitis, whereas surgeons who decide to remain conservative, will find their decision justified by spontaneous relief of symptoms. The treatment of this entity is also controversial because of the high recurrence rate after conservative management. We have studied 60 patients with a clinical and US diagnosis of spontaneously resolving appendicitis who were primarily treated conservatively. The follow-up period varied from 60–580 weeks with a median period of 297 weeks. A total of 23 out of 60 patients (38%) had recurrent appendicitis. Histology of the subsequently removed appendix demonstrated acute appendicitis in all 23 cases. Apart from a slightly higher chance of recurrence in men, in case of an appendiceal diameter of ≥8 mm, and in the absence of enlarged mesenteric lymph nodes, no clinical or US features, could predict a higher or lower chance of recurrence. The presence of enlarged mesenteric lymph nodes was associated with a lower chance of recurrence. One could argue that these lymph nodes were in fact associated with another bowel condition, such as infectious ileocecitis or Crohn's disease. In these conditions however, we would have expected to visualize the conspicuous wall thickening in the ileum and cecum as well (Puylaert et al. 1997). A possible explanation for the lower chance of recurrence in the group with enlarged lymph nodes is the existing theory (Rosai 1996) that obstructive appendicitis can be secondary to lymphoid hyperplasia in the appendiceal wall. If a patient has lymphoid hyperplasia, this will also be reflected by enlarged mesenteric lymph nodes. One could assume that transient lymphoid hyperplasia, as a cause of obstructive appendicitis, has a lower tendency for recurrence than other causes of mechanical obstruction.

It is thus difficult to give therapeutic recommendations with a recurrence rate of 38% after spontaneously resolving appendicitis. Many surgeons will indeed consider a 38% chance of recurrence an indication to operate immediately on any patient with spontaneously resolving appendicitis. Furthermore, in the subgroup of men with an appendiceal diameter of ≥8 and no enlarged mesenteric lymph nodes, the expected recurrence rate of 60% appears as a fair indication for immediate surgery. Nevertheless, patients who are completely free of symptoms may be reluctant to let themselves be operated. In view of the fairly high recurrence rate, patients who opt for conservative management must be warned to seek immediate medical help in case of recurrent symptoms.

If patients, despite clearly improving symptoms, are operated immediately, histology confirms acute inflammation, indiscernible from ordinary acute appendicitis. If conservative management is opted, there is a recurrence rate of almost 40% (Cobben et al. 2000), usually within 1 year. With each episode of recurrent appendicitis, the appendiceal wall might become more damaged and vulnerable, and it is probable that each attack implies a higher chance of perforation for the next episode. In our study, one of our 23 patients with recurrent appendicitis had indeed perforated appendicitis at the time of operation. This consideration, in combination with the high recurrence rate, plus the fact that the next attack may come at a more inconvenient time, is the reason why in our hospital almost all patients with a spontaneous resolving appendicitis, including those patients who are entirely free of symptoms again, undergo immediate appendectomy. In some cases an appendectomy "*à froid*" (i.e., interval appendectomy) is planned within a period of weeks. Although both patient and surgeon may favor appendectomy at a more convenient time, immediate appendectomy has the advantage that histological proof of acute inflammation is obtained. Another reason to perform immediate appendectomy is that recurrent appendicitis not infrequently occurs within the interval time in case of interval appendectomy. We have also observed that patients who claim to be entirely symptom free, in fact were probably dissimulating and progressed to an appendiceal abscess. The treatment of appendiceal abscess is further discussed

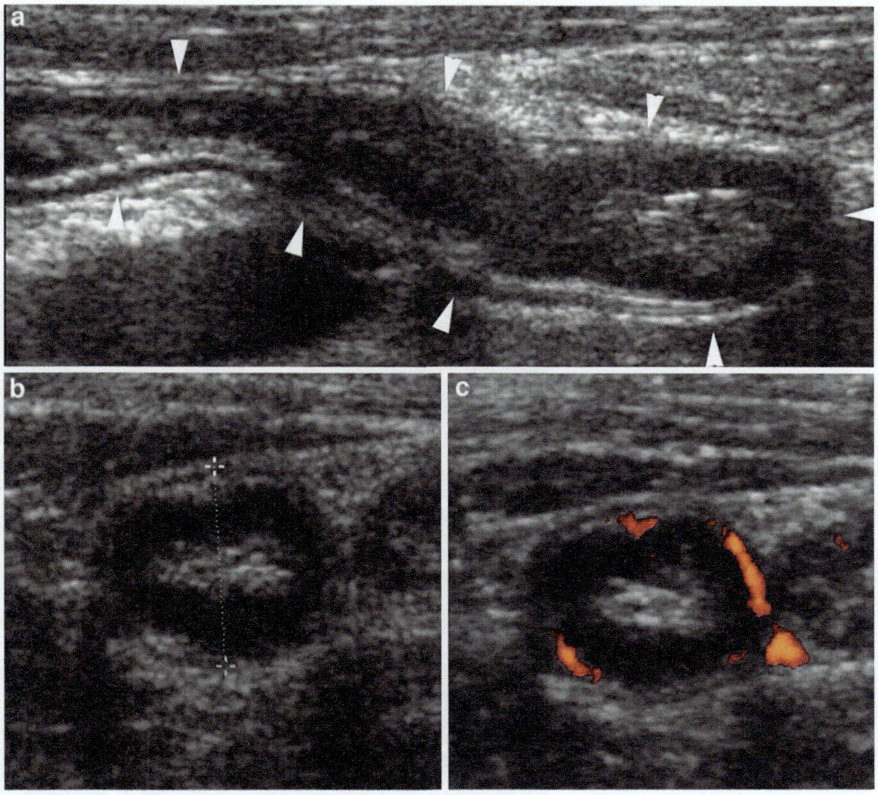

Fig. 4 Normal appendix with lymphoid hyperplasia of the appendix in a 8 year-old boy suspected of having appendicitis. Longitudinal (**a**) and transverse (**b**) US images show an enlarged appendix of 8 mm and power doppler (**c**) showed some reactive hyperemia in the appendiceal serosa. The layers of the appendix were intact. The appendix was not at the point of maximum tenderness and there were no signs of periappendicitis at all. Several enlarged mesenteric lymph nodes were seen and the patient was diagnosed as having mesenteric lymphadenitis. During follow-up no appendicitis developed

in "Treatment of Appendiceal Perforation" by Almoudaris and Faiz.

3 False-Positive Diagnoses of Spontaneously Resolving Appendicitis

A false-positive diagnosis can be made if the normal appendix is mistaken for an inflamed one. Of all normal appendices, 5% is larger than 7 mm. This is especially true in children due to lymphoid hyperplasia (Fig. 4) and in adults due to fecal impaction (Fig. 5). Apart from the clinical presentation, US features as appendiceal compressibility, the absence of hyperemia, and the absence of inflamed fat are the most important findings for deciding whether the appendix is normal or inflamed. If the appendix can be visualized over its entire length and all layers are preserved, and there is doubt whether it is inflamed or not, follow-up US the next day is a safe policy. An appendix with these features will not rupture overnight.

Mistaking a normal appendix for an inflamed one may also occur if there is secondary thickening of the appendix associated with cecal carcinoma. In the latter case, the appendiceal lumen is obstructed giving rise to sterile accumulation of mucus in the lumen. The patient usually has remarkably mild symptoms and is usually managed conservatively under the erroneous clinical diagnosis of an appendiceal phlegmon. If the underlying tumor is small and overlooked or not recognized, and considered to represent an appendiceal phlegmon, this may lead to considerable delay in surgical treatment. The combination of a relatively large appendix with paradoxically mild and atypical symptoms should raise suspicion of underlying malignancy. Large, round mesenteric lymph nodes in the direct neighborhood and liver metastases may indicate the true diagnosis.

Other conditions which may cause secondary thickening of the appendix are perforated peptic ulcer, Crohn's disease, and sigmoid diverticulitis. Detection of the underlying condition by US or CT is then mandatory.

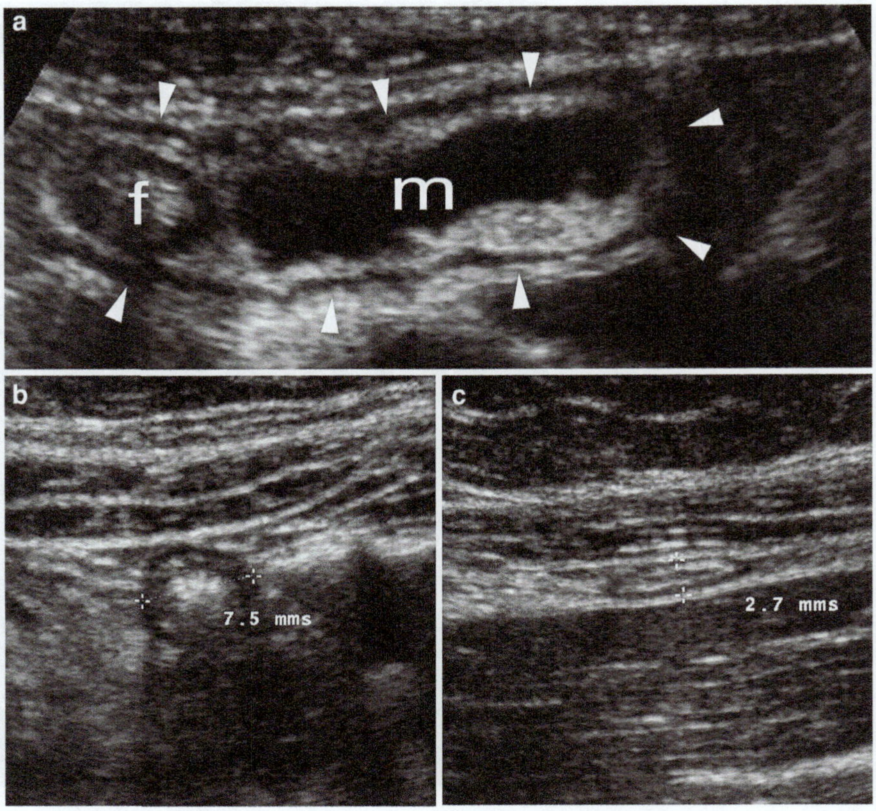

Fig. 5 Longitudinal (**a**) and transverse (**b**, **c**) US images show a normal appendix (*arrowheads*) filled with mucus (*m*) and feces (*f*) in a 45 year-old man who had an US study for surveillance of his abdominal aorta. The appendix was compressible, not painful and there were no signs of periappendicitis

4 Impact of the Diagnosis of Spontaneously Resolving Appendicitis on Study Results

Spontaneously resolving appendicitis is a clinical entity that could have an impact on the reported performances of diagnostic techniques. The negative laparotomy rate reflects the number of false-positive diagnoses and the perforation rate reflects the number of false-negative diagnoses. The perforation rate is defined as the number of perforated appendices divided by the total number of acutely inflamed appendices that are removed during an emergency procedure. Perforation is defined as a per-operatively confined, macroscopical defect in the appendiceal wall and/or the presence of pus or feces in the abdominal cavity (Rosai 1996). Surgeons tend to favor early surgery in an attempt to avoid perforation of the appendix and subsequent morbidity and mortality, but this result in a number of unwarranted operations. Diagnostic accuracy may be increased by a conservative attitude to surgery in uncertain cases (Thomson and Jones 1986). This strategy is criticized, however, for giving an increased perforation rate. Walled off perforations with development of an appendiceal mass usually will be treated conservatively, so no confirmation of the diagnosis in these patients is obtained.

Almost all studies on diagnostic accuracy deliberately leave out patients with an appendiceal mass and deal only with the results of emergency appendectomy. This implies that the actual perforation rates could be much higher than reported in these studies. In others, the diagnosis of appendicitis can be overestimated clinically at surgery because histological confirmation is not always present or accurate, and this can influence the calculated perforation rate (Andersson et al. 1994). The pathological criteria for acute appendicitis is the presence of polymorphic granulocytes throughout the appendiceal wall including the muscularis (Rosai 1996). All other pathologic diagnoses such as chronic fibrosis, parasitic infestation, and coprostasis are considered as normal. The natural course of non-perforating appendicitis is not known. Many surgeons regard acute appendicitis as a progressive inflammation, but spontaneous resolution may occur (Cobben et al. 2000; Migraine et al. 1997), and microscopy of excised appendices may show signs of healed inflammation. A high rate of exploratory laparoscopy in suspected appendicitis increases the number of confirmed cases (Howie 1964), presumably by adding cases of self-limiting inflammation which otherwise would have escaped detection. Inflammation without symptoms, which is seen in up to 35% of incidentally removed appendices (Pieper et al. 1982), may also be erroneously diagnosed at laparoscopy as appendicitis. The observed incidence of non-perforating appendicitis will therefore be influenced by a willingness to perform exploratory laparoscopy in cases of suspected appendicitis.

It is obvious that acute appendicitis, spontaneously resolving appendicitis, recurrent appendicitis, and non-operated appendiceal infiltrate or abscess all play a role in these difficult statistical analyses evaluating the outcome and effect of clinical imaging in patients suspected of having appendicitis.

References

Andersson R, Hugander A, Thulin A, Nystrom PO, Olaison G (1994) Indications for operation in suspected appendicitis and incidence of perforation. BMJ 308:107–110

Barber MD, McLaren J, Rainey JB (1997) Recurrent appendicitis. Br J Surg 84:110–112

Cobben LP, de Mol van Otterloo AM, Puylaert JB (2000) Spontaneously resolving appendicitis: frequency and natural history in 60 patients. Radiology 215:349–352

Crabbe MM, Norwood SH, Robertson HD, Silva JS (1986) Recurrent and chronic appendicitis. Surg Gynecol Obstet 163:11–13

Ferrier PK (1972) Acute appendicitis in university students: a twenty year study of 1028 cases. J Am Coll Health Assoc 20:287–290

Howie JG (1964) Too few appendicectomies? Lancet 1: 1240–1242

Jeffrey RB, Laing FC, Townsend RR (1988) Acute appendicitis: sonographic criteria based on 250 cases. Radiology 167:327–329

Lewis FR, Holcroft JW, Boey J, Dunphy E (1975) Appendicitis; a critical review of diagnosis and treatment. Arch Surg 110:677–684

Mattei P, Sola JE, Yeo CJ (1994) Chronic and recurrent appendicitis are uncommon entities often misdiagnosed. J Am Coll Surg 178:385–389

Migraine S, Atri M, Bret PM, Lough JO, Hinchey JE (1997) Spontaneously resolving acute appendicitis:clinical and sonographic documentation. Radiology 205:55–58

Ooms HWA, Koumans RMJ, Ho Kang You PJ, Puylaert JBCM (1991) Ultrasonography in the diagnosis of appendicitis. Br J Surg 78:315–318

Pieper R, Kager L, Nasman P (1982) Acute appendicitis: a clinical study of 1,018 cases of emergency appendectomy. Acta Chirurgica Scandinavica 148:51–62

Puylaert JBCM (1986) Acute appendicitis:US evaluation using graded compression. Radiology 158:355–360

Puylaert JBCM, Rutgers PH, Lalisang RI, de Vries BC, van der Werf SD, Dorr JP, Blok RA (1987) A prospective study of ultrasonography in the diagnosis of appendicitis. N Eng J Med 317:666–669

Puylaert JBCM, Van der Zant FM, Mutsaers JA (1997) Infectious ileocecitis caused by Yersinia, Campylobacter, and Salmonella: clinical, radiological and US findings. Eur Radiol 7:3–9

Rioux M (1992) Sonographic detection of the normal and abnormal appendix. AJR 158:773–778

Rosai J (1996) Chapter 11: Appendix. In: Ackerman's surgical pathology. St Louis: Mosby 711–716

Thomson HJ, Jones PF (1986) Active observation in acute abdominal pain. Am J Surg 152:522–525

Wangensteen OH, Bowers WF (1937) Significance of obstructive factor in the genesis of acute appendicitis: experimental study. Arch Surg 34:496–526

Imaging of Primary Appendiceal Neoplasms

Theodora A. Potretzke and Perry J. Pickhardt

Contents

T. A. Potretzke · P. J. Pickhardt (✉)
Department of Radiology,
University of Wisconsin School of Medicine
and Public Health, E3/311 Clinical Science Center,
600 Highland Ave, Madison, WI 53792-3252, USA
e-mail: ppickhardt2@uwhealth.org

Abstract

Primary appendiceal neoplasms are relatively uncommon but are being detected with increasing frequency as an incidental finding at cross-sectional imaging. Clinical presentation of acute appendicitis related to tumoral obstruction represents the other major clinical manifestation of primary appendiceal neoplasms. In either case, radiologists should be vigilant for imaging findings suggestive of underlying tumor. Mucoceles resulting from mucinous cystic neoplasms account for the majority of appendiceal neoplasms detected at cross-sectional imaging, whether manifesting as a symptomatic lesion or as an incidental finding. Other primary tumor types that may be encountered include colonic-type adenocarcinoma, carcinoid tumors (classic, tubular, or goblet cell varieties), and non-Hodgkin's lymphoma, among others. In addition, non-neoplastic processes may mimic a tumor at imaging. This chapter will review the salient clinical and imaging features of primary appendiceal neoplasms.

1 Introduction

Primary appendiceal neoplasms are relatively uncommon, present in approximately 0.5–1.0% of appendectomy specimens at pathologic evaluation (Connor et al. 1998; Deans and Spence 1995; Hananel et al. 1998), but they may occasionally present with clinical symptoms that lead to abdominal imaging or represent an incidental finding. Primary appendiceal neoplasms may be benign or malignant; the reported incidence of

C. Keyzer and P. A. Gevenois (eds.), *Imaging of Acute Appendicitis in Adults and Children*, Medical Radiology. Diagnostic Imaging, DOI: 10.1007/174_2011_227, © Springer-Verlag Berlin Heidelberg 2011

malignant tumors is 0.12 cases per 1,000,000 people per year (McCusker et al. 2002). There is a spectrum of tumor cell types and consequently a wide spectrum of affected patient demographics, clinical presentations, management, and outcomes. Primary appendiceal neoplasms include mucinous epithelial, colonic-type epithelial, classic carcinoid, tubular carcinoid, goblet cell, signet ring, lymphoma, and other tumor types which are exceeding rare and include gastrointestinal stromal tumors, smooth muscle tumors, and other rare entities. Mucoceles that result from cystic mucinous neoplasms account for the majority of appendiceal tumors detected at imaging, whether as a symptomatic lesion or an incidental finding, but other tumor types may also be encountered.

With the exception of carcinoid tumors, most appendiceal neoplasms are seen in adults who are middle-aged or older. Primary appendiceal neoplasms most often represent an incidental imaging and/or pathologic finding but up to 30–50% of non-carcinoid tumors may present with a clinical picture of acute appendicitis in published series (Connor et al. 1998; Pickhardt et al. 2002a; Carr et al. 1995). Other clinical presentations including a palpable mass, intussusception, gastrointestinal bleeding, ureteral obstruction or hematuria, torsion, and increasing abdominal girth from rupture of a malignant mucocele resulting in pseudomyxoma peritonei have also been reported (Hebert and Pickhardt 2007; Pickhardt et al. 2003). The remainder of this chapter will review the various types of primary appendiceal neoplasms, including the typical clinical and imaging manifestations.

2 Epithelial Neoplasms

Epithelial neoplasms of the appendix may be either benign (adenomas) or malignant (adenocarcinomas). Most are mucin-rich but non-mucinous adenomas and adenocarcinomas that are characteristic of non-appendiceal colorectal neoplasia are occasionally seen. Although epithelial neoplasms are less common than appendiceal carcinoid tumors in surgical pathology series, data from the National Cancer Institute's Surveillance, Epidemiology, and End-Results (SEER) program shows that malignant epithelial tumors are actually more common than malignant carcinoid tumors, with age-adjusted incidence rates of 1.3 and 0.63 per 1,000,000, respectively (McCusker et al. 2002; McGory et al. 2005). Mucinous adenocarcinoma represents the most common malignant appendiceal tumor overall. Compared with carcinoid tumors, which generally have a benign clinical course that elude diagnosis, epithelial neoplasms are more likely to be symptomatic due to their larger size, mucin production, and higher rate of complications.

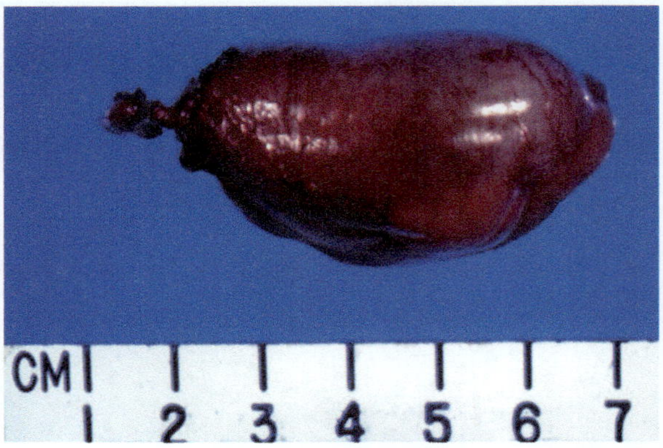

Fig. 1 Appendiceal mucocele from mucinous adenoma. Photograph of gross pathologic specimen shows ballooning dilatation of the vermiform appendix from luminal mucin

2.1 Mucinous Epithelial Neoplasms

Most epithelial tumors of the appendix are mucin-rich, demonstrate circumferential mucosal involvement, and have a strong propensity to form mucoceles (Carr et al. 1995). The term mucocele is simply a macroscopic description of an appendix that is grossly distended by mucus (Fig. 1). As such, it does not constitute a pathologic diagnosis and can be caused by a variety of non-neoplastic, benign neoplastic and malignant conditions. Although mucinous neoplasms of the appendix are by far the most common cause of mucoceles, the terms mucinous neoplasm and mucocele cannot be used interchangeably. Interestingly, mucoceles resulting from non-neoplastic occlusion (simple retention cysts) rarely exceed 2 cm in diameter (Carr et al. 1995; Carr and Sobin 1996). Mucoceles larger than 2 cm that are initially diagnosed as simple mucoceles are more likely to represent benign neoplasms that have been under sampled.

Unlike adenomas seen elsewhere in the large intestine, adenomas of the appendix are typically composed of mucin-rich epithelium and demonstrate

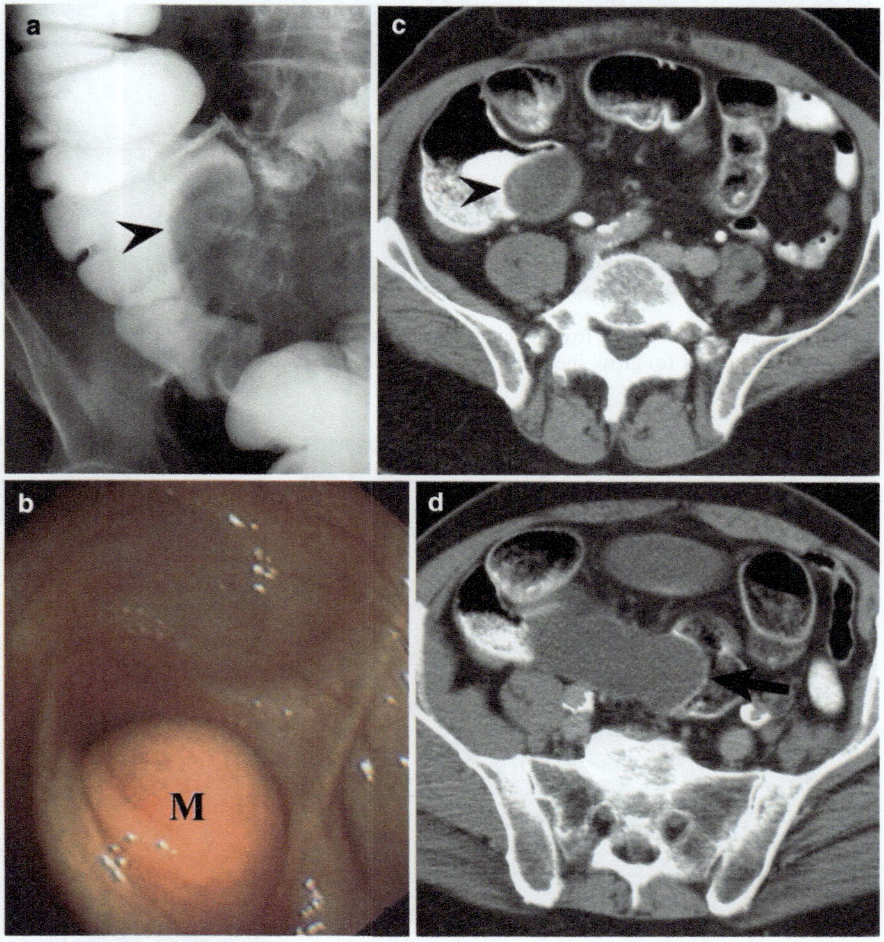

Fig. 2 Asymptomatic appendiceal mucocele from mucinous adenoma. Radiograph from single-contrast barium enema (**a**) shows a smooth broad-based impression (*arrowhead*) at the expected region of the appendiceal orifice. Image from optical colonoscopy (**b**) shows a smooth rounded mass (*M*) protruding into the cecum. Contrast-enhanced CT images (**c**) and (**d**) show not only the cecal filling defect (*arrowhead*) but also the low-attenuation contents and the entire extent of the mucocele (*arrow*) (Pickhardt et al. 2002a)

a villous architecture (Carr et al. 1995; Carr and Sobin 1996). Moreover, these neoplasms tend to be low-grade with circumferential involvement of the appendix. As these lesions grow, the villi become shorter and demonstrate more of an undulating growth pattern. Progressive growth to mucocele formation results in wall thinning and fibrosis of the submucosa, lamina propria, and muscularis propria.

The presence of invasive neoplastic cells beyond the muscularis mucosae is diagnostic for adenocarcinoma. The presence of acellular mucin within the appendiceal wall is not in itself diagnostic for malignancy and can be seen with some adenomas. Mucinous lesions that cannot be classified as clearly benign or malignant are considered to have uncertain malignant potential. A mucinous adenocarcinoma can be distinguished pathologically from the rarer colonic-type adenocarcinoma of the appendix in that at least 50% of the lesion is composed of mucin (Carr et al. 1995; Carr and Sobin 1996). Whether mucinous or non-mucinous, most adenocarcinomas of the appendix probably evolve through an adenoma-carcinoma sequence, similar to other colonic neoplasms (Carr and Sobin 1996).

2.1.1 Clinical Presentation

2.1.1.1 Benign Mucoceles due to Mucinous Adenomas

Most benign mucoceles due to mucinous adenomas are relatively asymptomatic and are found incidentally at abdominal imaging or, less likely, at physical examination as a palpable mass. Symptomatic manifestations from superinfection of a mucocele can be clinically indistinguishable from nontumoral acute appendicitis. However, mucinous neoplasms are less likely to manifest with acute appendicitis than are most other appendiceal neoplasms (Pickhardt et al. 2002a),

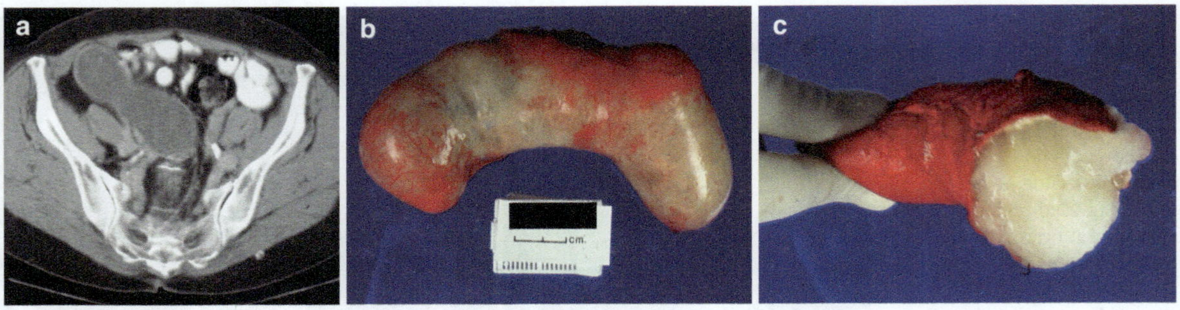

Fig. 3 Appendiceal mucocele from mucinous adenoma. Contrast-enhanced CT image (**a**) shows a large mucocele. Photographs of the uncut (**b**) and cut (**c**) gross specimen show the morphology and the intraluminal mucin

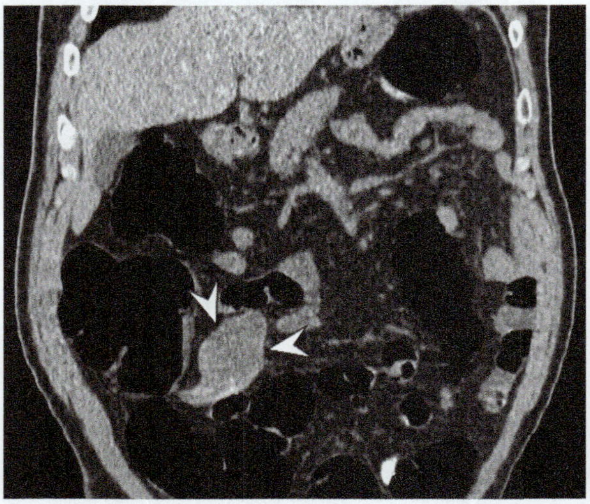

Fig. 4 Appendiceal mucinous adenoma detected incidentally at screening CT colonography. Coronal CT image from screening colonography shows bulbous distention of the appendix (*arrowheads*) with low-attenuation material. Note how the base of the appendix tapers to normal caliber, rendering the luminal appearance normal

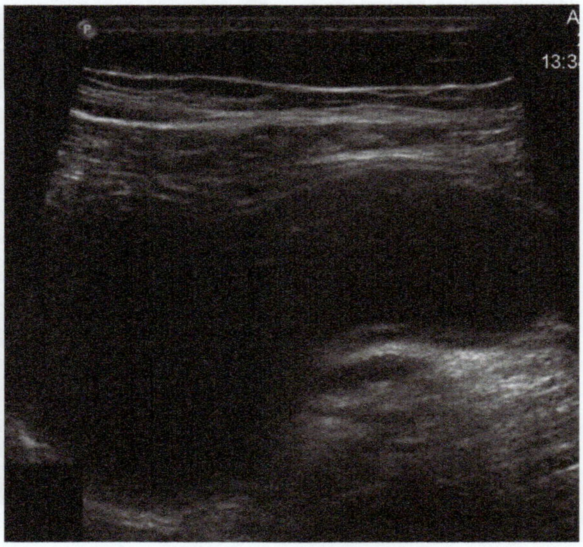

Fig. 5 Sonographic appearance of a mucocele of the appendix. US image of the right lower abdomen shows a non-compressible drumstick-shaped cystic structure containing diffuse low-level echoes

which may be related to the fact that mucoceles result from chronic luminal obstruction, such that acute presentation of these lesions generally requires superinfection. Other symptomatic manifestations include intussusception, torsion, and right ureteral obstruction (Deans and Spence 1995; Hebert and Pickhardt 2007; Pickhardt et al. 2003).

2.1.1.2 Mucinous Adenocarcinoma

Unlike mucinous adenomas, the majority of mucinous adenocarcinomas produce symptoms that lead to their eventual diagnosis (Deans and Spence 1995; Rutledge and Alexander 1992). Clinical manifestations may have any of the causes listed previously for benign neoplastic mucoceles, but malignancy-related causes such as direct invasion of an adjacent organ or increasing abdominal girth from tumor extension into the peritoneal cavity (pseudomyxoma peritonei) (Carr and Sobin 1996; Hinson and Ambrose 1998).

When used in an unqualified manner, the term pseudomyxoma peritonei is fraught with ambiguity (Pickhardt et al. 2003; Carr and Sobin 1996). It generally describes intraperitoneal accumulation of gelatinous material from mucin-producing cells, typically as a diffuse process, but is sometimes used to describe localized collections of acellular mucin from rupture of a benign mucocele. However, the diffuse

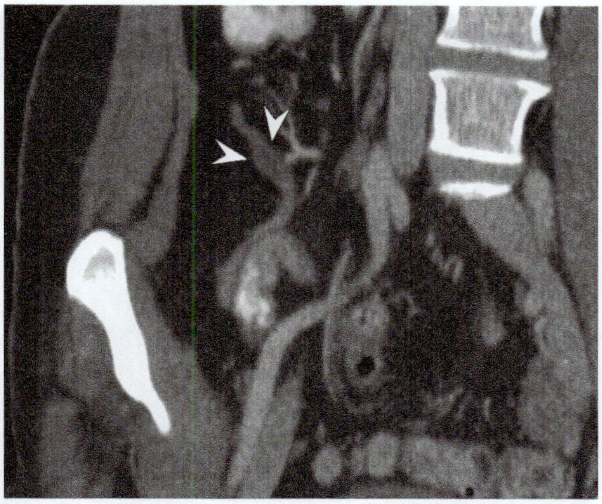

Fig. 6 Small incidental mucocele from mucinous adenoma. Curved reformatted CT image shows mild fusiform dilation of the appendix (*arrowheads*), which measured up to 9 mm in diameter. Subtle central low attenuation is present. Benign mucinous cystadenoma was confirmed at appendectomy

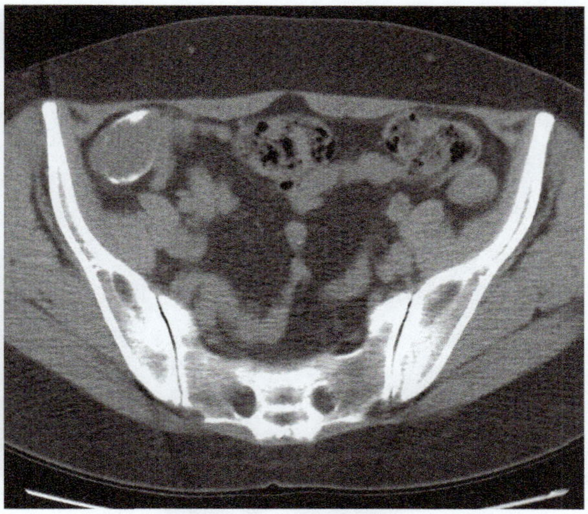

Fig. 7 Mural calcification of incidental appendiceal mucocele. Noncontrast CT image shows a cystic lesion in the right lower quadrant in the expected location of the appendix with coarse curvilinear mural calcification, which was confirmed to be a benign mucinous adenoma of the appendix

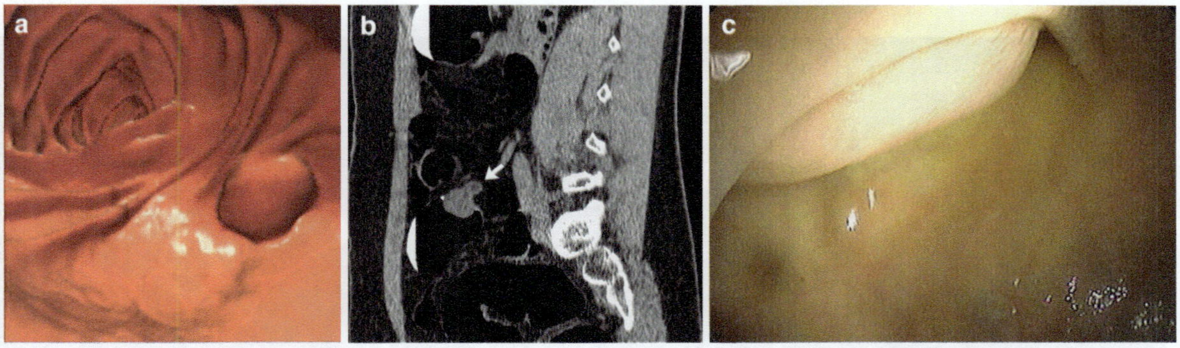

Fig. 8 Asymptomatic appendiceal mucocele from mucinous adenoma detected at screening CT colonography. 3D endoluminal (**a**) and 2D sagittal (**b**) images from screening CT colonography show a cystic appendiceal mass at the base of the cecum (*arrow*) which protrudes into the cecal lumen. Subsequent endoscopic image (**c**) shows only the endoluminal mass effect. The endoscopic impression was "inverted appendiceal stump". In this case, the cross-sectional imaging findings and lack of appendectomy history led to further intervention. An asymptomatic appendiceal mucocele from mucinous adenoma was confirmed at subsequent surgery

form involves proliferation of viable neoplastic cells throughout the peritoneum and implies a malignant cause (Carr and Sobin 1996). Some investigators posit that nearly all true cases of pseudomyxoma peritonei are appendiceal in origin and that associated ovarian lesions represent metastatic disease, although this is controversial (Carr and Sobin 1996; Hinson and Ambrose 1998). The clinical course of diffuse pseudomyxoma peritonei is typically insidious and unrelenting, with a 5 year survival rate approaching 65% (Carr and Sobin 1996). Treatment usually consists of surgical debulking with appendectomy, omentectomy, and, in women, bilateral oophorectomy. Intraperitoneal chemotherapy may be of benefit to some patients (Hinson and Ambrose 1998).

2.1.2 Imaging Features

The imaging diagnosis of mucinous neoplasms hinges primarily on detection of the resulting mucocele. Abdominal radiography may suggest a soft-tissue

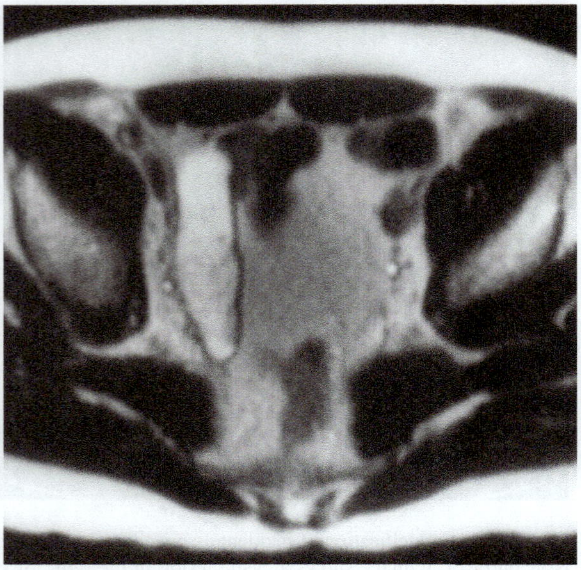

Fig. 9 MR appearance of a benign mucocele. T2-weighted MR image through the pelvis shows a high signal intensity blind-ending lesion consistent with an appendiceal mucocele, which was confirmed to be a benign mucinous adenoma

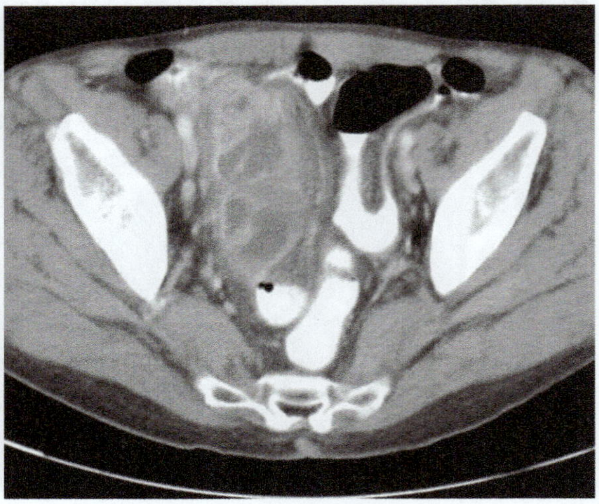

Fig. 10 Mucinous cystadenocarcinoma. Contrast-enhanced axial CT image shows a complex mixed attenuation lesion in the right lower quadrant with both solid and cystic components and areas of irregular wall thickening, which was confirmed to be a mucinous adenocarcinoma

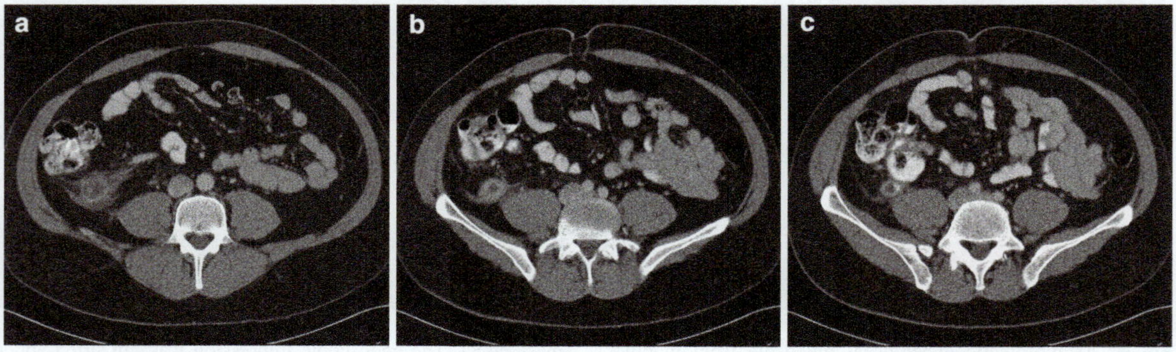

Fig. 11 Mucinous adenocarcinoma presenting as acute appendicitis. Contrast-enhanced axial CT images show a thick-walled dilated appendix with periappendiceal infiltration. These findings could be seen with severe non-neoplastic appendicitis but this lesion was confirmed to be a mucinous adenocarcinoma

mass in the right lower quadrant, but sensitivity and specificity are increased when calcification is identified. Curvilinear mural calcification is highly suggestive of the diagnosis but is identifiable at radiography in only a minority of cases (Dachman et al. 1985; Madwed et al. 1992). At luminal contrast examination, mucoceles cause a smooth impression on the medial aspect of the cecum, a finding that suggests an extramucosal or extrinsic process (Fig. 2). However, the typical location of the filling defect will usually favor an appendiceal process. Analogous findings are seen at endoscopy but, as with contrast enema examination, the overall size and morphologic features cannot be assessed (Fig. 2). Cross-sectional imaging (CT, ultrasonography [US], or magnetic resonance [MR] imaging) is useful for evaluating the full extent of the lesion in this setting (Figs. 2 and 3). Furthermore, some mucoceles will spare the base of the appendix (Fig. 4) and therefore not be visible at all at strictly luminal examinations.

At US, an ovoid cystic mass with or without acoustic shadowing from dystrophic mural calcifications is

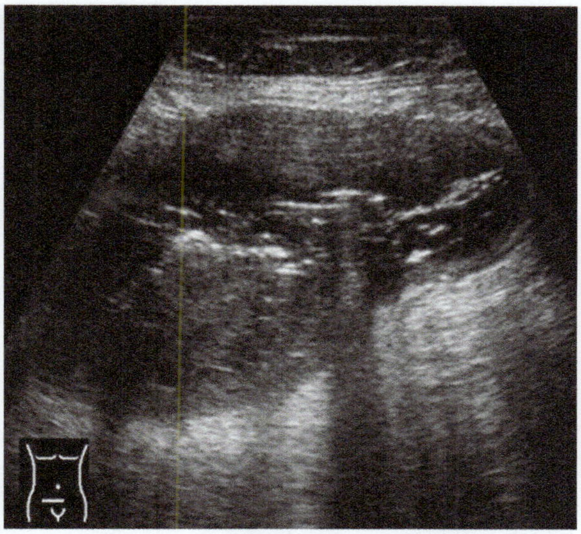

Fig. 12 Mucinous adenocarcinoma with superinfection presenting as appendicitis. Transabdominal US image at the right lower quadrant shows a complex cystic mass with scattered internal echogenic foci with shadowing due to intraluminal gas bubbles from superinfection of a mucinous adenocarcinoma

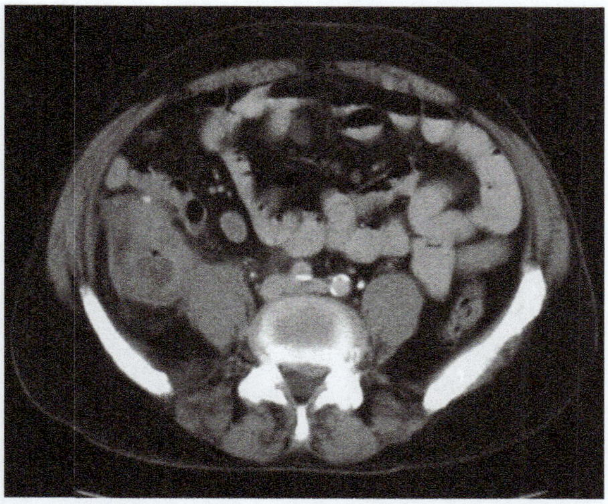

Fig. 13 Mucinous adenoma with superinfection presenting as appendicitis. Contrast-enhanced CT image shows a complex soft-tissue lesion in the right lower quadrant with atypical features including marked irregular wall thickening and stranding in the surrounding fat suggestive of malignancy. At pathology this lesion was found to be a benign mucinous adenoma with superinfection

characteristic of mucoceles from mucinous neoplasms (Fig. 5) (Kim et al. 1998). The intraluminal echotexture can have a variable appearance, but an anechoic appearance or low-level internal echoes are most typical. A pear-shaped or chicken drumstick appearance may be appreciated in some cases due to lesser dilatation of a portion of the appendix (Fig. 5). Identification of a separate right ovary in women is crucial for excluding processes such as cystic ovarian neoplasm or tubo-ovarian abscess. The differential diagnosis might also include periappendiceal abscess, enteric duplication cyst, mesenteric cyst, and hydrosalpinx.

CT is ideal for evaluating mucoceles of the appendix and has certain advantages over other imaging modalities. The anatomic relationship between the elongated cystic mass and the cecum is usually more apparent on CT than at US, and CT is more sensitive than conventional radiography in detecting smaller tumors (Fig. 6) and mural calcification (Fig. 7). With the increasing utilization of cross-sectional imaging, incidental detection of asymptomatic mucoceles is on the rise (Figs. 6–8). Inadequate opacification of the ileocecal region with positive enteric contrast material has been cited in the past as a cause of false-positive and false-negative findings at CT (Madwed et al. 1992). MR imaging recapitulates the CT finding of a cystic mass (Fig. 9), but calcification will be less apparent (Koga 1995). Atypical cross-sectional imaging features may reflect a secondary complication, malignancy, or an unusual pathologic variation. Soft-tissue thickening and irregularity of the mucocele wall and surrounding fat are nonspecific findings that suggest malignancy (mucinous adenocarcinoma), secondary inflammation, or both (Figs. 10, 11, 12, 13) (Lim et al. 1999). Intraluminal gas bubbles or an air–fluid level within a mucocele are generally diagnostic for superinfection, which can complicate both benign and malignant mucoceles (Figs. 12 and 13).

Myxoglobulosis is a rare mucocele variant consisting of multiple intraluminal pearly spherules that may be apparent at radiography or CT if they are calcified (Gonzalez et al. 1988). Intussusception into the colon is an uncommon but well-recognized manifestation of appendiceal mucoceles. Imaging findings suggestive of intussusception may be apparent on abdominal radiography (Fig. 14). Intussusception and the lead mass can be identified at contrast enema (Fig. 15) or US (Fig. 16) examination, but intussusception related to

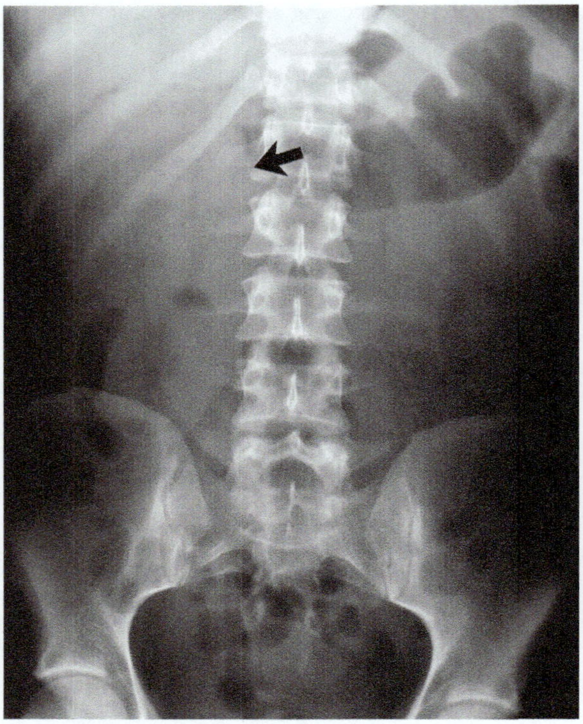

Fig. 14 Intussusception of an appendiceal mucocele at abdominal radiography. Abdominal radiograph shows abrupt cut-off of the transverse colon air column (*arrow*), a finding that suggests intussusception. Intussusception of an appendiceal mucocele was confirmed at CT (*not shown*) and surgery

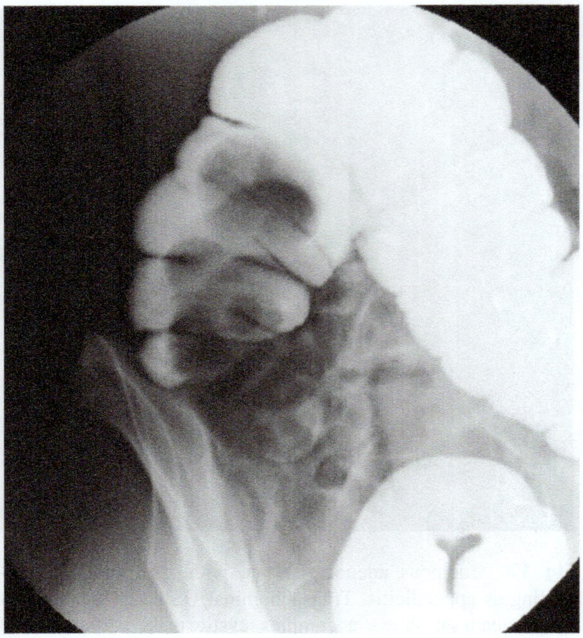

Fig. 15 Intussusception of an appendiceal mucocele at contrast enema. Single image from a contrast enema examination shows a well-defined filling defect in the ascending colon, including a rounded lead mass. Intussusception of an appendiceal mucocele was confirmed at CT (*not shown*) and surgery

the cystic lead mass is most readily identifiable at CT (Fig. 16). Mucocele torsion is a rare complication but one that can also be recognized on CT (Fig. 17). Genitourinary symptoms such as right ureteral obstruction or bladder compromise may result in an atypical genitourinary manifestation.

Finally, a substantial subset of patients with mucinous cystadenocarcinoma will present with slowly increasing abdominal girth from pseudomyxoma peritonei caused by prior mucocele rupture or transmural extension. Typical imaging features, especially with more long-standing disease, include widespread heterogeneous peritoneal locules that displace and distort the hollow viscera and produce a scalloping effect on the solid organs (Fig. 18) (Walensky et al. 1996). Linear or punctuate septal calcifications may be apparent at CT (Figs. 18 and 19). In most cases of pseudomyxoma, the primary appendiceal tumor will either not be clearly identifiable on imaging or will already be surgically absent, but occasionally the primary tumor or at least a remnant of it will still be apparent (Figs. 19, 20, 21). Rarely, the extraluminal mucinous collection will extend into retroperitoneal fascial planes instead of the peritoneal spaces, giving rise to "pseudomyxoma retroperitonei" (Fig. 21).

2.2 Colonic-Type (Non-Mucinous) Epithelial Neoplasms

The typical non-mucinous adenomas and adenocarcinomas that are characteristic of colorectal neoplasia rarely occur in the appendix. In one large pathology series, the relative frequency of colonic-type appendiceal neoplasms was 2 and 7% among adenomas and adenocarcinomas, respectively; the remaining tumors were mucinous (Carr et al. 1995). For malignant lesions, other studies have reported up to a 2:1 ratio of mucinous to colonic-type adenocarcinomas (Rutledge and Alexander 1992). The recent SEER data suggest an even higher frequency of colonic-type adenocarcinoma, although mucinous adenocarcinomas were still more common among

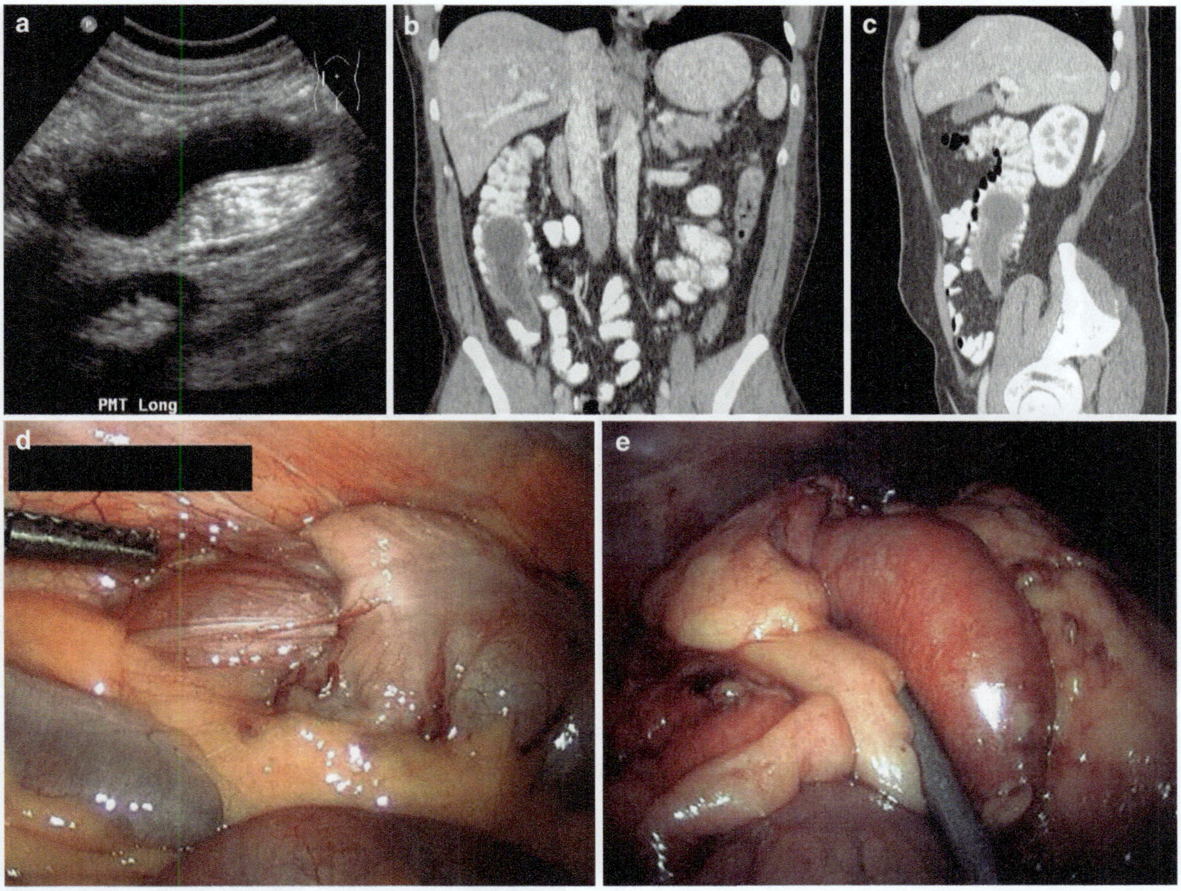

Fig. 16 Intussusception of an appendiceal mucocele at US and CT. Transabdominal longitudinal US image (**a**) shows a cystic lesion with a "chicken drumstick" appearance. The right kidney is seen in the inferior aspect of the image. Contrast-enhanced curved reformatted coronal (**b**) and sagittal (**c**) CT images confirm an appendiceal mucocele which has intussuscepted into the ascending colon. Photographs from laparoscopy show the intussusception (**d**) and offending mucocele (**e**)

the 2,514 cases of appendiceal malignancies reported (McGory et al. 2005).

Colonic-type (non-mucinous) adenocarcinomas of the appendix are defined as malignant tumors in which less than 50% of the lesion is composed of mucin (Carr et al. 1995). These lesions are rare within the appendix and appear as cuboidal or columnar neoplastic cells that form infiltrating glands resembling the typical adenocarcinomas of the colon and rectum (Carr et al. 1995). These non-mucinous tumors are typically more focal in nature than mucinous neoplasms and tend not to form mucoceles.

2.2.1 Clinical Presentation

Unlike mucinous neoplasms, most colonic-type epithelial neoplasms manifest clinically as acute appendicitis related to luminal obstruction (Pickhardt et al. 2002a; Rutledge and Alexander 1992). The mean age of diagnosis for these tumors is 63 years (McGory et al. 2005). Because the incidence of acute inflammatory appendicitis decreases with age, suspicion for an appendiceal colonic-type adenocarcinoma should increase in those presenting with symptoms of acute appendicitis who are over age 60. In a study of patients presenting with acute appendicitis (Todd et al. 2004), 34 of 131 cases were age >60. Of these 34 patients, 8 (24%) were found to have an appendiceal tumor, all but one of which was colonic-type adenocarcinoma or classified as a mixed "adenocarcinoid" variant. Of the 97 patients <60 years, only a single appendiceal tumor was diagnosed. Although the presence of right lower quadrant pain and fever did not differ between those with tumor and those without, abnormally long duration of symptoms

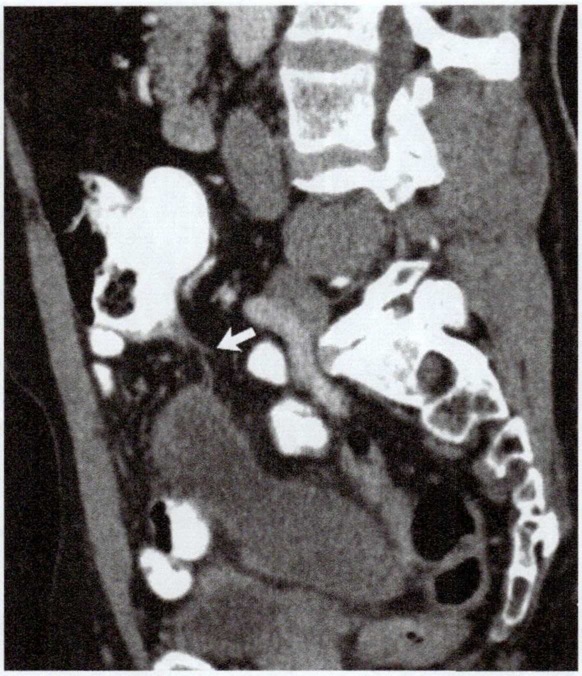

Fig. 17 Symptomatic torsion of an appendiceal mucocele. Curved reformatted sagittal image from contrast-enhanced CT shows a large appendiceal mucocele which has torsed or twisted. Note the narrowing and twisting at the base of the appendix (*arrow*) and stranding within the surrounding fat

(>2 days) and abnormally low hematocrit (<38%) were present in the majority of cancers in the study. In our experience, a neoplastic cause of appendicitis is quite rare, even among the elderly.

2.2.2 Imaging Features

Relatively little information exists on the imaging appearance of colonic-type neoplasms of the appendix. In our experience, the majority of cases detected at imaging will be malignant (adenocarcinoma), usually in the setting of suspected appendicitis in an older individual as discussed above (Pickhardt et al. 2002a; Todd et al. 2004). At CT, a focal or diffuse soft-tissue mass that involves the appendix without dominant mucocele formation is most characteristic (Figs. 22 and 23), a finding that underscores the dissimilarity between mucinous and non-mucinous neoplasms. A subtle infiltrative appendiceal mass with surrounding periappendiceal infiltration may be mistaken for nontumoral appendicitis (Fig. 22). Direct invasion of adjacent organs may manifest as clinical symptoms in some cases (Fig. 24). We have also detected asymptomatic non-mucinous adenocarcinomas in patients undergoing CT colonography screening (Fig. 25).

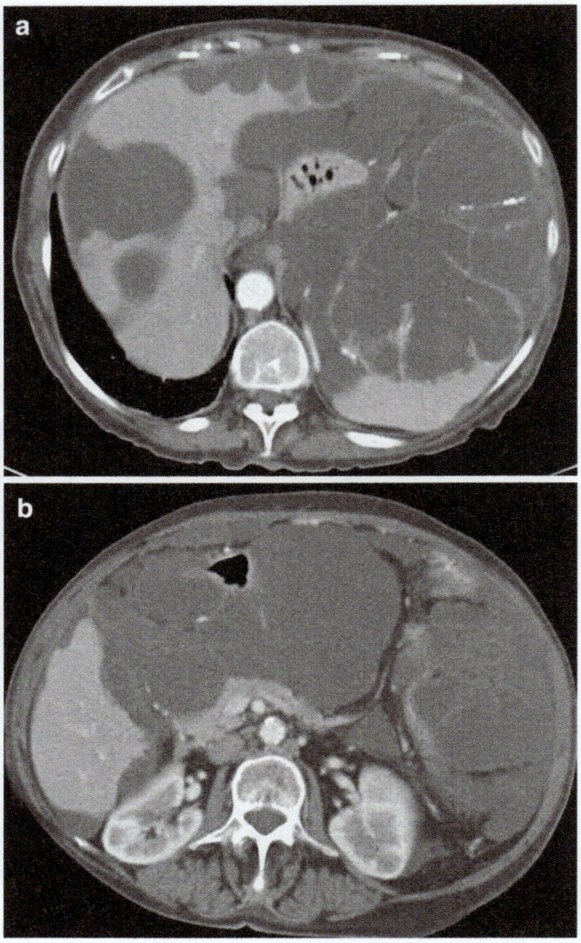

Fig. 18 Pseudomyxoma peritonei from mucinous adenocarcinoma of the appendix. Contrast-enhanced axial CT images (**a**) and (**b**) show extensive multiloculated low-attenuation material throughout the peritoneum with multiple septations and scattered septal calcifications. There is scalloping of adjacent solid organs and mass effect without evidence of bowel obstruction. Patient had a 20 year history of pseudomyxoma peritonei from mucinous appendiceal neoplasm

2.3 Signet Ring

A third histologic type of epithelial appendiceal cancer is the signet ring cell adenocarcinoma. This tumor type is far less common than either the mucinous or the typical non-mucinous colonic-type,

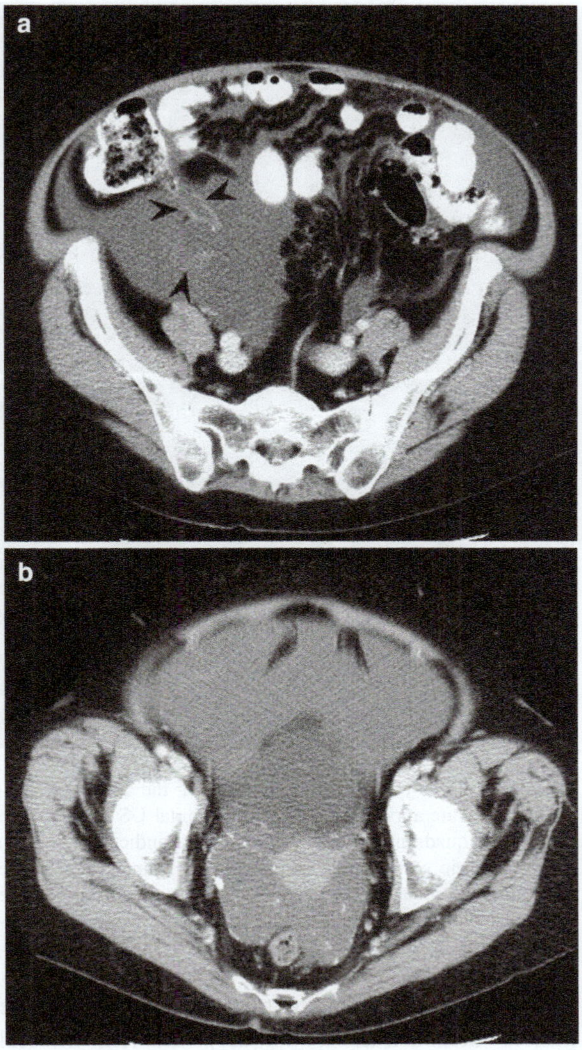

Fig. 19 Pseudomyxoma peritonei from mucinous adenocarcinoma of the appendix. Contrast-enhanced axial CT images (**a**) and (**b**) show peritoneal "fluid" in the abdomen and pelvis with scattered septal calcifications at the inferior peritoneal reflections. This was detected incidentally and proved to be mucinous/myxoid material due to pseudomyxoma peritonei from a ruptured mucinous adenocarcinoma of the appendix, which is subtly noted in the right lower quadrant (*arrowheads*)

accounting for only 4% of cases of malignant appendiceal neoplasms in the SEER database, and is associated with a poor prognosis (McCusker et al. 2002; McGory et al. 2005). The 5 year survival rate is the lowest of the malignant appendiceal neoplasms at 18% (5 year survival rates with mucinous and colonic-type being 46 and 42%, respectively) and it is more likely than not to show distant metastatic

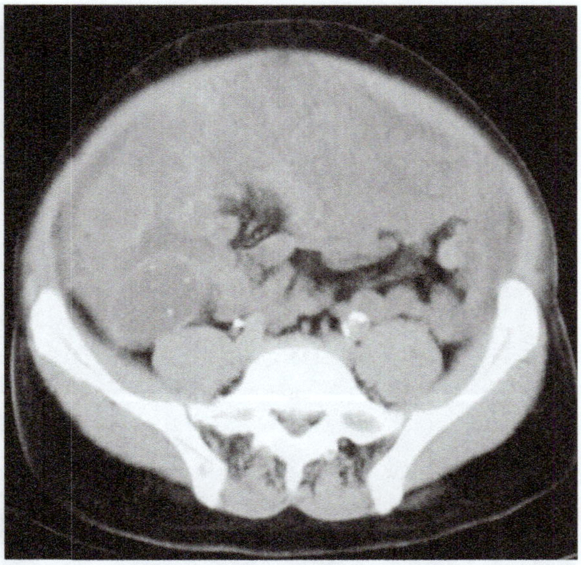

Fig. 20 Pseudomyxoma peritonei from mucinous adenocarcinoma of the appendix. CT image shows complex material filling the peritoneal cavity. The primary appendiceal mucocele (mucinous adenocarcinoma) remains apparent in the right lower quadrant, with punctuate luminal calcifications that may represent limited myxoglobulosis

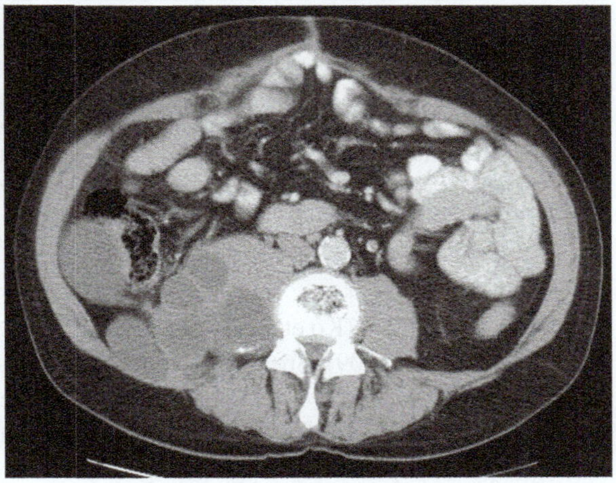

Fig. 21 Psuedomyxoma retroperitonei from mucinous adenocarcinoma of the appendix. Contrast-enhanced axial CT image shows multicystic extension along the right retroperitoneal fascial planes with septal calcifications from pseudomyxoma retroperitonei due to primary mucinous adenocarcinoma. The primary tumor remains apparent on this image

disease at presentation (60%) (McGory et al. 2005). Clinical presentation has been reported to include gradually increasing abdominal distention, abdominal pain and emesis, and colonic obstruction secondary to

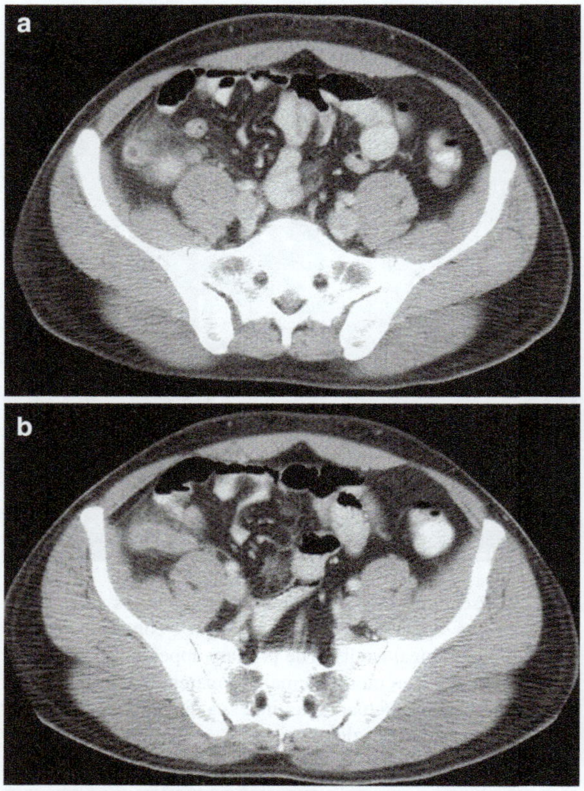

Fig. 22 Colonic-type adenocarcinoma of the appendix presenting as acute appendicitis. Contrast-enhanced CT images (**a**) and (**b**) show the typical changes of acute appendicitis including a dilated, thick-walled appendix and stranding within the surrounding fat. Note however the increased soft-tissue at the distal appendix. Colonic-type adenocarcinoma with periappendiceal infiltration was confirmed at pathology

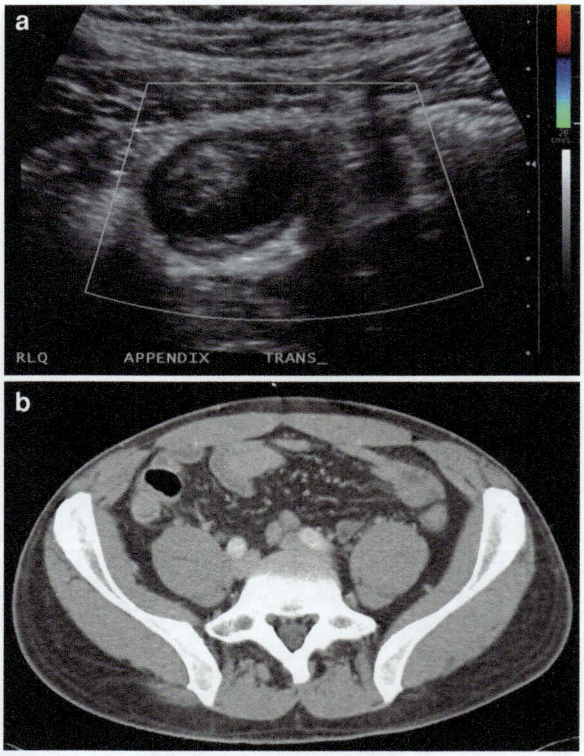

Fig. 23 Colonic-type adenocarcinoma of the appendix presenting as acute appendicitis. Transabdominal US image at the right lower quadrant (**a**) shows a dilated appendiceal base with focal eccentric soft-tissue mass. Contrast-enhanced CT image (**b**) confirms a focal eccentric soft-tissue mass at the base of the appendix causing obstructive appendicitis, which was confirmed to be colonic-type adenocarcinoma

lower abdominal mass (Ko et al. 2008; Mastoraki et al. 2010; Suzuki et al. 2009). Specific imaging characteristics have not been well established due to its rare nature. In our experience, this tumor demonstrates an infiltrative growth pattern at imaging (Fig. 26).

3 Carcinoid Tumor

3.1 Classic Carcinoid

Classic carcinoid tumors of the appendix derive from subepithelial neuroendocrine cells and may represent up to 80% of all appendiceal neoplasms (Deans and Spence 1995; Sandor and Modlin 1998). It remains unclear why the appendix is the most common site for gastrointestinal carcinoid tumors and why these tumors demonstrate a uniquely indolent clinical course in this location (5 year-survival rate >90%) compared with carcinoid tumors elsewhere along the gastrointestinal tract. Although all carcinoid tumors are considered potentially malignant, metastatic disease and carcinoid syndrome with an appendiceal primary site are exceedingly rare. Studies have shown that tumor size correlates well with prognosis and that simple appendectomy is sufficient for most carcinoid tumors less than 1.5–2.0 cm in size (Moertel et al. 1987). Current treatment recommendations state that for carcinoid tumors between 1 and 2 cm, appendectomy may be performed if the tumor is at the tip or mid-appendix, whereas right hemicolectomy should be performed for tumors at the base, if there is mesoappendiceal invasion, or in the presence of metastatic disease (McGory et al. 2005). Tumors greater than 2 cm should be considered malignant until

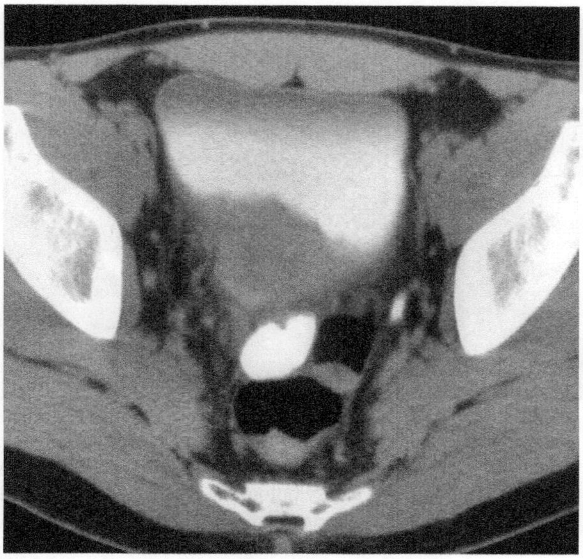

Fig. 24 Direct bladder invasion by colonic-type adenocarcinoma of the appendix. Contrast-enhanced CT image shows an irregular eccentric soft-tissue mass involving the bladder base related to direct invasion from a colonic-type adenocarcinoma of the appendix

proven otherwise and generally require right hemicolectomy (Deans and Spence 1995; McGory et al. 2005; Moertel et al. 1987).

The histologic features of classic carcinoid tumors are small cells with uniform round nuclei that contain stippled chromatin but are without prominent nucleoli. There is usually no significant mitotic activity, cytologic atypia, or nuclear pleomorphism (Buck and Sobin 1990).

3.1.1 Clinical Presentation

Unlike with most other primary appendiceal neoplasms, the discovery of an appendiceal carcinoid tumor at surgery is most often serendipitous. Even in the setting of acute appendicitis, a coexisting carcinoid tumor is the obstructing cause in only 25% of cases, reflecting the fact that over 70% are found in the distal third of the appendix (away from the base) and are less than 1 cm in size (Deans and Spence 1995; Moertel et al. 1987).

3.1.2 Imaging Findings

The relative paucity of imaging findings in the majority of appendiceal carcinoid tumors reflects the typical small size, confinement to the distal appendix, and low complication rate of these tumors (Fig. 27). A symptomatic obstructing carcinoid tumor near the base of the appendix will usually manifest both clinically and at imaging as appendicitis (Fig. 28); the tumor itself may not always be appreciated, even retrospectively (Hermans et al. 1993). Mucocele formation may also occur but is a very rare finding (Buck and Sobin 1990). The tumor itself may be discernible on imaging studies when it is of sufficient size or demonstrates calcification, which may mimic a non-tumoral appendicolith (Fig. 28).

Appendiceal carcinoid tumors sometimes demonstrate a diffuse infiltrative pattern that manifests as diffuse mural thickening at cross-sectional imaging (Fig. 29). Although rare, metastatic disease has CT features similar to those of small bowel carcinoid tumors, with mesenteric extension toward the root of the mesentery characteristic (Fig. 29).

3.2 Tubular Carcinoid

Tubular carcinoid tumor is a rare variant of the classic carcinoid tumor. However, the distinction between the two is purely histologic, as their clinical behavior is quite similar (Carr and Sobin 1996). At histologic analysis, tubular carcinoids are characterized by small, uniform groups of cells that form tubular structures within an abundant stroma (Carr and Sobin 1996). These lesions can generally be treated as classic carcinoid tumors.

3.2.1 Clinical Presentation

Tubular carcinoid tumors are usually seen in younger patients and tend to be small and localized to the appendiceal tip. They rarely metastasize and have a favorable prognosis.

3.2.2 Imaging Findings

The imaging findings in tubular carcinoid are not well documented. However, due to the aforementioned features, these tumors should generally resemble small classic carcinoid tumors.

3.3 Goblet Cell Carcinoid

Goblet cell carcinoid tumors are unusual tumors that are nearly exclusive to the appendix and likely represent an entity that is intermediate between

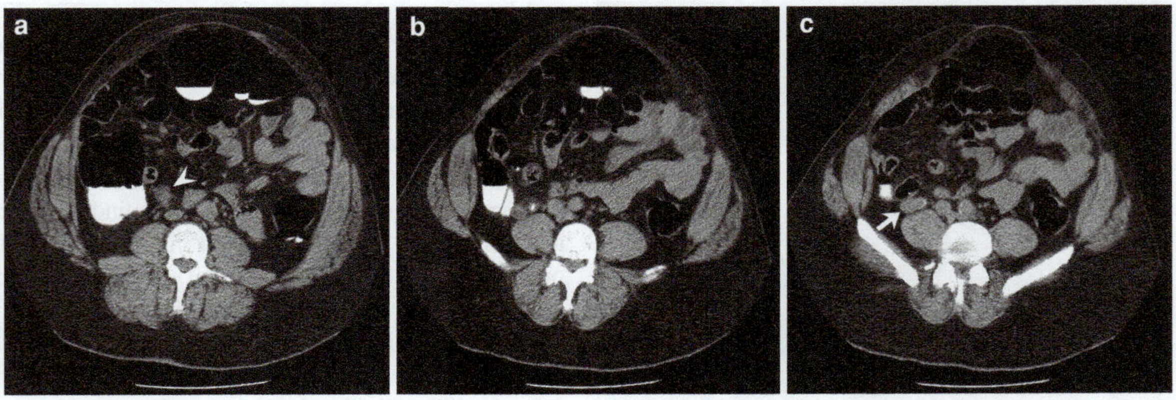

Fig. 25 Asymptomatic colonic-type adenocarcinoma of the appendix detected at CT colonography screening. CT images from screening CT colonography show (**a**) ileocecal lymphadenopathy (*arrowhead*), (**b**) a patent contrast-filled proximal appendiceal lumen with dilated and obstructed tip, and (**c**) an expansile polypoid soft-tissue lesion in the mid-appendix (*arrow*). This lesion was asymptomatic and confirmed to be a colonic-type adenocarcinoma

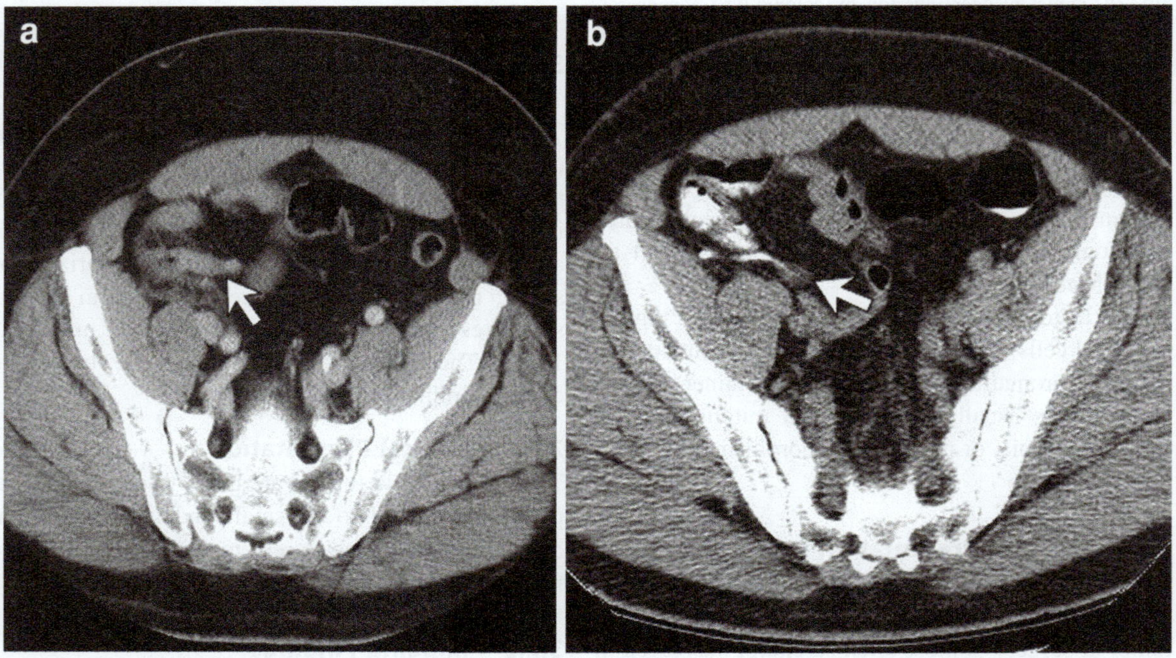

Fig. 26 Signet ring adenocarcinoma of the appendix presenting with acute appendicitis. Contrast-enhanced axial CT image (**a**) shows diffusely thickened appendix (*arrow*) with periappendiceal soft-tissue infiltration. At laparoscopic appendectomy and subsequent right hemicolectomy, a primary appendiceal signet ring adenocarcinoma with mesenteric tumor infiltration was identified. Image from screening CT colonography (**b**) of same patient performed 5 yrs earlier shows only subtle thickening at the tip of the contrast-filled appendix (*arrow*)

adenocarcinoma and classic carcinoid tumor (Carr and Sobin 1996). The terms *adenocarcinoid* and *goblet cell carcinoid* have been used interchangeably in the past. However, the former term has been omitted from the World Health Organization (WHO) classification scheme because it also applies to tubular carcinoid tumors, which are clinically and pathologically distinct. Goblet cell carcinoid tumors are best considered a low-grade malignancy, such that most patients will undergo right hemicolectomy. At gross

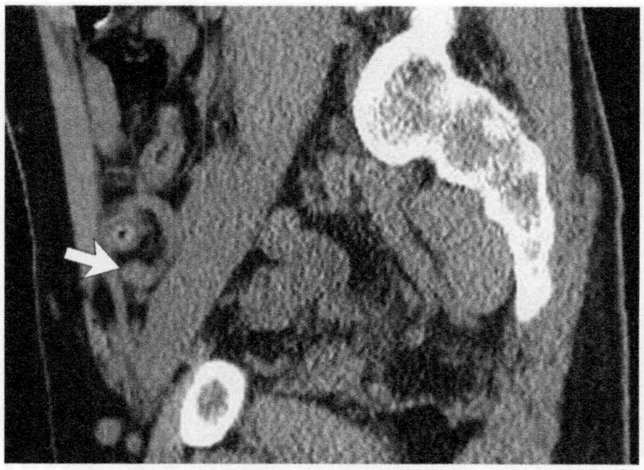

Fig. 27 Incidental sub-cm carcinoid tumor at the appendiceal tip. Sagittal CT image shows bulbous enlargement at the tip of the appendix (*arrow*), which was asymptomatic and proved to be a small carcinoid tumor at surgical resection

pathologic examination, goblet cell carcinoid tumors are infiltrative and typically involve the entire appendix circumferentially. If no discrete tumor nodules or mass is evident, the diagnosis can often be made only at microscopic examination. Not infrequently, frank mucinous adenocarcinoma will develop within a goblet cell carcinoid tumor (Carr et al. 1995). Metastatic spread is most often due to direct peritoneal extension (Carr and Sobin 1996). Histologically, goblet cells are characterized by the accumulation of mucinous secretory granules, which appear as abundant clear mucin-filled cytoplasm (Carr and Sobin 1996). Small groups of these cells in the form of clusters or strands diffusely infiltrate the appendiceal wall, often circumferentially. Smaller number of endocrine cells are present among these clusters of goblet cells and are best demonstrated with immunoexpression of neuroendocrine markers.

3.3.1 Clinical Presentation

In one series of 57 patients with goblet cell carcinoid, 70% presented with right lower quadrant pain mimicking acute appendicitis (Pham et al. 2006). Twenty-five percent had a right lower quadrant or pelvic mass (Pham et al. 2006). The average age at presentation is 52 years (McCusker et al. 2002; McGory et al. 2005), closer to that of adenocarcinoma than typical carcinoid tumors.

3.3.2 Imaging Findings

Cross-sectional imaging findings will typically reflect the infiltrative nature of the tumor, with diffuse mural thickening. The propensity of advanced tumors to metastasize to the ovaries and peritoneum has also been demonstrated at cross-sectional imaging (Fig. 30).

4 Lymphoma

Although the gastrointestinal tract is the most common site for extranodal non-Hodgkin's lymphoma, appendiceal lymphoma is rare (Muller et al. 1997; Tsujimura et al. 2000). Typically, non-Hodgkin's lymphoma of the appendix manifests as diffuse circumferential mural infiltration by monotonous-appearing lymphocytes. In our experience, mantle cell lymphoma and diffuse large B-cell lymphoma are the most common forms (Pickhardt et al. 2002b).

4.1 Clinical Presentation

Although rare, when lymphoma does involve the appendix, it tends to cause symptoms (Pickhardt et al. 2002b). The most common clinical manifestation is acute appendicitis, which may be the first and only indicator of disease. The appendix can become massively enlarged but typically maintains its vermiform appearance (Pickhardt et al. 2002b). To our knowledge, all reported cases of appendiceal lymphoma have proved to be non-Hodgkin's lymphoma.

4.2 Imaging Findings

The existing literature on the imaging appearance of appendiceal lymphoma is mainly limited to case reports (Carpenter 1991; Krepel et al. 1996). In our experience, however, all cases have demonstrated prominent enlargement of the appendix with relative maintenance of its vermiform appearance (Fig. 31) (Pickhardt et al. 2002b). If its blind-ending nature is not appreciated, the abnormal appendix could be mistaken for an abnormal small bowel loop or an extraintestinal process such as lymphadenopathy (Figs. 31 and 32). Diffuse mural thickening is typically hypoechoic at US and has fluid or soft-tissue attenuation at CT (Figs. 31 and 32). The hypoechoic appearance at US may mimic

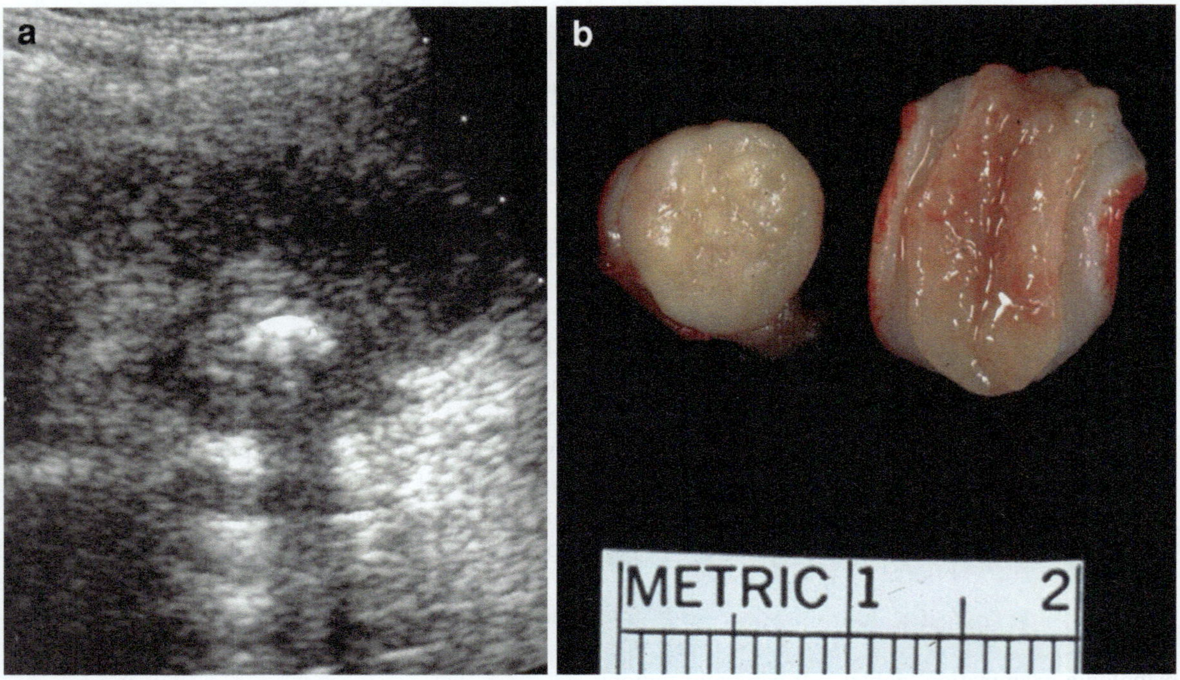

Fig. 28 Carcinoid tumor at appendiceal base presenting with obstructive appendicitis. US image (**a**) shows a shadowing focus of calcification at the appendiceal base with associated wall thickening, which was presumed to represent appendicitis secondary to obstructive appendicolith but found to be a carcinoid tumor at the base of the appendix with intra-tumoral calcifications. Photograph of the gross specimen (**b**) shows the obstructing tumor at left

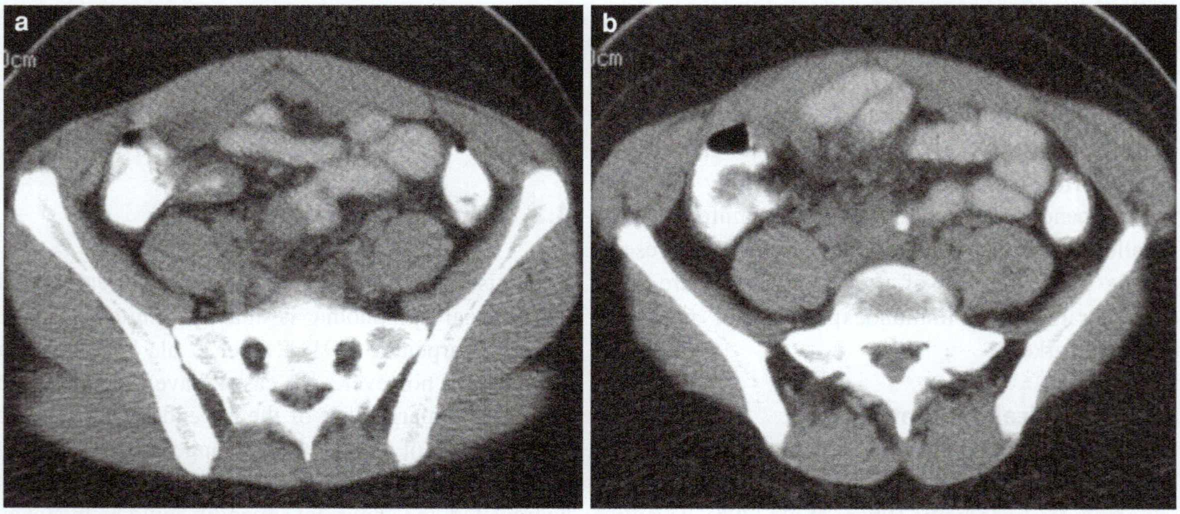

Fig. 29 Metastatic appendiceal carcinoid tumor. Contrast-enhanced CT images show (**a**) diffuse appendiceal wall thickening and (**b**) infiltrative soft-tissue and focus of eccentric calcification located near the root of the mesentery from primary appendiceal carcinoid tumor with mesenteric spread. (Pickhardt et al. 2002a)

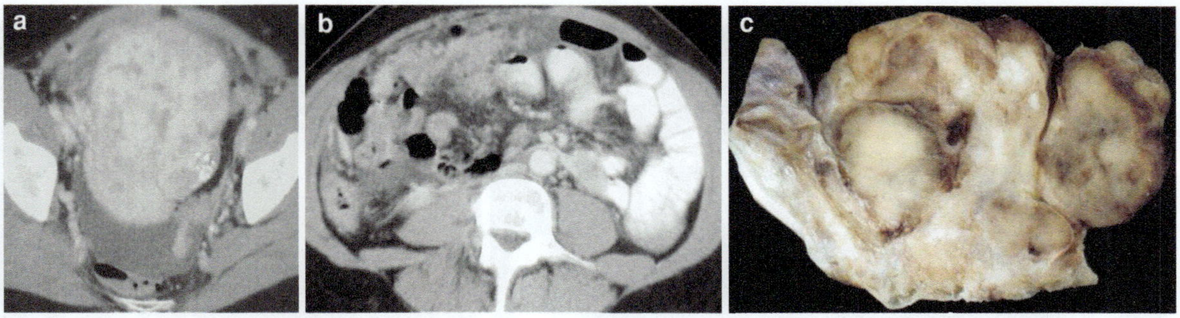

Fig. 30 Metastatic goblet cell carcinoid tumor of the appendix. Contrast-enhanced CT image shows (**a**) a large, heterogeneously enhancing pelvic mass that encases the ovaries, making determination of appendiceal origin difficult. A more cephalad image (**b**) demonstrates intraperitoneal spread. Photograph of gross specimen (**c**) confirmed to be metastatic goblet cell carcinoid of the appendix. (Pickhardt et al. 2002a)

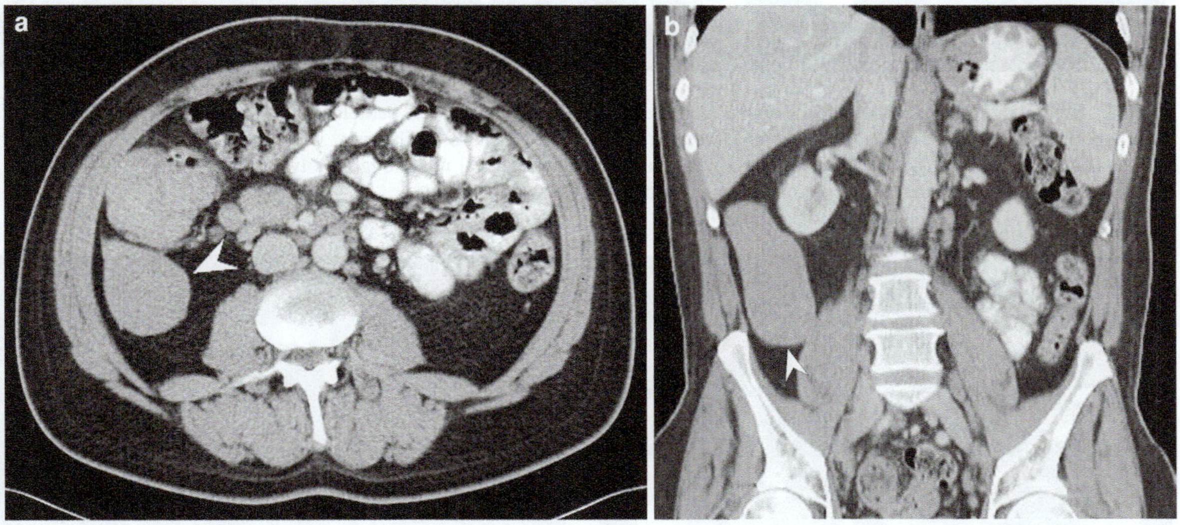

Fig. 31 Non-Hodgkin's lymphoma of the appendix. Contrast-enhanced transverse (**a**) and coronal (**b**) CT images show massive vermiform soft-tissue enlargement of the appendix (*arrowheads*). Mesenteric lymphadenopathy is also noted in this case

the cystic dilatation seen in mucoceles of the appendix. Circumferential mural soft-tissue thickening with preservation or even aneurysmal dilatation of the appendiceal lumen may be an important associated finding that is analogous to small bowel lymphoma (Fig. 33) (Pickhardt et al. 2002b). Coexisting lymphadenopathy is sometimes seen in the setting of appendiceal lymphoma (Fig. 31).

5 Other Neoplasms

Neuroendocrine tumors of the appendix beyond the carcinoid variants described above are rare but include ganglioneuromas and paragangliomas (van Eeden et al. 2000). Diffuse ganglioneuromatosis has been associated with neurofibromatosis type 1 (Lockhart et al. 2000). Mesenchymal tumors of the appendix are rare and are typically benign. Smooth muscle tumors involving the appendix have been reported, with leiomyomas affecting the appendix more often than leiomyosarcomas; the opposite is true for the remainder of the colon (Hatch et al. 2000). Neurofibromas and schwannomas also may rarely arise in the appendix (Collins 1955; Miettinen and Sobin 2001). Recently, however, it has been suggested that gastrointestinal stromal tumors may represent the most common mesenchymal tumor of the appendix (Miettinen and Sobin 2001). It is likely that many of the appendiceal smooth muscle tumors

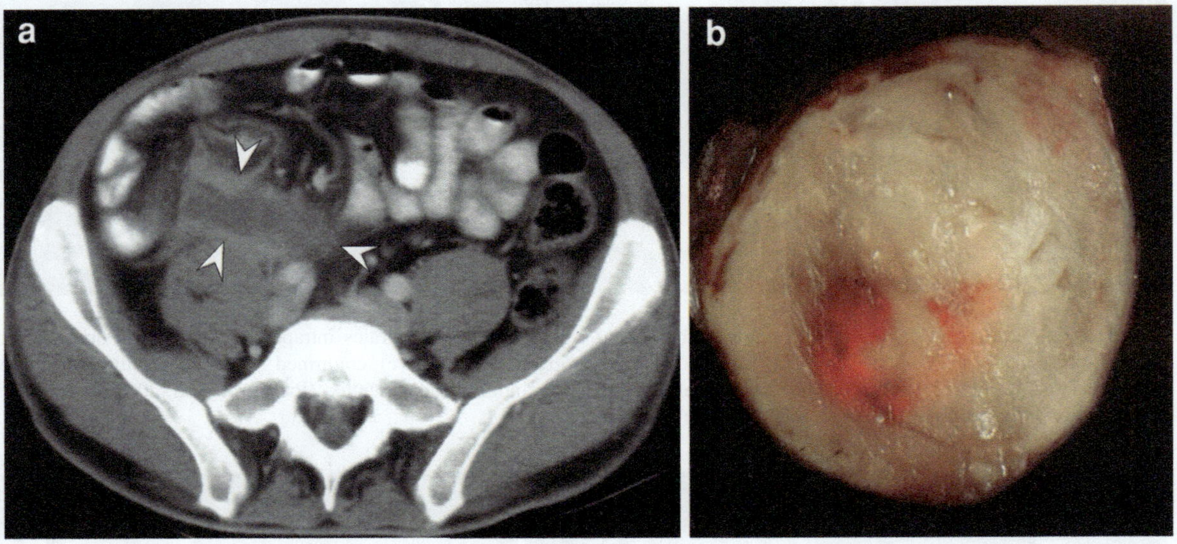

Fig. 32 Non-Hodgkin's lymphoma of the appendix presenting with appendicitis. Contrast-enhanced CT image shows a large tubular low-attenuation structure in the right lower quadrant (*arrowheads*) from circumferential mural lymphomatous infiltration. Gross pathology (**b**) shows enlarged appendix with diffuse mural infiltration, which was confirmed to be primary appendiceal non-Hodgkin's lymphoma

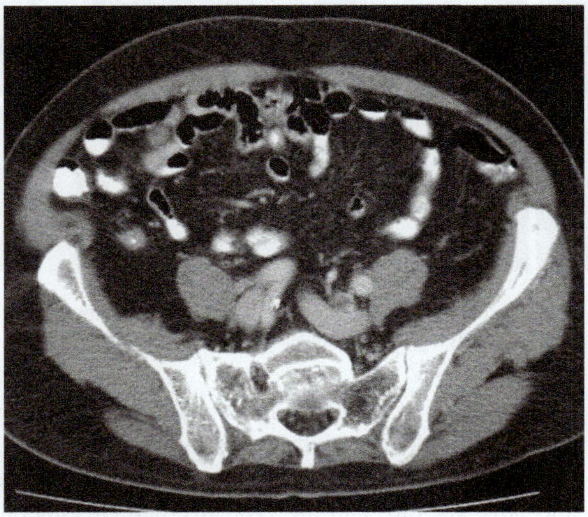

Fig. 33 Mantle cell lymphoma presenting as acute appendicitis. Contrast-enhanced CT image shows circumferential soft-tissue thickening of the appendix with preservation of luminal patency as demonstrated by the oral contrast opacification. There is only minimal periappendiceal infiltration. Diffuse Mantle cell lymphomatous infiltration was confirmed at pathology

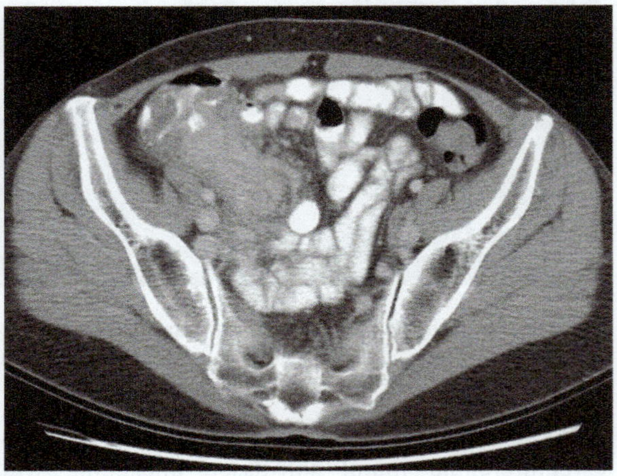

Fig. 34 Chronic appendicitis mimicking an appendiceal neoplasm. Contrast-enhanced CT image acquired preoperatively for suspected appendiceal neoplasm that was initially detected at screening CT colonography (*not shown*) shows an irregular infiltrating soft-tissue mass involving or replacing the appendix. At pathology these changes were all chronic inflammatory and fibrotic rather than neoplastic

reported in older literature would now be reclassified as gastrointestinal stromal tumors at modern immunohistochemical analysis. Kaposi sarcoma of the appendix has been reported in patients with acquired immunodeficiency syndrome (AIDS) (Zebrowska and Walsh 1991). Compared with that of AIDS-related lymphoma, the growth pattern of Kaposi sarcoma is more focal and nodular, but distinguishing between

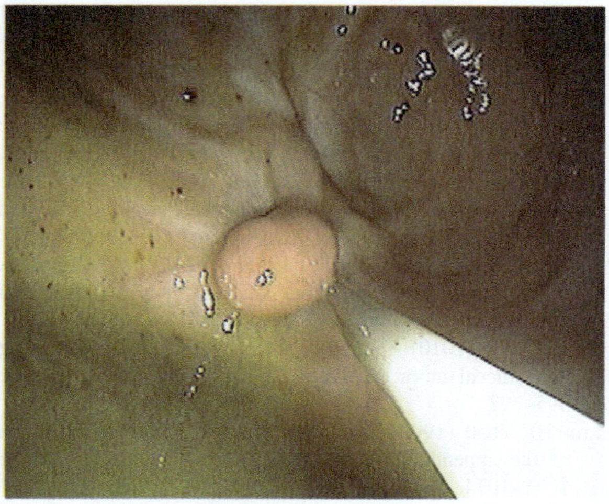

Fig. 35 Inverted appendiceal stump. A polypoid cecal lesion initially seen at screening CT colonography (*not shown*) and favored to be an inverted appendiceal stump was further evaluated with optical colonoscopy, where it was felt to be a true mucosal lesion and snared. Benign inverted appendiceal stump was confirmed at pathology

these two entities at imaging may be difficult. Although extrapulmonary small cell carcinoma is rare (comprising approximately 2.5% of all small cell carcinomas), primary appendiceal small cell carcinoma has been reported, manifesting as massive appendiceal enlargement with metastatic disease (O'Kane et al. 2008). Benign mesothelioma arising from the appendix has also been reported as an incidental finding at surgery (Bansal and Zakhour 2006).

6 Pitfalls in Imaging Suspected Appendiceal Neoplasms

The primary pitfall when there is suspicion of primary appendiceal neoplasm on radiologic or endoscopic imaging is the non-neoplastic mimic. These mimics primarily include complicated appendicitis and fibrous obliteration of the appendix (Fig. 34). An inverted appendiceal stump may mimic a cecal polyp or appendiceal tumor at endoluminal evaluation (Figs. 35 and 36), but the specific location, surgical history, and lack of extracecal appendiceal mass at 2D CT generally allow for exclusion of an appendiceal neoplasm. Patient age, clinical presentation, and surgical history should influence the radiologist's level of suspicion. Appendiceal actinomycosis, a chronic infectious disease more commonly reported to mimic acute appendicitis, has also been found to mimic appendiceal tumor (Lee et al. 2010). Involvement of the appendix by endometriosis may also mimic appendicitis and underlying tumor.

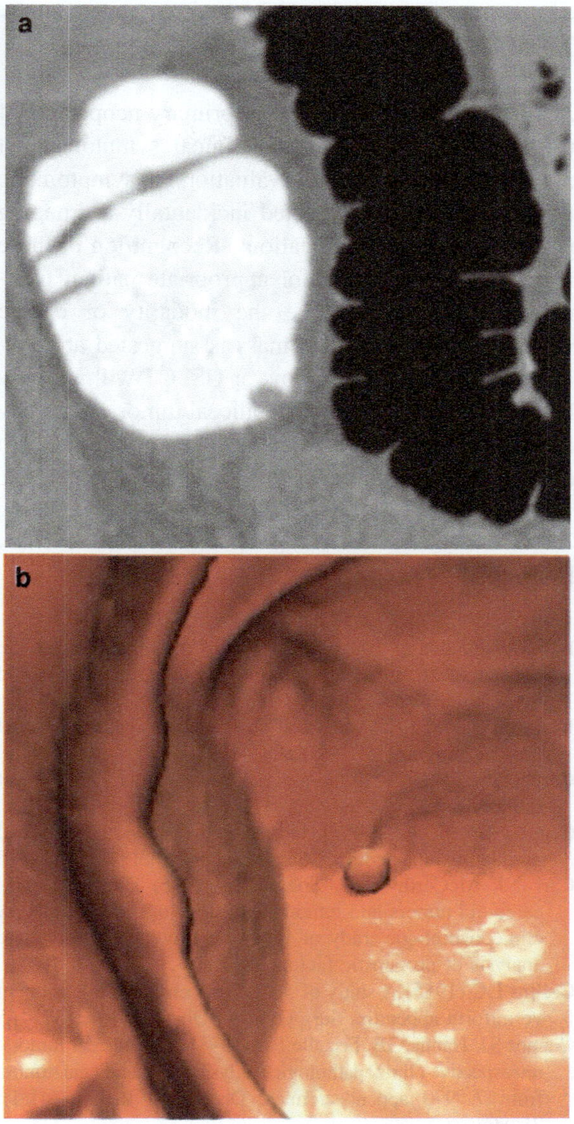

Fig. 36 Inverted appendiceal stump. 2D coronal (**a**) and 3D endoluminal (**b**) images from CT colonography screening show a polypoid cecal lesion at the expected location of the appendiceal orifice, which represents an inverted appendiceal stump

7 Conclusions

Although they are uncommon, primary neoplasms of the appendix often produce clinical symptoms that may lead to imaging evaluation. Asymptomatic tumors may also be detected incidentally at imaging performed for other indications. Recognition of these neoplasms is important for appropriate patient treatment. CT appears to be the modality of choice whenever an appendiceal mass is suggested at physical examination, endoscopy, or US. CT will not only help rule out or confirm appendiceal tumor, but it may also suggest a more specific diagnosis and help effectively direct therapy.

References

Bansal A, Zakhour HD (2006) Benign mesothelioma of the appendix: an incidental finding in a case of sigmoid diverticular disease. J Clin Pathol 59(1):108–110

Buck JL, Sobin LH (1990) Carcinoids of the gastrointestinal tract. Radiographics 10(6):1081–1095

Carpenter BW (1991) Lymphoma of the appendix. Gastrointest Radiol 16(3):256–258

Carr NJ, Sobin LH (1996) Unusual tumors of the appendix and pseudomyxoma peritonei. Semin Diagn Pathol 13(4):314–325

Carr NJ, McCarthy WF, Sobin LH (1995) Epithelial non-carcinoid tumors and tumor-like lesions of the appendix. A clinicopathologic study of 184 patients with a multivariate analysis of prognostic factors. Cancer 75(3):757–768

Collins DC (1955) A study of 50, 000 specimens of the human vermiform appendix. Surg Gynecol Obstet 101(4):437–445

Connor SJ, Hanna GB, Frizelle FA (1998) Appendiceal tumors: retrospective clinicopathologic analysis of appendiceal tumors from 7, 970 appendectomies. Dis Colon Rectum 41(1): 75–80

Dachman AH, Lichtenstein JE, Friedman AC (1985) Mucocele of the appendix and pseudomyxoma peritonei. Am J Roentgenol 144(5):923–929

Deans GT, Spence RA (1995) Neoplastic lesions of the appendix. Br J Surg 82(3):299–306

Gonzalez JE, Hann SE, Trujillo YP (1988) Myxoglobulosis of the appendix. Am J Surg Pathol 12(12):962–966

Hananel N, Powsner E, Wolloch Y (1998) Adenocarcinoma of the appendix: an unusual disease. Eur J Surg 164(11): 859–862

Hatch KF et al (2000) Tumors of the appendix and colon. World J Sur 24(4):430–436

Hebert JJ, Pickhardt PJ (2007) MDCT diagnosis of an appendiceal mucocele with acute torsion. Am J Roentgenol 189(1):W4–W6

Hermans JJ et al (1993) Appendicitis caused by carcinoid tumor. Radiology 188(1):71–72

Hinson FL, Ambrose NS (1998) Pseudomyxoma peritonei. Br J Surg 85(10):1332–1339

Kim SH et al (1998) Mucocele of the appendix: ultrasonographic and CT findings. Abdom Imaging 23(3):292–296

Ko YH et al (2008) Primary signet ring cell carcinoma of the appendix: a rare case report and our 18 year experience. World J Gastroenterol 14(37):5763–5768

Koga H et al (1995) Appendiceal mucocele: sonographic and MR imaging findings. Am J Roentgenol 165(6):1552

Krepel VM, van Erp WF, Vlasveld LT (1996) Lymphoma of the appendix: sonographic findings. Am J Roentgenol 167(1):286

Lee SY et al (2010) Actinomycosis of the appendix mimicking appendiceal tumor: a case report. World J Gastroenterol 16(3): 395–397

Lim HK et al (1999) Primary mucinous cystadenocarcinoma of the appendix: CT findings. Am J Roentgenol 173(4): 1071–1074

Lockhart ME et al (2000) Appendiceal ganglioneuromas and pheochromocytoma in neurofibromatosis type 1. Am J Roentgenol 175(1):132–134

Madwed D, Mindelzun R, Jeffrey RB Jr (1992) Mucocele of the appendix: imaging findings. Am J Roentgenol 159(1):69–72

Mastoraki A et al (2010) A case of signet ring carcinoma of the appendix: dilemmas in differential diagnosis and management. J Gastrointest Cancer 41(2):141–144

McCusker ME et al (2002) Primary malignant neoplasms of the appendix: a population-based study from the surveillance, epidemiology and end-results program, 1973–1998. Cancer 94(12):3307–3312

McGory ML et al (2005) Malignancies of the appendix: beyond case series reports. Dis Colon Rectum 48(12):2264–2271

Miettinen M, Sobin LH (2001) Gastrointestinal stromal tumors in the appendix: a clinicopathologic and immunohistochemical study of four cases. Am J Surg Pathol 25(11):1433–1437

Moertel CG et al (1987) Carcinoid tumor of the appendix: treatment and prognosis. N Engl J Med 317(27):1699–1701

Muller G et al (1997) Leukaemia and lymphoma of the appendix presenting as acute appendicitis or acute abdomen. Four case reports with a review of the literature. J Cancer Res Clin Oncol 123(10):560–564

O'Kane AM et al (2008) Small cell carcinoma of the appendix. World J Surg Oncol 6:4

Pham TH et al (2006) Surgical and chemotherapy treatment outcomes of goblet cell carcinoid: a tertiary cancer center experience. Ann Surg Oncol 13(3):370–376

Pickhardt PJ et al (2002a) Primary neoplasms of the appendix manifesting as acute appendicitis: CT findings with pathologic comparison. Radiology 224(3):775–781

Pickhardt PJ et al (2002b) Non-Hodgkin's lymphoma of the appendix: clinical and CT findings with pathologic correlation. Am J Roentgenol 178(5):1123–1127

Pickhardt PJ et al (2003) Primary neoplasms of the appendix: radiologic spectrum of disease with pathologic correlation. Radiographics 23(3):645–662

Rutledge RH, Alexander JW (1992) Primary appendiceal malignancies: rare but important. Surgery 111(3):244–250

Sandor A, Modlin IM (1998) A retrospective analysis of 1570 appendiceal carcinoids. Am J Gastroenterol 93(3): 422–428

Suzuki J et al (2009) Signet ring cell carcinoma of the appendix manifesting as colonic obstruction and ovarian tumors: report of a case. Surg Today 39(3):235–240
Todd RD et al (2004) Incidence and predictors of appendiceal tumors in elderly males presenting with signs and symptoms of acute appendicitis. Am J Surg 188(5):500–504
Tsujimura H et al (2000) Involvement of the appendix in a relapsed case of primary nasal NK/T-cell lymphoma. Leuk Lymphoma 37(5–6):633–634
van Eeden S et al (2000) Gangliocytic paraganglioma of the appendix. Histopathology 36(1):47–49
Walensky RP et al (1996) Pseudomyxoma peritonei. Am J Roentgenol 167(2):471–474
Zebrowska G, Walsh NM (1991) Human immunodeficiency virus-related Kaposi's sarcoma of the appendix and acute appendicitis. Report of a case and review of the literature. Arch Pathol Lab Med 115(11):1157–1160

Impact of Imaging on Negative Appendectomy Rate

Courtney A. Coursey and Ricardo D. Moreno

Contents

C. A. Coursey (✉)
Department of Radiology, Emory Healthcare,
1364 Clifton Road NE, Atlanta, GA 30322, USA
e-mail: courtney.coursey@emoryhealthcare.org

R. D. Moreno
Department of General Surgery,
The Southeast Permanente Medical Group,
2004 Peachtree Road, NW Suite 100,
Atlanta, GA 30309, USA

Abstract

A negative appendectomy is defined as the removal of a normal appendix during an urgent appendectomy performed because of suspected acute appendicitis. In this chapter, we will trace the historical acceptability of a negative appendectomy rate, negative appendectomy rates in the pre-CT era, and negative appendectomy rates in the CT era. Gender differences in the impact of CT on negative appendectomy rates will be reviewed. Controversies related to the role of CT in lowering negative appendectomy rates will be discussed. Acceptable rates of negative appendectomy in the CT era will be addressed. The impact of ultrasound on negative appendectomy rates and the impact of imaging on negative appendectomy rates in children also will be discussed.

1 Historical Acceptability of a Negative Appendectomy Rate

Making the diagnosis of acute appendicitis is not always clear clinically as the classic clinical history of umbilical pain that migrates to the right lower quadrant may only be present in half of patients (Kazarian et al. 1970). The specificities of right lower quadrant pain (53%), pain migration (82%), pain before vomiting (64%), anorexia (36%), and vomiting (45%) for the diagnosis of acute appendicitis are well short of 100% (Wagner et al. 1996). If the diagnosis of acute appendicitis is missed and the appendix perforates, morbidity and mortality rates increase (Kazarian et al. 1970;

C. Keyzer and P. A. Gevenois (eds.), *Imaging of Acute Appendicitis in Adults and Children*,
Medical Radiology. Diagnostic Imaging, DOI: 10.1007/174_2011_228, © Springer-Verlag Berlin Heidelberg 2011

Table 1 Negative appendectomy rates in the pre-CT era, 1937–1973

	Publication year	Study years	*n*	Overall neg appy rate (%)	Male neg appy rate (%)	Female neg appy rate (%)
Barnes et al. (1962)	1962	1937–1959	5800	18	na	na
Hobson and Rosenman (1964)	1964	1957–1962	820	21	na	na
Kazarian et al. (1970)	1970	1961–1965	539	17	10	26
Chang et al. (1973)	1973	1969–1972	183	33	21	46
Lewis et al. (1975)	1975	1963–1973	1000	20	12	34

Egdahl 1964; Hobson and Rosenman 1964; Barnes et al. 1962; Lewis et al. 1975).

Historically the removal of a normal appendix in a patient preoperatively suspected to have acute appendicitis (a "negative appendectomy") was considered acceptable so long as the operating surgeon's overall rate of negative appendectomies was within reasonable limits. As stated by Cantrell and Stafford of The Johns Hopkins Hospital (Baltimore, MD, USA) in 1955, "An exact diagnosis [of acute appendicitis] will frequently be impossible; yet if we are to eliminate perforation, we must accept the removal of a certain number of normal appendices." (Cantrell and Stafford 1955) The authors proposed 20–25% as an acceptable rate of negative appendectomy (Cantrell and Stafford 1955).

2 Historical Studies Reporting Pre-CT Rates of Negative Appendectomy

A 15–25% rate of negative appendectomy was cited as acceptable in the medical literature in the mid and latter half of the twentieth century before the widespread use of computed tomography (Detmer et al. 1981; Korner et al. 1997) (Table 1). Negative appendectomy rates for several large series of patients treated between 1937 and 1973 are reported in Table 1.

Higher rates of negative appendectomy of up to 40% were considered acceptable in women of reproductive age due to gynecologic conditions which can confound the diagnosis (Borgstein et al. 1997) (Table 1). For example, Lewis et al. (1975) reported that 48% of women who underwent negative appendectomy were ultimately diagnosed with pelvic inflammatory disease or other gynecologic pathology as the etiology of abdominal pain (Lewis et al. 1975). Alternatively, in men in the same series who underwent a negative appendectomy, mesenteric adenitis was the most common alternate etiology of abdominal pain (Lewis et al. 1975).

Similarly, Barnes et al. (1962) reported mesenteric adenitis, ovarian cyst pathology, and pelvic inflammatory disease as the most common alternative diagnoses in patients who underwent negative appendectomy. Kazarian et al. (1970) also reported pelvic inflammatory disease, ruptured ovarian cyst, and mesenteric adenitis as the most common etiologies of abdominal pain in patients who underwent negative appendectomies.

Other alternative diagnoses in patients who underwent negative appendectomies included gastroenteritis, diverticulitis, Meckel's diverticulitis, peptic ulcer disease, and renal and ureteral pathology (Kazarian et al. 1970; Barnes et al. 1962; Lewis et al. 1975). It should be noted that these alternative diagnoses, in addition to acute appendicitis, are often readily diagnosed at CT.

3 Introduction of CT for the Diagnosis of Acute Appendicitis

In the early to mid-1980s, several articles were published describing the utility of CT in diagnosing appendiceal disorders (Fish et al. 1981; Jones et al. 1983; Gale et al. 1985; Balthazar et al. 1986). In 1991, Balthazar et al. (1986) reported a 98% sensitivity, 83%

Table 2 Sensitivity, specificity, and accuracy of CT for the diagnosis of acute appendicitis, early reports

	Publication year	*n*	Number of detectors	Contrast material	Sensitivity (%)	Specificity (%)	Accuracy (%)
Balthazar et al. (1986)	1991	100	single	oral, IV	98	83	93
Malone et al. (1993)	1993	211	single	none	87	97	93
Lane et al. (1999)	1999	300	single	none	96	99	97

Table 3 Studies comparing overall negative appendectomy rates in patients who did and did not undergo preoperative CT

	Year	*n*	Neg. appy rate with CT (%)	Neg. appy rate without CT (%)	*p*
Weyant et al. (2000)	1995–1999	625	12	19	<.05
Brandt and Wahl (2003)	1999–2002	330	7	18	.009
Chooi et al. (2007)	2000–2004	380	11	22	.006
Augustin et al. (2009)	2000–2005	445	8	18	.003
Rhea et al. (2005)	2001	753	3	6	0.326
Musunuru et al. (2007)	2002–2004	411	8	14	0.09
Morse et al. (2007)	2003–2006	439	9	24	<0.001
Kim et al. (2008)	2009	339	7	21	<0.05

specificity, and 93% accuracy for the CT diagnosis of acute appendicitis. This study was performed with a single slice CT scanner and intravenous and oral contrast material (Balthazar et al. 1986).

Multiple publications were to follow over the next nearly 20 years which reported similarly high sensitivities, specificities, and accuracies for the CT diagnosis of acute appendicitis. A sampling of these publications is listed in Table 2. For a more exhaustive discussion of the accuracy of CT in the diagnosis of acute appendicitis and best CT techniques, the reader is referred to "Imaging of Acute Appendicitis in Adults: Computed Tomography" by Keyzer and "Imaging of Acute Appendicitis in Children: Computed Tomography Including Radiation Issues" by Spencer in this volume.

4 CT and the Negative Appendectomy Rate

Given that the clinical diagnosis of acute appendicitis is not always clear and CT is a highly accurate test for the diagnosis of acute appendicitis, it is not surprising that increased use of preoperative CT has been associated with lower rates of negative appendectomy. A number of publications have documented a convincing reduction in negative appendectomy rates in the CT era. The majority of these publications (1) compare negative appendectomy rates in patients who underwent preoperative CT to rates in patients who did not undergo preoperative CT or (2) evaluate changes in negative appendectomy rates with increased use of preoperative CT. Many studies have also investigated gender differences in negative appendectomy rates with increased use of preoperative CT.

For a review of studies comparing negative appendectomy rates in patients who did or did not undergo preoperative CT, the reader is referred to Table 3. When interpreting studies of this design, it is important to remember that patients who did not undergo preoperative CT when CT was readily available would be expected to have a low rate of negative appendectomy. Clinical suspicion of acute appendicitis would be expected to be very high for patients who did not undergo preoperative CT when CT was readily available.

Table 4 Studies reporting overall negative appendectomy rates with increased use of preoperative CT

	n	Initial Year(s)	Later Year(s)	Initial rate of preop CT (%)	Later rate of preop CT (%)	Initial rate of neg. appendectomy (%)	Later rate of neg. appendectomy (%)	*p*
Flum et al. (2001)	10382	1987	1998	na	na	15	16	na
Raja et al. (2010)	1608	1990–1994	2003–2007	1	98	23	2	<0.0001
Rao et al. (1999)	702	1992–1995	1997	0	59	20	7	<.001
Perez et al. (2003)	218	1994	2000	11	48	12	18	.317
Wagner et al. (2008)	1425	1995–1999	2000–2007	32	95	16	8	.005
Raman et al. (2008)	1081	1996	2006	20	85	24	3	.001
Naoum et al. (2002)	194	1998	2001	32	84	25	6	<.05
Coursey et al. (2010)	925	1998	2007	19	94	17	9	<0.0001
Frei et al. (2008)	2714	1998	2004	12	84	16	8	0.072
Jones et al. (2004)	389	2000	2002	52	86	17	2	.001

Nevertheless, even with this limitation all studies reported in Table 3 found a reduction in the negative appendectomy rate in patients who underwent preoperative CT as compared to those who did not undergo preoperative CT. For example, Kim et al. (2008) found a negative appendectomy rate of 7% in patients who underwent preoperative CT as compared to a negative appendectomy rate of 21% in patients who did not undergo preoperative CT (Table 3). Morse et al. (2007) found a negative appendectomy rate of 9% in patients who underwent preoperative CT as compared to a negative appendectomy rate of 24% in patients who did not undergo preoperative CT (Table 3).

These differences in negative appendectomy rates were statistically significantly different for all studies except Rhea et al. (2005). Rhea et al. (2005) found a negative appendectomy rate of 3% in patients who underwent preoperative CT as compared to 6% in patients who did not undergo preoperative CT (Table 3). However, this difference was not statistically significantly different ($p = 0.326$).

Next, a number of publications have also reported a convincing decrease in negative appendectomy rates with increased use of preoperative CT (Table 4). The design of these studies was to trace rates of preoperative CT in patients with suspected acute appendicitis and also trace rates of negative appendectomy for each corresponding year. The vast majority of these publications found a decrease in negative appendectomy rates with increased use of preoperative CT (Table 4).

As seen in Table 4, initial rates of preoperative CT ranged from 0 to 52%, and later rates of preoperative CT ranged from 48 to 98%. For the publications that reported a decrease in negative appendectomy rates with increased use of preoperative CT, initial negative appendectomy rates (when preoperative CT use was relatively lower) ranged from 16 to 25% (Table 4). In these same publications, later rates of negative appendectomy (when preoperative CT use was relatively higher) ranged from 2 to 9% (Table 4). For example, Raja et al. (2010) found that from 1990 to 1994, 1% of patients who underwent urgent appendectomy also underwent preoperative CT. However, by 2003–2007 the percentage of patients with suspected acute appendicitis who underwent preoperative CT had increased to 98%. During 1990–1994, the rate of negative appendectomy was 23%, and during 2003–2007 the rate of negative appendectomy was 2%. This difference in negative appendectomy rates was statistically significantly different. Numerous similar studies with similar findings are reported in Table 4 and provide convincing evidence that the increased use of preoperative CT has been associated with an overall decrease in negative appendectomy rates.

However, publications by Frei et al. (2008); Perez et al. (2003); Flum et al. (2001) found no statistically significant change in negative appendectomy rates. Frei et al. (2008) reported that the negative appendectomy rate at their institution was 16% in 1998 when 12% of patients underwent CT prior to appendectomy. In 2004 when 84% of patients underwent CT prior to appendectomy, the negative appendectomy rate was 8%. These numbers appear to indicate a decrease in the negative appendectomy rate with increased use of preoperative CT. However, the authors report that when the negative appendectomy rates were looked at on a year-by-year basis from 1998 to 2004, the negative appendectomy rates did not differ by year ($p = 0.072$) although the year-to-year differences did approach statistical significance.

Perez et al. (2003) reported that the negative appendectomy rate went from 12% in 1994 when 11% of patients underwent CT prior to appendectomy to 18% in 2000 when 48% of patients underwent CT prior to appendectomy. Perez et al. also reported that at their institution CT accuracy rates for the diagnosis of acute appendicitis were 81–82% and CT specificities for the diagnosis of acute appendicitis were 17–18%. All of these values are well below other published values (please see "Imaging of Acute Appendicitis in Adults: Computed Tomography" by Keyzer and "Imaging of Acute Appendicitis in Children: Computed Tomography Including Radiation Issues" by Spencer in this volume). The reported specificity values are so low in Perez et al. because their study population included only those patients who underwent non-incidental appendectomy for suspected acute appendicitis. To accurately compute CT accuracy and specificity, the authors should have also included those patients who underwent CT scan for suspected acute appendicitis but were found not to have appendicitis at CT and at final clinical analysis, a limitation which the authors acknowledge. Perez et al. posit that one reason the results at their institution differ from other published results is because the radiologists at their institution were not emergency radiology specialists.

As Flum et al. (2001) is widely cited as evidence that increased CT utilization has not resulted in a decrease in negative appendectomy rates, it will be discussed in detail below in the next section.

Finally, a number of publications have compared gender differences in changes in the negative appendectomy rate with increased use of preoperative CT (Table 5). In women, these studies largely found a decrease in the negative appendectomy rate with increased use of preoperative CT. For example, Rao et al. (1999) reported a baseline negative appendectomy rate of 35% in women which decreased to 11% with increased use of preoperative CT, a difference which was statistically significant.

That negative appendectomy rates in women would be lowered with increased use of preoperative CT is not surprising since before the CT era these rates ranged from 26 to 46% (Table 1). Presumably rates of negative appendectomy are lower in women with increased use of preoperative CT because preoperative CT either diagnosed acute appendicitis, identified an alternate etiology of abdominal pain, or identified a normal appendix.

Published results for men are more mixed (Table 5). For example, Chooi et al. (2007) and Raja et al. (2010) found a statistically significant reduction in negative appendectomy rates in men with increased use of preoperative CT. However, the other articles reported in Table 5 did not find a statistically significant reduction in the negative appendectomy rate in males.

Why these conflicting results? In several articles which did not find a decrease in negative appendectomy rates in men with increased use of preoperative CT, the initial male negative appendectomy rate was quite low (3–7%) (Coursey et al. 2010; Bendeck et al. 2002; Fuchs et al. 2002). Although CT is a highly accurate test for the diagnosis of acute appendicitis, it is not 100% perfect. Therefore, it would be difficult to

Table 5 Studies reporting rates of negative appendectomy for women and men with increased use of preoperative CT

	Women				Men			
	n	Baseline rate of neg. appy (%)	Rate of neg. appy w/increased CT (%)	*p*	*n*	Baseline rate of neg. appy (%)	Rate of neg. appy w/increased CT (%)	*p*
Rao et al. (1999)	234	35	11	<.001	280	11	5	.114
Bendeck et al. (2002)	117	28	7	.005	168	3	5	.368
McGory et al. (2005)	24901	15	9–13	.001–.056	31970	5–9	5–9	.47–.87
Raja et al. (2010)	515	30	2	<.0001	456	16	2	<.0001
Coursey et al. (2010)	399	43	7	.0001	526	7	12	na
Chooi et al. (2007)	167	34	17	.024	213	17	6	.009
Fuchs et al. (2002)	66	24	5	.07	55	4	7	1

reduce an already low negative appendectomy rate of 3% in male patients with a test that is 95% accurate. The studies that did report a significant negative appendectomy rate reduction in male patients with increased use of preoperative CT found higher male baseline rates of negative appendectomy ranging from 16 to 17% (Chooi et al. 2007; Raja et al. 2010). It is reasonable to assume that it would be possible to improve on these baseline rates of negative appendectomy with a test that is 95% accurate.

4.1 Controversies Regarding CT and Reductions in Rates of Negative Appendectomy

Despite the now overwhelming evidence that increased use of computed tomography has coincided with a decrease in negative appendectomy rates, the literature on this topic is sometimes misquoted in the lay press and health policy literature (Grumbach 2002; Brownlee 2008). For example, journalist Shannon Brownlee wrote in her 2008 book "Overtreated: why too much medicine is making us sicker and poorer" that "Astonishingly enough, however, the rate of negative appendectomies probably hasn't budged in the two decades since belly CT scans became commonplace" Brownlee (2008) citing a 2001 Journal of the American Medical Association Article (JAMA) by Flum et al. (2001).

Similarly, writing in a 2002 *Health Affairs* article entitled "The ramifications of specialty-dominated medicine", Dr. Kevin Grumbach, a family and community medicine physician, states "Many patients with clinical findings suggestive of possible appendicitis who formerly went straight to the operating room now make a detour to the radiology suite for a diagnostic sonogram or computed tomography (CT) scan of the abdomen. However, a statewide study of appendectomies in Washington State over the past decade found no reduction in rates of removal of normal appendices (Flum et al. 2001). Elliott Fisher and Gilbert Welch have cogently discussed the general case for 'how might more be worse' in health care" (Grumbach 2002).

As both of these authors use the 2001 JAMA publication by Flum et al. (2001) to support their arguments that preoperative CT does not lower the rate of negative appendectomy, this article by Flum et al. (2001) warrants close reading.

Flum et al. analyzed data obtained from the Washington State Comprehensive Hospital Abstract Reporting System database covering the years 1987–1998. Patients who underwent non-incidental appendectomy ($n = 63{,}707$) were identified by searching the database for the International Classification of Diseases, Ninth revision (ICD-9) procedure codes for non-incidental appendectomy (for example, code 47.0 = appendectomy excludes incidental). This group of patients identified as having undergone non-incidental appendectomy was then evaluated by searching for the ICD-9 diagnostic codes for appendiceal pathology (for example, code 540 = acute appendicitis). Based on these codes, Flum et al. reported rates of negative appendectomy (i.e., number of patients who had an ICD-9 procedure code indicating a non-incidental appendectomy but did not have an ICD-9 diagnostic code reflecting acute appendicitis divided by the number of patients who had an ICD-9 procedure code indicating a non-incidental appendectomy) per year from 1987 to 1998. Reported rates of negative appendectomy ranged from 15.2% in 1987 to 15.5% in 1998. Flum et al. interpreted these results as indicating that the increased availability of CT did not result in a decrease in the misdiagnosis of acute appendicitis.

A major limitation of Flum et al. is that the authors did not identify which patients in their study actually underwent preoperative CT. The authors state that the "availability of CT… to aid in diagnosis of appendicitis has increased dramatically over the last decade", but present no information about the number of patients who actually underwent preoperative CT during the years of their investigation. A number of articles report low rates of preoperative CT in appendectomy patients in the early to mid-1990s. As an example, a leading academic institution reported that they were not performing appendiceal CT between 1992 and 1995 at their institution (Rao et al. 1999). Therefore, it is highly possible that the underlying premise of Flum et al. is incorrect. In other words, preoperative CT use for the diagnosis of acute appendicitis may not have increased significantly during the years of their study (1987–1998).

In addition, technology used for CT data acquisition and image interpretation has significantly improved since the time period (1987–1998) studied by Flum et al. (2001). For example, the introduction of multi-detector CT scanners has resulted in the generation of CT images with improved image resolution and fewer motion artifacts. The shift from single-detector CT to multi-detector CT and the use of decreasing section thickness has been shown to correlate with a reduction in false-positive CT diagnoses of acute appendicitis (Coursey et al. 2010). The ability to generate data sets composed of isotropic voxels has also made possible the generation of high quality coronal reformations. In general, these isotropic data sets are possible with multi-detector CT machines that are capable of acquiring 16 or more slices at a time. Coronal reformations have been shown to improve confidence in visualization of the appendix and in the diagnosis or exclusion of acute appendicitis (Paulson et al. 2005).

Furthermore, a follow-up study by the Surgical Care and Outcomes Assessment Program (SCOAP) which investigated statewide hospital data in the same state during 2006–2007 contradicts. This more recent article published by SCOAP found that the prevalence of negative appendectomy was 9.8% in patients who had no imaging and 4.5% in patients who underwent preoperative CT (SCOAP 2008). The authors report that CT/US use increased from 80 to 90% during the time period of the study, and that the prevalence of negative appendectomy decreased significantly during the same time period ($p = 0.01$) (SCOAP 2008). Importantly, the negative appendectomy rates reported in the SCOAP publication (4.5 and 9.8%) are both lower than the negative appendectomy rate reported by Flum et al. (15%) for the same state nearly a decade earlier.

As Flum et al. does not reflect the most up to date CT technology, the underlying premise of the article is likely flawed, and a more recent publication looking at statewide data from the same state found different results, Flum et al. should no longer be cited without qualification in discussions of the impact of CT on the negative appendectomy rate.

4.2 Does CT Use Delay Diagnosis and Increase Perforation Rates?

Is there a tradeoff between reductions in the negative appendectomy rate and increases in the appendiceal perforation rate with increase in use of preoperative CT? As images of the abdomen and pelvis can be acquired in as few as 5–10 s on a 64-slice multidetector CT scanner, scan times should not result in an increase in perforation rates. Wait times of 1 h are adequate to allow for the transit of oral contrast material through the small intestine (Hebert et al.

2006). Not surprisingly then, time between CT order and CT scan completion was found to be 172 min for patients undergoing CT with oral contrast material and 104 min for patients undergoing CT without oral contrast material ($p < 0.001$) in one series (Huynh et al. 2004).

Numerous articles in the surgical literature support the notion of a 3–10 h observation period for patients who present with questionable findings of acute appendicitis (Jones 2001; Graff et al. 1991; Andersson et al. 2000). Given that such an observation period has been shown to not result in a higher rate of appendiceal perforation, it is doubtful that the 1–1.5 h increase in the time interval before a CT scan is performed with oral contrast material would result in a significant increase in the rate of appendiceal perforation. Delays in presentation of greater than 12 h are associated with increased risks of perforation (Colson et al. 1997; Eldar et al. 1997). See also "Appendicitis Perforation Rates and Time Interval Between Symptom Onset and Surgery" by Menes.

Several articles have reported that increased rates of preoperative CT are not associated with increased appendiceal perforation rates (Rao et al. 1999; Raman et al. 2008). For example, Rao et al. (1999) found that perforation rates decreased from 22 to 14% with the availability of CT. Raman et al. (2008) report that the rate of appendiceal perforation decreased from 18 to 5% as the rate of preoperative CT increased from 20 to 93%.

For a more complete discussion of whether oral contrast material is necessary for the CT diagnosis of acute appendicitis, the reader is referred to the "Imaging of Acute Appendicitis in Adults: Computed Tomography" by Keyzer and "Imaging of Acute Appendicitis in Children: Computed Tomography Including Radiation Issues" by Spencer in this volume.

4.3 How Low Can We Go? What is an Acceptable Negative Appendectomy Rate in the CT Era?

In the CT era in which we now live with more than 90% of patients undergoing CT prior to appendectomy at many institutions (Raman et al. 2008; Coursey et al. 2010), what is an acceptable rate of negative appendectomy? The two primary variables that will likely prevent an idealized negative appendectomy rate of 0% include (1) limitations in the CT diagnosis of acute appendicitis and (2) limitations in the pathology diagnosis of acute appendicitis.

While the reported accuracy of CT is very high in the diagnosis of acute appendicitis, it is not 100% perfect. Reasons for CT misdiagnosis include overlap in the appearance of the normal and diseased appendix and difficulty in identifying the appendix at CT.

Overlap in the appearances of normal and acutely inflamed appendices can be a source of diagnostic error. In an investigation of asymptomatic patients undergoing CT evaluation as potential renal donors, Johnson et al. (2005) found that the mean diameter of collapsed normal appendices was 5 mm (range 3–7 mm). Mean diameter of normal air-distended appendices was 7 mm (range 4–10 mm). Based on this data, if a radiologist were to rely solely on an appendiceal diameter measurement to diagnose acute appendicitis, the radiologist would surely issue false positive reports if an appendiceal diameter cutoff of 6–8 mm is used. In addition, Johnson et al. identified minimal periappendiceal stranding in 3% of asymptomatic patients who did not have acute appendicitis based on clinical findings.

In addition, the appendix cannot always be visualized at CT. For example, a normal appendix can be relatively more difficult to identify in patients with scant intra-abdominal fat and/or a low body mass index (Keyzer et al. 2008). Nonvisualization of the appendix has been shown to exclude the diagnosis of acute appendicitis in 98% of patients (Ganguli et al. 2006; Nikolaidis et al. 2004). Based on these publications, nonvisualization of the appendix does not entirely exclude the diagnosis of acute appendicitis.

Also, beyond the accuracy of the final CT report, other variables which could impact the negative appendectomy rate in a patient who undergoes preoperative CT include (1) whether the surgeon or treating physician believes the CT report when factoring in clinical data and (2) perhaps the role of preliminary reports issued by radiology residents in academic training programs. A minority of published studies report what the negative appendectomy rate would have been if the CT report were acted on as if it were accurate. In other words, presumably there are occasions when a surgeon feels so strongly that a patient has acute appendicitis based on clinical grounds that he or she will remove the patient's appendix even in the setting of a normal CT report.

In terms of the effect of resident preliminary reports, it has been the custom at many training institutions in the United States (although this is an area where workflow is in flux at some institutions) for radiology trainees to issue preliminary reports that are often acted upon before the staff radiologist issues the final radiology report. The role of such preliminary reports and their impact on negative appendectomy rates is largely not addressed in the published literature which analyzes results based on the final radiology report.

In addition to limitations in the CT diagnosis of acute appendicitis, pathologists do not agree 100% of the time on whether or not acute appendicitis is present. When two pathologists reviewed 415 appendectomy specimens, there was disagreement about whether or not acute appendicitis was present or absent at histology in 7% of cases (Riber et al. 1999). Furthermore, appendices removed because of preoperatively suspected acute appendicitis that appear histologically normal have been found to show increased cytokine expression as clear evidence of an inflammatory response (Wang et al. 1996). That there is less than 100% pathologist agreement on the presence or absence of acute appendicitis is a source of intrinsic variability in negative appendectomy rates.

Due to these multiple variables at work in diagnosing acute appendicitis preoperatively and at pathology, achieving a consistent negative appendectomy rate of 0% likely is not possible. Jones et al. (2004) proposed that appropriate utilization of CT should decrease the negative appendectomy rate to 2%. This figure may also be too optimistic, but a negative appendectomy rate of 5–10% for men and women would seem to be achievable.

5 Ultrasound and Negative Appendectomy Rate

As CT is frequently obtained if ultrasound (US) examinations are equivocal or negative and clinical suspicion for acute appendicitis remains high, it is difficult to isolate the impact of US on the negative appendectomy rate based on the available literature. Two studies which attempted to define the impact of US on negative appendectomy rates are described briefly below.

van Breda Vriesman et al. (2003) retrospectively evaluated the negative appendectomy rate in patients who underwent US ($n = 233$) followed by noncontrast CT ($n = 30$) if US results were equivocal. The negative appendectomy rate was 6.0% in this patient population. This negative appendectomy rate is lower than the historical negative appendectomy rate of 15–20% cited in the pre-US and CT era.

Styrud et al. (2000) retrospectively reviewed 610 patients who were evaluated with US and 114 patients evaluated with CT for suspected acute appendicitis. The negative appendectomy rate was 12% for patients who underwent preoperative CT or US as compared to 18% at the same institution before the use of preoperative US and CT.

Both of these studies indicate that preoperative US followed by preoperative CT when US is equivocal or negative can lower the negative appendectomy rate compared to historical controls at institutions with expertise performing appendiceal US. Please refer to "Ultrasonography Versus Computed Tomography: Evidence-Based Imaging" and "US Versus CT: Evidence-Based Medicine and Cost-Effectiveness in Imaging Acute Appendicities in Children" in this volume for a detailed discussion of the accuracy of ultrasound as compared to CT in the diagnosis of acute appendicitis.

6 Imaging, Negative Appendectomy Rate and Children

As compared to the adult literature, there are relatively fewer published articles addressing the effect of imaging on negative appendectomy rates in the pediatric population. Similar to the US literature, most pediatric articles describe a combined approach of US followed by CT if the initial US is negative or equivocal for acute appendicitis.

Applegate et al. (2001) reviewed 299 pediatric patients who underwent urgent appendectomy preceded by no imaging or preceded by preoperative CT and/or preoperative US. In the study population, the negative appendectomy rate without imaging was 14%. The negative appendectomy rate for patients who underwent preoperative US with or without CT was 17%, but this difference was not statistically significantly different as compared to the no imaging group. The negative appendectomy rate for patients who underwent CT with or without US was 7%, but this rate also was not statistically significant as compared to the rate with no imaging ($p = 0.10$). The negative appendectomy rate for patients who underwent CT only was 2%, and this rate was statistically significantly different as compared to the rate of negative appendectomy with no imaging ($p = 0.02$). The rate of negative appendectomy was also statistically significantly lower for preoperative CT only as compared to preoperative US ($p = 0.007$).

Smink et al. (2004) evaluated 272 pediatric patients who underwent urgent appendectomy in 1997 and also after the implementation of a clinical practice guideline in 2001 which established criteria for ordering preoperative US and CT in pediatric patients. In 1997, 52% of patients underwent preoperative CT and/or US (5% CT only, 38% US only, 9% CT and US), and the negative appendectomy rate was 10.6%. In 2001, 90% of patients underwent preoperative CT and/or US (60% CT only, 12% US only, 18% CT and US), and the negative appendectomy rate was 5.5%. This decrease in the negative appendectomy rate with increased preoperative imaging was statistically significantly different ($p = 0.03$). The authors do not report whether CT or US had more of an impact on the negative appendectomy rate but recommend CT as the imaging modality of choice for all boys and for girls younger than 11 years of age.

In a prospective study of 139 children and adolescents, Garcia Pena et al. (1999) compared negative appendectomy rates for those patients who did and did not undergo preoperative US with or without CT. The imaging protocol for this study was that all patients underwent US first. If US results were equivocal or negative, patients underwent CT with rectal contrast material. The negative laparotomy rate for patients who underwent the imaging protocol was 6% as compared to 12% for patients who did not undergo preoperative imaging.

Martin et al. (2004) evaluated 720 pediatric patients admitted with a diagnosis of appendicitis between 1998 and 2001. During this time period, preoperative US decreased from 20.0 to 7.0%, and preoperative CT increased from 17.6 to 51.3%. During this time period, the negative appendectomy rate decreased from 10.9 to 6.0%, but the authors report that this difference was not statistically significantly different.

In summary, the pediatric literature suggests a trend toward lower rates of negative appendectomy with increased preoperative imaging. For a more detailed discussion regarding the optimal preoperative imaging algorithm in pediatric patients, the reader is referred to the "US Versus CT: Evidence-Based Medicine and Cost-Effectiveness in Imaging Acute Appendicities in Children" in this volume.

7 Conclusion

In conclusion, there is convincing evidence in the medical literature documenting a decrease in overall negative appendectomy rates in adults as rates of preoperative CT have increased. Negative appendectomy rates in women have consistently been found to be lower with increased use of preoperative CT. Results for men have been more variable. In studies where initial male negative appendectomy rates were low, no change was found with increased use of preoperative CT. However, in studies where initial male negative appendectomy rates were higher, statistically significant decreases were found with increased use of preoperative CT. Increased rates of preoperative imaging have also been shown to be associated with reductions in negative appendectomy rates in children.

References

Andersson RE, Hugander A, Ravn H et al (2000) Repeated clinical and laboratory examinations in patients with an equivocal diagnosis of appendicitis. World J Surg 24: 479–485

Applegate KE, Sivit SJ, Salvator AE (2001) Effect of cross-sectional imaging on negative appendectomy and perforation rates in children. Radiology 220:103–107

Augustin T, Bhende S, Chavda K et al (2009) CT scans and acute appendicitis: a 5 year analysis from a rural teaching hospital. J Gastroin Surg 13:1306–1312

Balthazar EJ, Megibow AJ, Hulnick D et al (1986) CT of appendicitis. AJR 147:705–710

Barnes BA, Behringer GE, Wheelock FC et al (1962) Treatment of appendicitis at the Massachusetts General Hospital (1937–1959). JAMA 180:122–126

Bendeck SE, Nino-Murcia M, Berry GJ et al (2002) Imaging for suspected appendicitis: negative appendectomy and perforation rates. Radiology 225:131–136

Borgstein PJ, Gordijn RV, Eijsbouts QAJ et al (1997) Acute appendicitis—a clear-cut case in men, a guessing game in young women. Surg Endo 11:923–927

Brandt M-M, Wahl WL (2003) Liberal use of CT scanning helps to diagnose appendicitis in adults. Am Surg 69: 727–734

Brownlee S (2008) Overtreated: why too much medicine is making us sicker and poorer. Bloomsbury Publishing, New York

Cantrell JR, Stafford ED (1955) The diminishing mortality from appendicitis. Ann of Surg 141:749–756

Chang FC, Hogle HH, Welling DR (1973) The fate of the negative appendix. Am J Surg 126:752–754

Chooi WK, Brown JA, Zetler P et al (2007) Imaging of acute appendicitis and its impact on negative appendectomy and perforation rates: The St. Paul's experience. Can Assoc of Rad Jnl 58:220–224

Colson M, Skinner KA, Dunnington G (1997) High negative appendectomy rates are no longer acceptable. Am J Surg 174:723–726

Coursey CA, Nelson RC, Patel MB et al (2010) Making the diagnosis of acute appendicitis: Do more preoperative CT scans mean fewer negative appendectomies? A 10 year study. Radiology 254:460–468

Detmer DE, Nevers LE, Sikes ED (1981) Regional results of acute appendicitis care. JAMA 246:1318–1320

Egdahl RH (1964) Current mortality in appendicitis. Am J Surg 107:757–759

Eldar S, Nash E, Sabo E et al (1997) Delay of surgery in acute appendicitis. Am J Surg 173:194–198

Fish B, Smulewicz JJ, Barek L (1981) Role of computed tomography in diagnosis of appendiceal disorders. N Y State J Med 81:900–904

Flum DR, Morris A, Koepsell T et al (2001) Has misdiagnosis of appendicitis decreased over time? A population-based analysis. JAMA 286:1748–1753

Frei SP, Bond WF, Bazuro RK (2008) Appendicitis outcomes with increasing computed tomographic scanning. Am J Emerg Med 26:39–44

Fuchs JR, Schlamberg JS, Shortsleeve MJ et al (2002) Impact of abdominal CT imaging on the management of appendicitis: an update. J Surg Res 106:131–136

Gale ME, Birnbaum S, Gerzof SG et al (1985) CT appearance of appendicitis and its local complications. J Comput Assist Tomogr 9:34–37

Ganguli S, Raptopoulos V, Komlos F et al (2006) Right lower quadrant pain: value of the nonvisualized appendix in patients at multidetector CT. Radiology 241:175–180

Garcia Pena BM, Mandl KD, Kraus SJ et al (1999) Ultrasonography and limited computed tomography in the diagnosis and management of appendicitis in children. JAMA 282:1041–1046

Graff L, Radford MJ, Werne C (1991) Probability of appendicitis before and after observation. Ann Emerg Med 20:503–507

Grumbach K (2002) The ramifications of specialty-dominated medicine. Health Aff 21:155–157

Hebert JJ, Taylor AJ, Winter TC (2006) Comparison of colonic transit between polyethylene glycol and water as oral contrast vehicles in the CT evaluation of acute appendicitis. AJR 187:1188–1191

Hobson T, Rosenman LD (1964) Acute appendicitis—when is it right to be wrong? Am J Surg 108:306–312

Huynh LN, Coughlin BF, Wolfe J et al (2004) Patient encounter times intervals in the evaluation of emergency department patients requiring abdominopelvic CT: oral contrast versus no contrast. Am Soc Emergency Radiol 10:310313

Johnson PT, Eng J, Moore CJ et al (2005) Multidetector-row CT of the appendix in healthy adults. Emer Radiol 12: 248–253

Jones PF (2001) Management of suspected acute appendicitis. Br J Surg 88:1570–1577

Jones B, Fishman EK, Siegelman SS (1983) Computed tomography and appendiceal abscess: special applicability in the elderly. J Comput Assist Tomogr 7:434–438

Jones K, Pena AA, Dunn EL et al (2004) Are negative appendectomies still acceptable? Am J Surg 188:748–754

Kazarian KK, Roeder WJ, Mersheimer WL (1970) Decreasing mortality and increasing morbidity from acute appendicitis. Am J Surg 119:681–685

Keyzer C, Pargov S, Tack D et al (2008) Normal appendix in adults: reproducibility of detection with unenhanced and contrast-enhanced MDCT. AJR 191:507–514

Kim K, Lee CC, Song K-J et al (2008) The impact of helical computed tomography on the negative appendectomy rate: a multi-center comparison. J Emer Med 34:3–6

Korner H, Sondenaa K, Soreide JA et al (1997) Index of acute nonperforated and perforated appendicitis: age-specific and sex-specific analysis. World J Surg 21:313–317

Lane MJ, Liu DM, Huynh MD et al (1999) Suspected acute appendicitis: nonenhanced helical CT in 300 consecutive patients. Radiology 213:341–346

Lewis FR, Holcroft JW, Boey J et al (1975) Appendicitis: a critical review of diagnosis and treatment in 1,000 cases. Arch Surg 110:677–684

Malone AJ, Wolf CR, Malmed AS et al (1993) Diagnosis of acute appendicitis: value of unenhanced CT. AJR 160: 763–766

Martin AE, Vollman D, Adler B et al (2004) CT Scans may not reduce the negative appendectomy rate in children. J Pediatr Surg 39:886–890

McGory ML, Zingmond DS, Nanayakkara D et al (2005) Negative appendectomy rate: influence of CT scans. Am Surg 71:803–808

Morse BC, Roettger RH, Kalbaugh CA et al (2007) Abdominal CT scanning in reproductive-age women with right lower quadrant abdominal pain: does it reduce negative appendectomy rate and healthcare costs? Am Surg 73: 581–584

Musunuru S, Chen H, Rikkers LF et al (2007) Computed tomography in the diagnosis of acute appendicitis: definitive or detrimental? J Gastrointest Surg 11:1417–1422

Naoum JJ, Mileski WJ, Daller JA et al (2002) The use of appendiceal computed tomography scan decreases the frequency of misdiagnosis in cases of suspected appendicitis. Am J Surg 184:587–589

Nikolaidis P, Hwang CM, Miller FH et al (2004) The nonvisualized appendix: incidence of acute appendicitis when secondary inflammatory changes are absent. AJR 183:889–892

Paulson EK, Harris JP, Jaffe TA et al (2005) Acute appendicitis: added diagnostic value of coronal reformations from

isotropic voxels at multidetector row CT. Radiology 235:879–885
Perez J, Barone JE, Wilbanks TO et al (2003) Liberal use of computed tomography scanning does not improve diagnostic accuracy in appendicitis. Am J Surg 185:194–197
Raja AS, Wright C, Sodickson AD et al (2010) Negative appendectomy rate in the era of CT: an 18 year perspective. Radiology 256:460–465
Raman SS, Osuagwu FC, Kadell B et al (2008) Effect of CT on false positive diagnosis of appendicitis and perforation. NEJM 358:972–973
Rao PM, Rhea JT, Rattner DW et al (1999) Introduction of appendiceal CT: impact on negative appendectomy and appendiceal perforation rates. Ann Surg 229:344–349
Rhea JT, Halpern EF, Ptak T et al (2005) The status of appendiceal CT in an urban medical center 5 years after its introduction: experience with 753 patients. AJR 184:1802–1808
Riber C, Tonnesen H, Aru A et al (1999) Observer variation in the assessment of the histopathologic diagnosis of acute appendicitis. Scand J Gastroenterol 34:46–49
SCOAP (2008) Negative appendectomy and imaging accuracy in the Washington state surgical care and outcomes assessment program. Ann Surg 248:557–563
Smink DS, Finkelstein JA, Garcia Pena BM et al (2004) Diagnosis of acute appendicitis in children using a clinical practice guideline. J Ped Surg 39:458–463
Styrud J, Josephson T, Eriksson S (2000) Reducing negative appendectomy: evaluation of ultrasonography and computer tomography in acute appendicitis. Int J Qual Health Care 12:65–68
van Breda Vriesman AC, Kole BJ, Puylaert JBCM (2003) Effect of ultrasonography and optional computed tomography on the outcome of appendectomy. Eur Radiol 13:2278–2282
Wagner JM, McKinney WP, Carpenter JL (1996) Does this patient have appendicitis? JAMA 276:1589–1594
Wagner PL, Eachempatia SR, Soe K (2008) Defining the negative appendectomy rate: for whom is preoperative computed tomography making an impact? Surgery 144:276–282
Wang Y, Reen DJ, Puri P (1996) Is a histologically normal appendix following emergency appendectomy always normal? Lancet 347:1076–1079
Weyant MJ, Eachempati SR, Maluccio MA et al (2000) Interpretation of computed tomography does not correlate with laboratory or pathologic findings in surgically confirmed acute appendicitis. Surgery 128:145–152

Radiation Dose from MDCT Examinations for Suspected Acute Appendicitis

Denis Tack and Caroline Keyzer

Contents

Abstract

Multidetector computed tomography (MDCT) is frequently used in patients with right iliac fossa pain and enables confident positive and negative diagnoses of both acute appendicitis and alternative diseases. The radiation risk related to MDCT has however to be taken into account. In this chapter, we will review the background of radiation risks, dose descriptors available on CT scanners, strategies for limiting the dose per examination, and the latest technology improvements for dose optimization and reduction. We will provide dose values for optimized and low-dose acquisitions, suited for adults, adolescents, and children tending to a radiation dose delivered by MDCT reduced to that of an abdominal plain film examination with two views.

1 Introduction

Since its introduction in the late 80s, CT has revolutionized imaging of the abdomen. Single-detector CT (SDCT) units and, more recently, MDCT units have substantially increased the number of indications of CT. As a result, the number of CT examinations performed has increased dramatically as well as the average scanned volume per patient. The subsequent increase in the collective radiation dose has been of

D. Tack
Department of Radiology, Clinique Louis Caty, Hôpital RHMS, Rue Louis Caty 136, 7331 Baudour, Belgium

C. Keyzer
Department of Radiology, Hôpital Erasme, Université libre de Bruxelles, Route de Lennik 808, 1070 Brussels, Belgium

D. Tack (✉)
Clos du Mélèze, 17, 1420 Braine-L'Alleud, Belgium
e-mail: denis.tack@skynet.be

C. Keyzer and F. A. Gevenois (eds.), *Imaging of Acute Appendicitis in Adults and Children*, Medical Radiology. Diagnostic Imaging, DOI: 10.1007/174_2011_229, © Springer-Verlag Berlin Heidelberg 2011 concern to radiologists, medical physicists, and governmental regulatory authorities, and it has been claimed that the radiation dose delivered by CT was excessive (Rogers 2001; Berrington de González et al. 2009; Little et al. 2009).

The radiation dose delivered to patients undergoing diagnostic radiologic examinations by CT is generally in the order of 1–24 mSv per examination for adults (UNSCEAR 2000) and 4–10 mSv for children (Shrimpton et al. 2003). These average effective doses represent a lifetime risk of cancer induction and can be classified as low (Tubiana et al. 2009), even though they are invariably greater than those resulting from conventional radiography. Typically, an abdominal radiographic examination with two views delivers 0.4–1.0 mSv. In contrast, a standard-dose MDCT delivers up to 15 mSv per acquisition, which is equal to a 15-fold risk of death by cancer according to current model. In other words, one death by cancer is expected for every 30,000 abdominal X-rays and every 2,000 MDCT examinations (ICRP 1991). Most importantly, more than one-half of the collective radiation dose delivered by diagnostic-imaging procedures is due to CT examinations (Golding and Shrimpton 2002). Although CT is an imaging technique that uses relatively high-radiation doses, it should be noted that it has replaced other techniques—such as barium enema and small bowel follow through—that delivered equivalent or even higher doses. Nevertheless, a further step in reducing the radiation dose is needed, as CT has become the main source of the radiation delivered by medical procedures. Therefore, particular attention has to be paid to dose optimization and reduction. Radiologists and medical physicists should be aware of their responsibility in achieving the appropriate balance between the image quality required for diagnostic purposes and the amount of radiation dose delivered to patients (Golding and Shrimpton 2002). In the rapidly evolving field of MDCT, the quest for the highest image quality has often obscured possible issues regarding the radiation. In this chapter, we will first review the technical basis for the assessment of radiation delivered by CT. We will then review the interactions between the image quality, diagnostic performances, and radiation dose. Furthermore, we will specifically focus on clinical advances in dose reduction in abdominal CT and in particular in those performed in adults and children to rule out acute appendicitis.

2 Assessment of Radiation Dose

The issue of increased delivery of radiation is compounded by the fact that younger and thus more radiation-sensitive patients are being scanned with increasing frequency (e.g., for right iliac fossa pain) (Hricak et al. 2010). The resulting public concerns have stimulated the publication of guidelines for maximum dose levels administered by CT. The European Guideline for Quality in Computed Tomography (European Commission 1999) defines such dose levels for all organs. The following paragraphs will focus on the factors that determine dose delivery in abdominal CT and on the relationship between radiation dose and image quality.

2.1 Measurement of Radiation Dose

Several methods are currently in use to quantify the delivery of ionizing radiation to the patient. The fact that there are several methods attests the complexity of this issue and may also present an obstacle to the understanding of radiation dose assessment. The most important parameters for radiation dose assessment, together with brief explanations, are summarized in Table 1 (Nagel 2007; Christner et al. 2010).

2.2 Technical Factors Influencing Dose Delivery

Dose delivery and image quality are substantially influenced by scanner technology. The following parameters are of practical importance.

2.2.1 Scanner Geometry

To decrease the centrifugal forces of the tube during rotation, manufacturers tend to move the tube closer to the isocenter of the scanner. At fixed mAs settings, this substantially increases the patient dose, notably the skin entry dose.

2.2.2 Focal Spot Tracking

Slightly widening the prepatient collimation ("overbeaming") was used in early MDCT units to compensate for subtle alterations of the focal spot size during tube rotation. Overbeaming has now been

Table 1 Parameters frequently used in the calculation of dose

Parameter	Abbreviation	Comment
CT dose index	CTDI	Integral under the dose profile of a CT section
Weighted CT dose index	CTDIw	Average radiation dose across the diameter of a phantom. Corresponds to the sum of one-third of the dose in the center and two-thirds of the dose in the periphery of the phantom
Volume CT dose index	CTDIvol	Corresponds to CTDIw divided by the pitch factor. Indicates average local dose to a patient within the scan volume. Allows for direct comparison of the radiation dose from different scan parameter settings, even between scanners. Directly reflects image quality
Dose-length product	DLP	Corresponds to CTDIvol multiplied by the length of the scan. At identical CTDIvol, scans covering longer anatomic areas will deliver more dose than those covering shorter areas. Reflects the dose per acquisition, and is summed for all acquisitions, the dose per examination
Effective dose	E	Computed parameter used to estimate the radiation risk to the population. Does not provide precise radiation risk for the individual patient, but is rather an index of risk for a particular scanner and examination

Note
E can be calculated from the DLP: E = DLP × Cf,
where Cf is a conversion factor specific to abdomen CT and equals 0.015 mSv/mGy cm (7)

replaced by focal spot tracking that adjusts the collimator setting and is a standard feature in the latest generation scanners.

2.2.3 Geometric Efficiency

The geometric efficiency of a detector is determined by the amount of radiation that reaches the detector relative to the amount of radiation that leaves the patient. Geometric efficiency depends on width, spatial orientation, absorption of the septa-separating detectors, and width of the dose profile in the z-direction.

2.2.4 Detector Efficiency

Solid-state detectors have up to 30% higher quantum yield than older xenon gas detectors. Using solid-state detectors, the same image noise can thus be achieved with a considerably lower dose compared with xenon detectors. Newly developed Gemstone detectors have a high sensitivity but also are very fast and allow dual energy imaging with one CT source.

2.2.5 Image Noise

Image noise appears as a mottle aspect in CT images and is measured through the standard deviation of CT numbers. Noise depends on scanner characteristics and among them on tube current and reconstructions algorithms (kernels). Noise can be substantially reduced by increasing image thickness on raw data and on multiplanar reformations (MPR), by using soft reconstructions algorithms, and by the newly-developed iterative reconstruction algorithms. These denoising tools are the key factors for dose optimization and reduction because they reduce the dose necessary for making image quality acceptable.

2.2.6 Tube Current Time Product

Radiation dose is proportional to the tube current time product and is expressed in mAs. Optimization of CT dose includes reduction of this parameter. Drawback of this approach is the produced image noise that will limit reduction. Mean tube current time product is part of the DICOM information in each CT image reconstructed from the raw data.

2.2.7 Tube Voltage (U)

In CT, increased tube voltages are used preferentially for improvements in tube loading and image quality. Contrary to the tube current time product, the consequences of variations in U cannot easily be assessed or predicted. There are therefore very few recommendations for the use of lower U settings as those currently used for standard or even low-dose CT scanning (120 and 140 kV). The relationship between dose and tube potential U is not linear, but rather of an exponential nature which varies according to the specific circumstances. The radiation dose varies with U to the power of 3.5. If the tube potential is increased, e.g., from 120 to 140 kV, the electrical signal obtained from the detectors therefore changes by a factor 1.7. U at 140 kV should thus be used in conjunction with very low tube currents in order to keep CTDIvol within acceptable limits. This tube

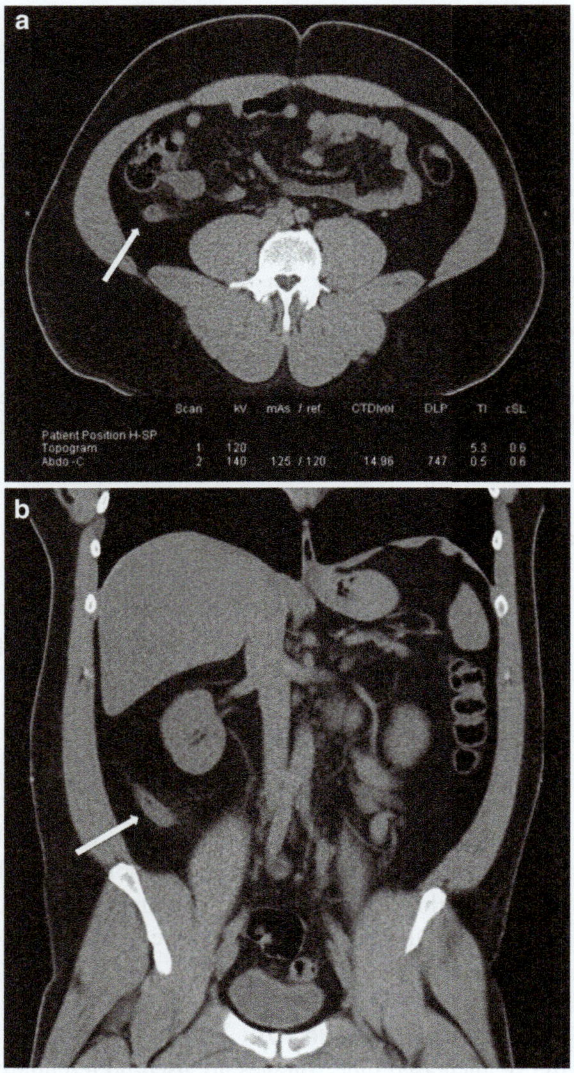

Fig. 1 Optimized dose MDCT in an obese patient weighing 135 kg, with acute appendicitis. Tube potential at 140 kV is used. Dose-length product is as high as 747 mGy cm. Transverse abdominal diameters are of 37 (P-A) and 43 (lateral) cm. *Arrows* in **a** (axial plane) and **b** (coronal plane) show enlarged appendix and fat stranding

potential may be appropriate in obese patients as shown in Fig. 1, but a priori not in children unless with extremely low tube currents.

Image noise generated by reduction in tube potential is less appearing as compared to the equivalent dose reduction obtained by lowering the tube current. Recently, Guimaraes et al. (2010) assessed the maximum patient diameter for acquiring CT with 80 kV: 35 cm should be considered as the maximum with the most recently developed CT generation. This indicates that U as low as 80 kV could be used in children but also in adults. Thus, as long as the patient is not obese, lowered kV settings can be used when imaging the abdomen: U at 100 kV can be recommended in non-traumatic emergencies such as suspected acute appendicitis in patients weighing 80 kg or less. In children under the age of 10, with a body weight lower than 40 kg, U at 80 kV can be recommended. Examples of MDCT acquisitions at standard U (120 kV) and at lowered U (100 and 80 kV) are shown in Figs. 2, 3, 4, 5, 6, 7, 8, 9, 10, 11, in adults and/or children. If IV iodine contrast injection is mandatory, a reduced contrast volume and/or concentration could be used because the absorption of iodine at lower U is significantly increased (Nagel 2007). Note that reduced U at 80 and 100 kV is recommended for CT angiography (Paul and Abada 2007). Finally, for performing low-dose acquisitions in obese patients, tube potential may be high and set at 140 kV, but compensated by very low tube currents. Thanks to the natural contrast of fat separating abdominal organs, this technique enables excellent visualization of the appendix with reduced DLP values as shown in Fig. 12.

2.2.8 Tube Current Modulation: Automatic Exposure Control

Tube current modulation, also called automatic exposure control (AEC), has been developed because of substantial differences in absorption between the antero-posterior and the lateral orientations since these diameters of the body cross section differ in thickness (Kalra 2007; Mulkens et al. 2005). Lateral-abdominal diameter in a young women may reach 35 cm whereas the antero-posterior diameter is of 18 cm, only 50% of the lateral one. Attenuation follows an exponential function. Thus small changes in diameter will cause major differences in attenuation. AEC systems are able to measure this attenuation and to adapt the tube current in order to maintain image quality, mainly image noise, at a constant level. By adapting the tube current, and reducing it in the antero-posterior orientation in abdominal CT, AEC systems allow for overall dose reduction of 10–20% in mean without loss of image quality, as compared to fixed tube current. In addition to modulate the dose in the *x*–*y* plane, AEC systems also determine and adapt the highest and lowest mA in the *Z* axis and provide equalized image quality throughout

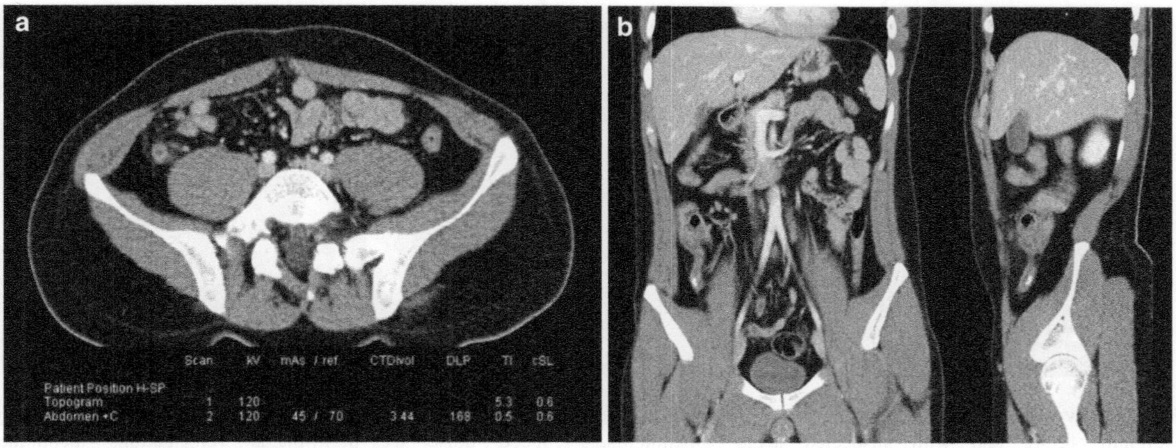

Fig. 2 Iodine-enhanced low-dose MDCT at 120 kV in a 20-year-old man with suspected appendicitis that was confirmed surgically. Noise in ROI obtained in psoas muscle is at 16 HU. Image quality can be considered as sufficient using CTDIvol at only 3.48 mGy for this 81 kg weighing patient (**a**). Note that Z-coverage includes lung bases and lower aspect of pubis bone and could have been reduced by 20–25% (**b**). Thus, actual DLP of 168 mGy cm that is in the range of low-dose MDCT could have been reduced to 140 mGy cm

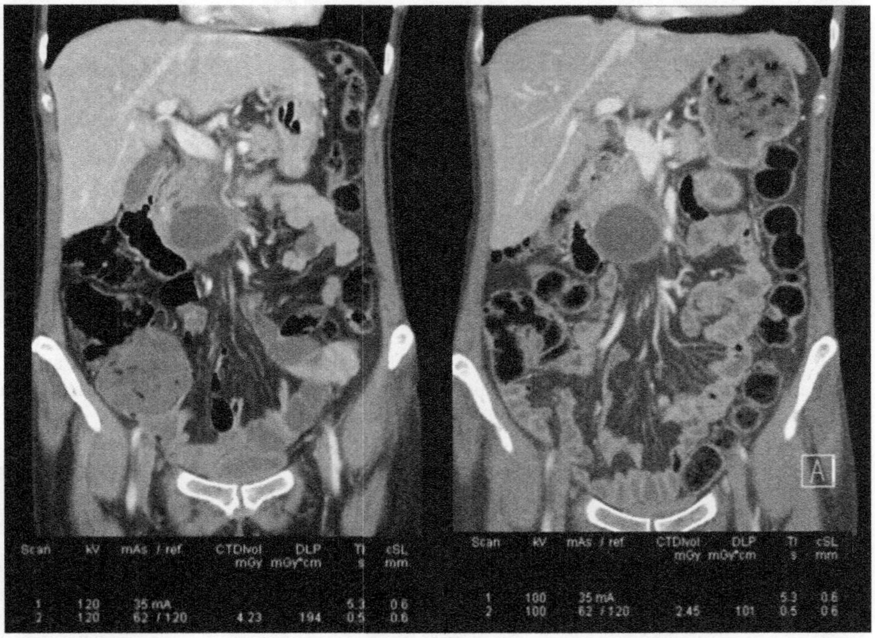

Fig. 3 Tube potential optimization: advantage of using 100 kV in a patient weighing <80 kg. Two consecutive optimized dose abdominal MDCT are obtained in a 36-year-old patient weighing 67 kg, for follow-up of acute pancreatitis with pseudocyst of the pancreatic head. Left coronal image is acquired at 120 kV and follow-up CT displayed is right coronal image is acquired at 100 kV. CTDIvol has been reduced from 4.23 to 2.46 and the DLP have been reduced from 194 to 101 mGy cm whereas image quality is preserved

the acquisition. Different technical solutions are currently applied to modulate the tube current according to the maximum and minimum patient size as determined by the scanogram (also named scout view or topogram). Using AEC, the dose delivered to the patient will depend on his body habitus, and as a consequence, the dose will be reduced in thin patients but conversely it will also be increased in large-frame and in obese patients (Mulkens et al. 2005). AEC systems are the only systems able to automatically adapt the mA (and the dose) to the patient's absorption. Thus, in abdominal MDCT, these systems should always be activated.

Because AEC systems differ from one manufacturer to the other, in particular when scanning small or obese patients, dose delivered to individuals by different scanners can only be compared and set up on standard-sized patients (approximately 70 kg weight and 1m70 tall).

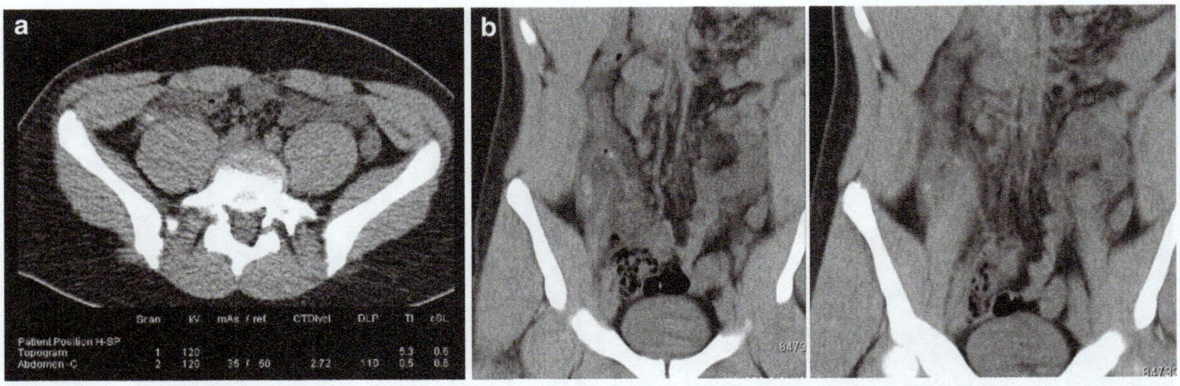

Fig. 4 Low-dose MDCT protocol in a 17-year-old male weighing 85 kg and with suspected acute appendicitis. **a** represents a 5 mm axial slice reconstructed without denoising algorithm. **b** represents two coronal views in the same patients, showing acute appendicitis and significantly reduced noise by multi-planar reformations technique. Appendicitis was confirmed surgically. MDCT delivered 110 mGy cm (1.6 mSv)

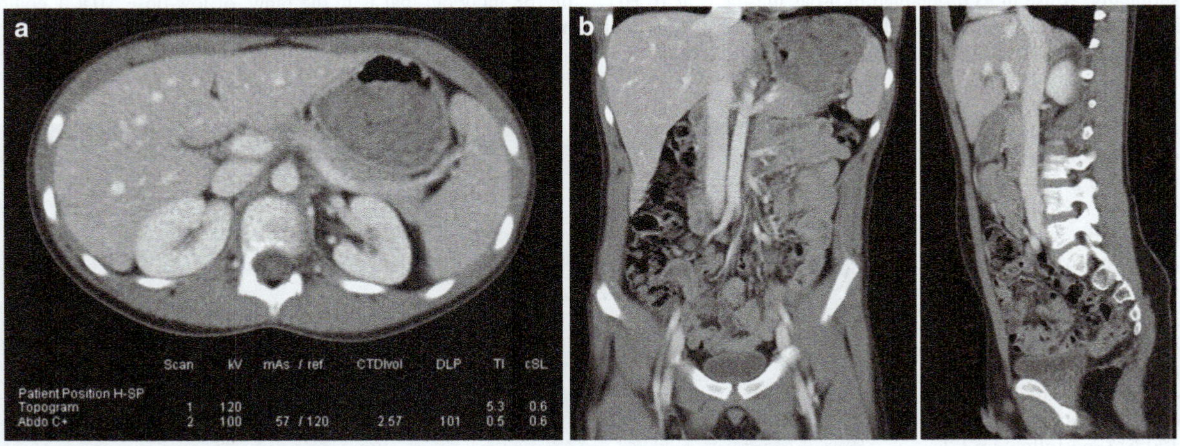

Fig. 5 Iodine enhanced abdominal MDCT in a 12-year-old boy weighing 45 kg. No sign of appendicitis was found by CT. Low-dose protocol with U at 100 kV was chosen for acquisition. DLP is at 101 mGy cm whereas image quality is excellent in axial (**a**) and in coronal or sagittal (**b**) orientations

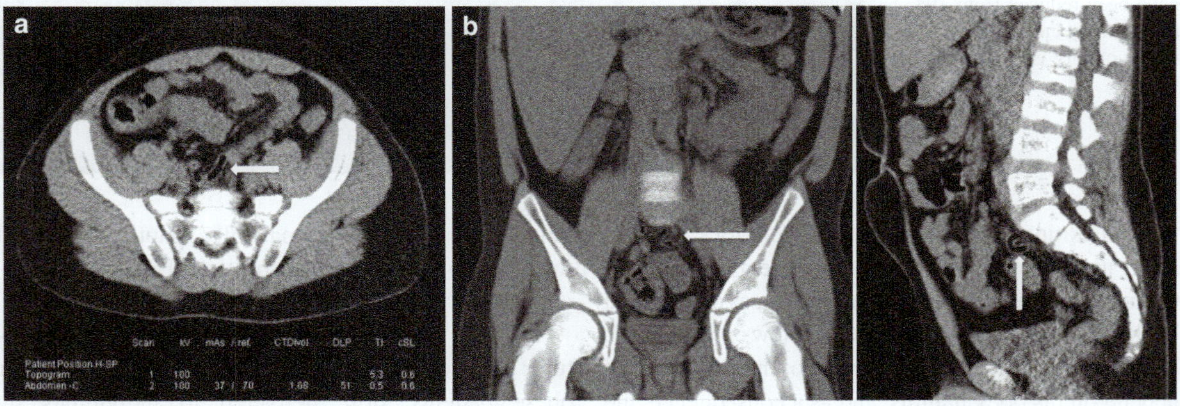

Fig. 6 Unenhanced MDCT obtained at 100 kV in a 12-year-old boy after two consecutive inconclusive (*or negative*) ultrasound examinations. **a** in axial orientation and **b** in coronal and sagittal orientations show a normal appendix (*arrows*). CTDIvol is at 1.68 mGy and DLP is at 51 mGy cm. This dose descriptor corresponds to the effective dose E of an abdominal plain film examination with 1–2 views

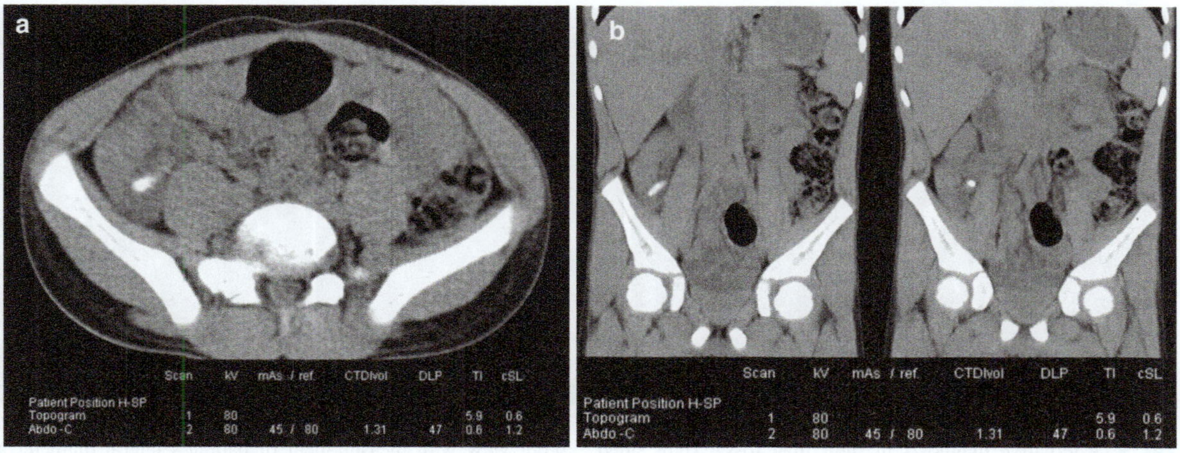

Fig. 7 Unenhanced MDCT obtained at 80 kV in a 9-year-old boy weighing 34 kg after inconclusive ultrasound examination. Acute appendicitis is demonstrated by MDCT while CTDIvol is at 1.38 mGy only and DLP is lower than 50 mGy cm

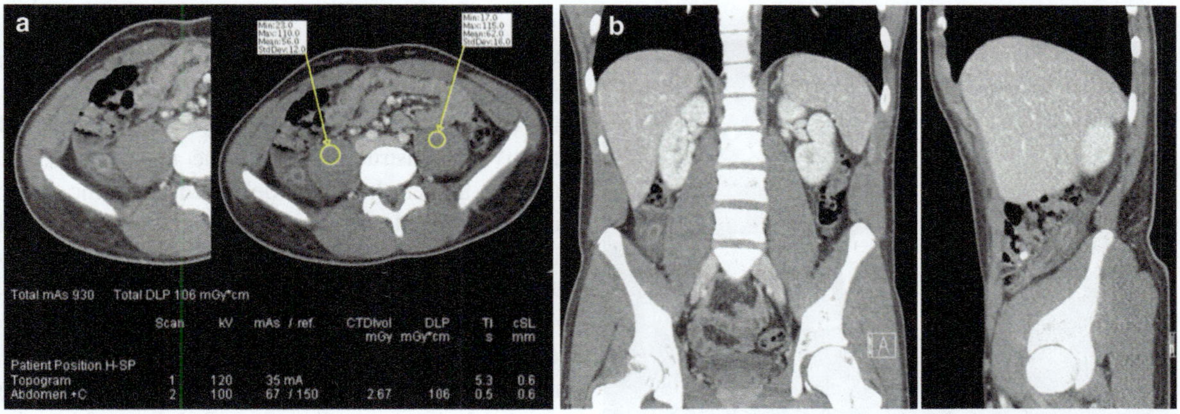

Fig. 8 Iterative reconstruction on standard-dose-enhanced MDCT in a 70 kg weighing female patient complaining of right lower quadrant pain. In axial 3 mm slice of **a** noise in psoas muscle is at 12 HU, a value that is in the range of standard-dose MDCT whereas the CTDIvol has been lowered to 2.67 mGy and the DLP to 101 mGy cm Appendicitis was confirmed surgically. Note that iterative reconstruction technique slightly reduces image sharpness in axial view (**a**) but not on coronal views generated with filter back projection reconstruction technique (**b**)

The amount of dose increase driven by AEC in obese patients is scanner dependant. It is highest with AEC systems that warrant a constant noise in images through the use of a noise index. CT scanners from General Electric and from Toshiba have this approach. In these scanners, protocols with higher noise index as compared to standard-sized patients are recommended for obese patients in order to avoid the dose to be unnecessarily excessively increased in obese. AEC systems from Philips and Siemens moderate the dose increase in obese patients. Further software versions of these AEC devices will enable the CT users to select the amounts of dose increase in obese depending on the body region.

One major drawback to the use of noise index for quantifying image quality is that the noise index also depends on the slice thickness and on the reconstruction algorithm. Therefore, recommendations for optimized dose levels cannot be expressed in noise index but only with volume computed tomography dose index (CTDIvol) and Dose-length product (DLP) values as presented in Tables 2, 3, 4. Optimized noise indexes for abdominal acquisitions using GE scanners can be found in the literature to be as high as 30

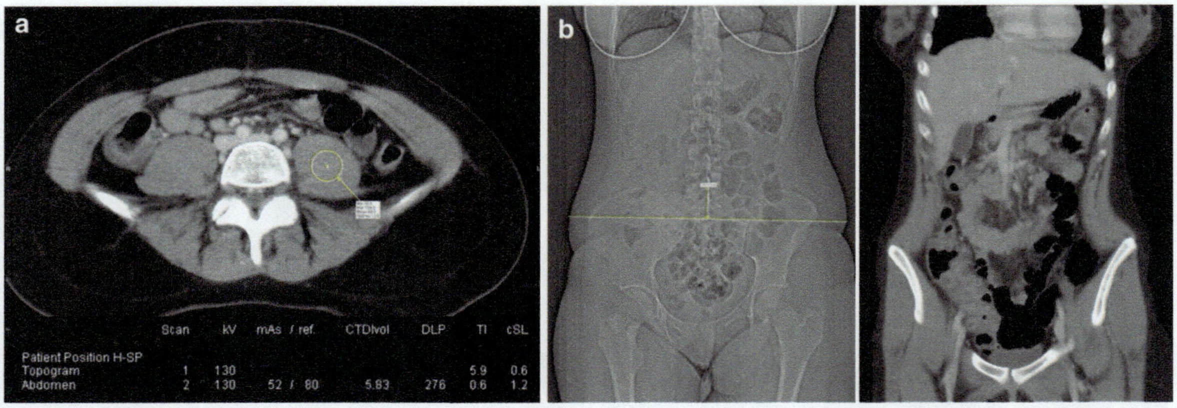

Fig. 9 Alternative diagnosis in right iliac fossa: right sided colitis. Optimized dose MDCT in a 28 year-old female patient weighing 78 kg and with right lower quadrant pain. **a** shows standard deviation of HU measurements within a ROI placed in psoas muscle, representing image noise at 12–16 HU. **b** shows scout view with measurement of patient's lateral diameter at 35 cm on the left and coronal view with right colon thickening indicating colitis. Radiation dose expressed in mean CTDIvol was 5.83 mGy and expressed in DLP was 276 mGy cm

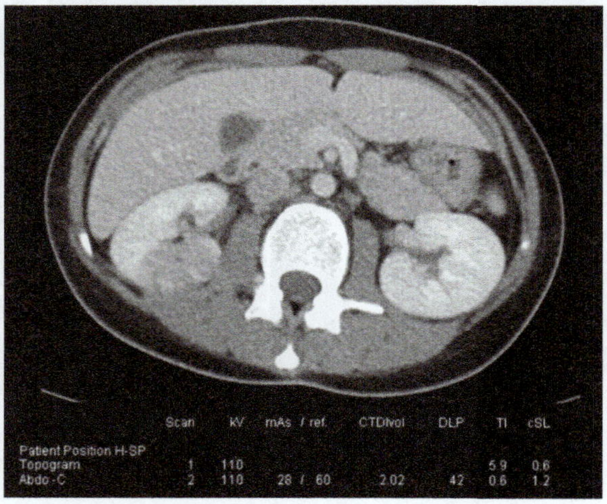

Fig. 10 Alternative diagnosis: pyelonephtitis. 16-year-old female patient weighing 50 kg, admitted to the emergency department with right-sided abdominal pain and fever. Low-Dose MCDT is performed with CTDIvol at 2 mGy

(Kambadakone et al. 2010) and depend on all the above-mentioned parameters.

2.3 Definition of Terms for Qualifying the Dose

Terms qualifying radiation dose are not strictly defined. As an example, the dose of a so-called "low-dose" protocol in one CT center could correspond to the one of a standard dose in another center. A typical confusion of this order can be seen when introducing iterative reconstructions in clinical practice (Singh et al. 2010). The low-dose achieved with iterative reconstructions by some researchers is as high or higher than that delivered by some others using optimized acquisitions and reconstructing with filtered back projection technique (Kambadakone et al. 2010; Allen et al. 2010; Leng et al. 2010). As a general rule outlined by Leng et al. (2010), iterative reconstruction should be applied on optimized doses hereafter defined as the lowest dose providing acceptable image quality. Specific effect of iterative reconstruction algorithm on the diagnosis of acute appendicitis has not yet been investigated. An example of iterative reconstruction is given in Fig. 8.

2.3.1 Standard Dose

The term "standard dose" refers to the dose usually recommended by CT manufacturers and often used in routine practice but that could be substantially reduced—to an optimized dose level—without deleterious effect on image quality. Typically, CTDIvol proposed by manufacturers in Europe range between 11 and 23 mGy in a standard-sized patient. At standard dose, noise in images (SD of ROI in a homogeneous area, e.g., aorta) is usually at 12 ± 3 HU. Standard dose may be considered as an acceptable technique in oncology and elderly patients. DLP for a standard abdomino-pelvic CT in a standard-sized patient should be lower than 800 mGy cm.

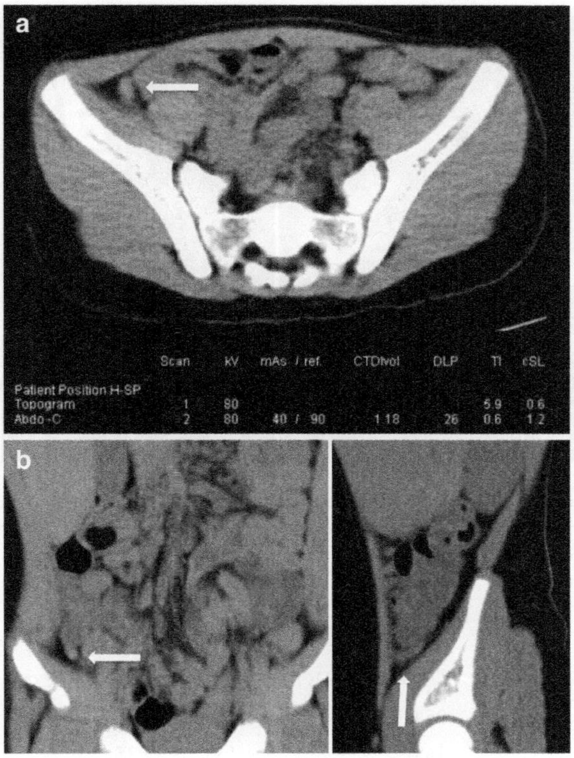

Fig. 11 Seven-year-old boy weighing 30 kg referred to MDCT for a suspected appendicitis. Unenhanced MDCT at 80 kV with CTDIvol at 1.18 mGy and DLP at 26 mGy cm. Appendix is normal—see arrows in axial view (**a**) and in coronal and sagittal views (**b**). No recurrence occurred for the next three following months

2.3.2 Optimized Dose

The term "optimized dose" should refer to a dose that provides adequate image quality but not with excessive radiation, and is the practical application of ALARA (As Low As Reasonably Achievable) principle. At optimized dose, noise in images ranges usually from 12 to 22 HU, depending on the image thickness, typically 15 HU in a 3 mm thick slice. Optimized dose is an acceptable technique in young adults and in non-oncology patients. DLP for an abdominal CT in an adult standard-sized patient with abdominal pain at optimized dose conditions should range between 200 and 400 mGy cm. Optimization process is per definition a process that eliminates the excess of radiation that does not provide significant increase in image quality. Optimized dose level for a given examination and on a given CT unit is not known, but has to be found out by the user who is responsible for this process (Golding 2010).

2.3.3 Low-Dose

The term "low dose" should be restricted to a CT delivered dose not higher than that delivered by a set of plain films investigating the considered condition. At low-dose, image quality is lower but diagnostic accuracy is preserved. At low-dose, noise in images ranges usually from 18 to 30 HU in 3 mm slices. Low-dose should be the preferred method for scanning young patients and patients with potentially recurring abdominal pain. DLP for an abdominal CT in a young standard-sized patient with abdominal pain at low-dose conditions should be around 100 mGy cm and lower than 200 mGy cm. Using a conversion factor of 0.015 mSv/mGy cm, the corresponding effective dose would be equal or lower than 3 mSv, a limit admitted as that of low-dose abdominal CT (Tack 2007).

3 Radiation Dose from MDCT in Patients with Suspected Appendicitis

According to ALARA principle, the dose delivered to the patient should be at the level below which the image quality would be insufficient to yield an accurate diagnosis. Practically, the delivered dose should be adapted first to the patient's size and second to the clinical indication. AEC systems adapt the dose to the patient's size. CT users are in charge of appropriate AEC parameters in order to choose the ALARA image quality depending on the CT signs that enable accurate diagnosis of appendicitis and alternative diagnoses. In this paragraph, we will discuss the impact of dose reduction, including acquisition length and number of acquisitions, on the CT findings and on CT diagnosis of acute appendicitis.

3.1 Dose Reduction Regarding the CT Signs and Diagnosis of Acute Appendicitis

3.1.1 Dose Reduction in Acute Abdominal Disorders with High Contrast Between Structures

Reduction in radiation dose was first investigated in diagnostic conditions characterized by high intrinsic contrast between structures, such as lung nodule screening (Rusinek et al. 1998), CT colonography,

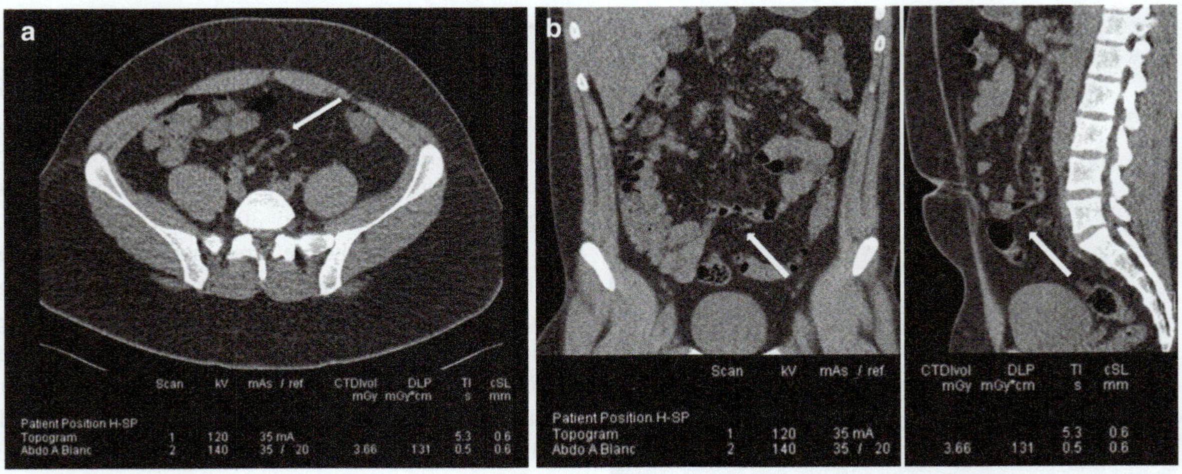

Fig. 12 Twenty-one year-old man weighing 105 kg referred to MDCT for a suspected appendicitis. Unenhanced MDCT at 140 kV with reduced mAs and CTDIvol at 3.66 mGy is obtained and perfectly delineates a normal appendix in axial (**a**), and in coronal and sagittal orientations (**b**). Because acquisition length has been optimized as well, DLP is at 131 mGy cm only, a value that represents a very low dose as compared to the one expected for the patient's body weight (105 kg)

Table 2 Reference diagnostic levels (RDLs) for abdominal MDCT including pelvis in average sized adults

Year	Origin	CTDIvol (mGy)	DLP (mGy cm)
1999	EUR	25.0	1,100
2002	Germany	14.6	635
2003	UK	15.3	534
2008	France	17.0	800
2010	Belgium	17.1	830

Note
Values are given for an average adult patient weighing 70–75 kg
RDLs correspond to the 75th percentile of observed dose values in survey
CTDIvol: in mGy is the computed tomography dose index volume (CTDIw/pitch)
DLP: in mGy cm is the dose-length product

Table 3 Recommended dose values for optimized and low-dose abdominal MDCT in an average size adult patient

Year	Origin/Reference	CTDIvol (mGy)	DLP (mGy cm)
2010/OD	Belgium P25	NA	415
2010/OD	Luxemburg P25	7.9	352
2009/OD	Seo et al. (2009)	6.0	240
2004/LD	Keyzer et al. (2004)	3.0	100–150
2009/LD	Keyzer et al. (2009)	2.0–3.0	80–150
2009/LD	Platon et al. (2009)	2.1	84 ± 10

Note
P25: 25th percentile of dose values as observed in nationwide surveys
Recommended levels for optimised dose (OD)
Recommended levels for low-dose (LD)
NA = nonavailable

and ureteral stones (Diel et al. 2000; Liu et al. 2000; Hamm et al. 2002; Tack et al. 2003; Kalra et al. 2005). In these early studies, it was suggested that alternative diagnoses can be made despite the reduced dose. Indeed, periureteric and perinephric fat stranding is still visible at low-dose CT (Heneghan

Table 4 MDCT parameters and dose descriptors in low-dose MDCT for acute appendicitis as a function of body weight

Patient's weight (Kg)	Tube potential (KV)	Example	CTDIvol (mGy)	DLP (mGy cm)
Optimized MDCT of the abdomen in adult patients				
>120	140	Fig. 1	12.0–15.0	600–1000
100–120	120	NA	8.0–12.0	400–600
80–100	120	Figs. 3, 9	4.0–8.0	300–400
60–80	100	Fig. 3	3.0–4.0	200–300
Low-dose MDCT of the abdomen in adult patients				
>120	140	NA	8.0–12.0	300–500
100–120	120	Fig. 12	4.0–6.0	200–300
80–100	120	Figs. 2, 4	2.0–4.0	150–200
60–80	100	Figs. 8, 10	1.5–3.0	100–150
Low-dose MDCT of the abdomen in small adults and in children				
40–60	100	Figs. 5, 6	1.5–3.0	50–100
<40 kg	80	Figs. 7, 11	1.0–2.0	25–50

Note
1. AEC current modulation should always be activated
2. Low-dose protocols suppose accepted higher noise levels as compared to routine optimized MDCT acquisitions
3. In adults, DLP values are given for an optimized acquisition length is of 30 cm, set from the top of the kidneys to the superior aspect of the symphysis pubis
4. In children, acquisition length is of 25 cm in those weighing <40 kg and is at 30 cm in all others
5. These protocols can be applied on most MDCT scanners
6. Using newly developed scanners (GE HD750, Siemens Definition, and Philips ICT) and using iterative reconstruction algorithms, noise can be reduced, enabling further significant dose reductions by 30–50%

et al. 2003) suggesting that any intra-abdominal fat stranding, as in numerous acute abdominal conditions, could also be detectable. These low intrinsic contrast conditions—also characterized by peritoneal and retroperitoneal fat stranding—are visible in acute colon diverticulitis and acute appendicitis.

3.1.2 Dose Reduction in Acute Abdominal Disorders with Low Contrast Between Structures as in Acute Appendicitis

Because of its high sensitivity and specificity in the diagnosis of acute appendicitis—even without intravenous injection of iodinated contrast material (Lane et al. 1999; Ege et al. 2002)—CT has been used more and more frequently in the past decade in order to increase the accuracy of clinical diagnosis. CT, especially without any contrast material, is rapid and causes little discomfort to the patient. Nevertheless, as many individuals suspected of acute appendicitis are young—with a mean age of 30 years (Flum et al. 2001)—the radiation dose should be reduced. Keyzer et al. (2004) compared unenhanced low-dose (30 mAs, 120 kVp) and standard-dose (100 mAs, 120 kVp) MDCT in adults with suspected acute appendicitis. The frequency of visualization of the appendix and the diagnostic performance were similar regardless of the radiation dose. Unenhanced low-dose and standard-dose MDCT achieve sensitivity and negative predictive values up to 97% or even more. These two performance values are the most important in patients suspected of acute appendicitis as this condition is potentially life-threatening but can be easily and efficiently treated by surgery (Krieg et al. 1975). Specificity and positive predictive values are lower than sensitivity and negative predictive values but they are not different between doses (Keyzer et al. 2004).

As in acute colon diverticulitis, fat stranding—i.e., periappendiceal fat stranding—is the most predictive sign of acute appendicitis whatever the dose. This was also shown in alternative disorders such as acute left colon diverticulitis (Tack et al. 2005). In addition, the ability to propose a correct alternative diagnosis is not influenced by the dose. Furthermore, a study based on a technique that simulates dose reduction has shown that dose reduction does not affect the correctness of the diagnosis at oral and/or IV-enhanced CT as at unenhanced CT (Keyzer et al. 2009). Early studies were first performed on scanners that were not equipped with AEC. In these studies, mAs presets were maintained constant whatever the patient's size. With 30 mAs eff. (effective mAs defined as tube current time product in mAs divided by the pitch factor), Keyzer et al. (2004) showed that for the visualization of the appendix and the diagnosis of acute appendicitis, standard-dose and low-dose CT have equivalent diagnostic performance in patients with a BMI greater than 30 kg/m^2. This observation can be explained by the fact that the negative effect of an increase in BMI could be, at least in part, balanced by the accumulation of intra-abdominal fat around the appendix. Other studies investigating dose reduction in patients suspected of acute appendicitis were in accordance with these first results as these were not able to elicit any upper threshold of BMI at which the diagnosis of acute appendicitis or the appendix visualization were hindered at low-dose (Keyzer et al. 2009; Seo et al. 2009). These observations should however be confirmed by studies focused on patients with extreme BMI categories (extremely obese patients) as their numbers were low in all these studies.

3.2 Acquisition Length and Number of Paths for Excluding Acute Appendicitis

3.2.1 Optimization of *Z*-Coverage (Acquisition Length)

With MDCT scanners, the ability to rapidly scan large volumes tempts the operator to increase this volume along the *z*-axis, and/or to use multiple-pass instead of single-pass CT. Concerning the acquisition length, there is very few information in the literature about the efficacy of limited *Z*-coverage with focus on the painful abdominal zone. One retrospective study by Kamel et al. (2000) showed that limiting CT acquisition to the pelvis would induce 7% of missed diagnoses, some of them necessitating rapid surgery. These authors showed that, by comparison to an abdomino-pelvic CT, the sensitivity of a focused pelvic CT would decrease from 96 to 82% for the identification of cases in need of immediate surgery. Alternative diagnoses that could be missed include among others, perforated gastric or duodenal ulcer, incarcerated hernias, pneumonias, pleural diseases, acute cholecystitis, pyelonephritis, ureteric stone disease (an exhaustive list of alternative diagnosis is given in Table 1 of chapter "Imaging of Acute Appendicitis in Adults: Computed Tomography"). The probable ideal acquisition length includes the root of diaphragms, easily seen on the scanogram and being at least 2 cm above the top of the kidneys, to the upper limit of pubic symphysis. Such an acquisition length includes the Douglas pouch and is of 32 cm in standard-sized men and 30 cm in standard-sized women while it ranges between 20 and 25 cm in children aged 8–13 years. Examples of acquisition length optimization can be shown in Fig. 2b (non-optimized acquisition length) and Fig. 4b (optimized acquisition length). Another example is given in Fig. 12 in an obese patient.

3.2.2 Optimization of the Number of Acquisitions

There is almost no discussion on the number of acquisitions needed for accurate CT diagnosis of appendicitis: one single acquisition and its subsequent radiation dose are sufficient in the vast majority of patients. The choice on the appropriate technique to be applied on adults with suspected acute appendicitis regarding the use of iodine injection and that of oral contrast is extensively discussed in the chapter "Imaging of Acute Appendicitis in Adults: Computed Tomography" by Keyzer. Whatever the contrast protocol, there is no need for scanning patients twice in the vast majority of cases. Unjustified multi-phasic screening the entire abdomen because of a "you never know" policy should thus be banished. Such policy is unacceptable, in particular in young patients who are at a low risk of having an incidental associated disease. Repeated acquisitions should thus not be performed in circumstances where they do not specifically yield additional information.

4 Methods for Optimizing and Reducing the Dose per Slice By Means of AEC Parameters

In this paragraph, we will address the methods for optimizing and reducing the radiation dose regarding the appropriate choice of AEC parameters that differ from manufacturer to manufacturer and between scanner generations, and the latest denoising algorithms based on iterative reconstruction techniques.

4.1 General Concept for Approaching Dose Optimization

Automatic modulation of the tube current as a function of the patient's absorption is now available on all modern CT scanners. Differences still exist between manufacturers regarding the methods used for this modulation and the dose reductions subsequently obtained. Detailed description, limitations, and results of the different AEC devices have been presented and discussed in the literature (Kalra 2007). The most important feature of these devices is that the radiation dose is adapted to the patient's weight and absorption. Consequently, the role of the CT user is not to adapt the tube current to the patient's weight but more to select appropriate tube potential and image quality to fit with the clinical indication of the CT examination. Examples of CTDIvol and DLP values depending on the patients' habitus are given in Table 4 and Figs. 1, 2, 3, 4, 5, 6, 7, 8, 9, 10, 11, 12. Pitfalls have to be avoided for successful optimization and are listed hereafter.

4.2 Step-by-Step Recommendations in Optimization Process

1. Do not use the RDLs from surveys as reference for dose optimization. These values listed in Table 2 represent the upper limits of acceptable practice, in other words, the limit of radiation malpractice.
2. Bear in mind the objective for optimization. For this, refer to Table 3 and in particular to the 25th percentile of surveys.
3. For imaging appendicitis with low-dose MDCT, refer to low-dose values in Table 4.
4. Read the dose reports generated by the CT scanner for each examination you interpret to become familiar with the CTDIvol and DLP values.
5. Take the appropriate time necessary for optimization.
6. Always keep your AEC switched "on."
7. Choose a standard-sized patient for optimization (1m70 and 70–75 kg).
8. Choose an appropriate kV setting as presented in Table 4.
9. Check parameters limiting AEC: On GE and Toshiba scanners, make sure that the mA window is widely opened enabling tube current to be significantly reduced in small individuals and increased in obese. For this purpose, reduce the lowest possible mA limit value to 20 mA, and increase as high as possible one to the upper limits of the scanner generator. Before acquisition, check the mA table in order to make sure that the AEC system is acting in varying the mA from slice to slice.
10. Adapt the index of image quality stepwise while decreasing the CTDIvol displayed on the CT screen. This index of image quality corresponds to the noise index with GE and Toshiba scanners, to the "*reference eff. mAs*" with Siemens scanners, and to the eff. mAs with Philips scanners.
11. Choose a slice thickness value slightly higher than the detector's nominal thickness, typically 1.5 mm for abdominal MDCT when acquired with 0.5, 0.6, or 0.625 mm.
12. Use smoother reconstruction algorithms if possible. Typically, with a Siemens scanner, use B10 or B20 and not B30 or B40.
13. Use slightly thickened slices for 3D display to eliminate noise from native images.
14. Compare with previous acquisitions in the same patient.
15. Discuss with your colleagues. If satisfied, process to a new optimization round. If not satisfied, check parameters such as collimation and reconstruction thickness, and prepare increasing the dose by 10%. If this dose level is not as those displayed in Table 4 and Figs. 1, 2, 3, 4, 5, 6, 7, 8, 9, 10, 11, 12, contact your manufacturer for further support.
16. In children, lower the kV settings to 100 if patient's weight ranges from 40 to 80 kg and down to 80 kV if weight is lower than 40 kg. Tube current time products should remain unchanged or slightly increased when lowering tube voltage for imaging appendicitis (Table 4).

4.3 Image Noise in Optimized and Low-Dose Abdominal MDCT

Noise accounts among the most important indicators of image quality and is directly linked to radiation dose through the tube current time product. Very few is known on noise levels requested in clinical practice for a given diagnosis or condition. For example, noise in a liver parenchyma for assessment of focal liver lesions is usually around 10 HU in a standard quality examination. In an optimized-dose CT, noise can be as high as 17 HU. In low-dose CT, noise in native images is as high as 30 but is reduced lower than 20 by MPR thickening.

The indication of each examination is very important to consider in order to select the required image quality and subsequently the lowest acceptable radiation dose. As an example, the dose delivered when searching for metastases or for imaging trauma can be higher than that for imaging acute abdominal pain. As explained above in the section defining the terms associated to the concept of CT dose, an optimized to standard dose setting is appropriate for imaging patient for follow-up of malignancies. For imaging recurrent abdominal disorders such as Crohn's disease, optimized dose or even low-dose techniques are more appropriate (Kambadakone et al. 2010; Allen et al. 2010; Leng et al. 2010).

5 MDCT for Suspected Appendicitis in Children

An extensive review of the current literature concerning the radiation risks for children is presented in "Imaging of Acute Appendicitis in Children: Computed Tomography Including Radiation Issues" by Spencer et al. In this paragraph, we aim to give some advice in optimization of MDCT parameters in small bodies such as in children. The dose from MDCT could be adapted to child's age, but important variations in body weight are observed in children. Thus, we recommend adapting the MDCT parameters to the body weight or the average diameter between lateral and antero-posterior orientations. The strategy for adapting the parameters for excluding appendicitis in children is similar to that in adults unless for tube potential that should be at 100 kV (typically in a 12-year-old child) or at 80 kV (typically in a 8–10 year old child) as listed in Table 4. Automatic exposure control should be switched on and index of image quality should be set up in order to generate images with at least 20 HU image noise. Examples of CT examinations in children at low-dose settings are given in Figs. 5, 6, 7, and 11. DLP values as low as 26–101 mGy cm, with *Z*-coverage ranging from the kidneys to the symphysis pubis can be used for excluding appendicitis in children who are 1.0–1.30 m tall. These dose descriptors correspond to effective dose values of less than 1 mSv, as dose frequently reported in plain film examinations of the abdomen including two views.

6 Conclusion

In a standard-sized individual (weighing 70–75 kg), MDCT for excluding appendicitis can be acquired with low-dose settings and delivers DLP values ranging from 70 to 150 mGy cm using a scanner with 16 or more detector-rows. This dose can be divided by 50% in children aged between 6 and 10 years and by 30% with the newest MDCT acquisitions techniques and/or with iterative reconstructions software.

References

Allen BC, Baker ME, Einstein DM, Remer EM, Herts BR, Achkar JP, Davros WJ, Novak E, Obuchowski NA (2010) Effect of altering automatic exposure control settings and quality reference mAs on radiation dose, image quality, and diagnostic efficacy in MDCT enterography of active inflammatory Crohn's disease. AJR 195:89–100

Berrington de González A, Mahesh M, Kim KP, Bhargavan M, Lewis R, Mettler F, Land C (2009) Projected cancer risks from computed tomographic scans performed in the United States in 2007. Arch Intern Med 169:2071–2077

Christner JA, Kofler JM, McCollough CH (2010) Estimating effective dose for CT using dose-length product compared with using organ doses: consequences of adopting International Commission on Radiological Protection publication 103 or dual-energy scanning. AJR 194:881–889

Diel J, Perlmutter S, Venkataramanan N, Mueller R, Lane MJ, Katz DS (2000) Unenhanced helical CT using increased pitch for suspected renal colic: an effective technique for radiation dose reduction? JCAT 24:795–801

Ege G, Akman H, Sahin A, Bugra D, Kuzucu K (2002) Diagnostic value of unenhanced CT in adult patients with suspected acute appendicitis. Br J Radiol 75:721–725

European Commission (1999) European guidelines on quality criteria for computed tomography, Report EUR 16262. Brussels: EC

Flum DR, Morris A, Koepsell T, Dellinger EP (2001) Has misdiagnosis of appendicitis decreased over time? A population-based analysis. JAMA 286:1748–1753

Golding SJ (2010) Radiation exposure in CT: what is the professionally responsible approach? Radiology 255: 683–685

Golding SJ, Shrimpton PC (2002) Radiation dose in CT: are we meeting the challenge? (Commentary). Br J Radiol 75:1–4

Guimaraes LS, Fletcher JG, Harmsen WS, Yu L, Siddiki H, Melton Z, Huprich JE, Hough D, Hartman R, McCollough CH (2010) Appropriate patient selection at abdominal dual-energy CT using 80 kV: relationship between patient size, image noise, and image quality. Radiology 257:732–742

Hamm M, Knopfle E, Wartenberg S, Wawroschek F, Weckermann D, Harzmann R (2002) Low dose unenhanced helical computerized tomography for the evaluation of acute flank pain. J Urol 167:1687–1691

Heneghan JP, McGuire KA, Leder RA, DeLong DM, Yoshizumi T, Nelson RC (2003) Helical CT for nephrolithiasis and ureterolithiasis: comparison of conventional and reduced radiation-dose techniques. Radiology 229:575–580

Hricak H, Brenner DJ, Adelstein SJ, Frush DP, Hall EJ, Howell RW, McCollough CH, Mettler FA, Pearce MS, Suleiman OH, Thrall JH, Wagner LK (2010) Managing radiation use in medical imaging: a multifaceted challenge radiology 101157; Published online 16 December 2010, doi: 10.1148/radiol.10101157

ICRP (1991) Recommendations of the international commission on radiological protection. Ann ICRP 21:1–201

Kalra MK (2007) Automatic exposure control in multidetectorrow computed tomography. In: Tack D, Gevenois PA (eds) Medical radiology: diagnostic imaging. Springer, NY, pp 117–128

Kalra MK, Maher MM, D'Souza RV, Rizzo S, Halpern EF, Blake MA, Saini S (2005) Detection of urinary tract stones at low-radiation-dose CT with Z-Axis automatic tube current modulation: phantom and clinical studies. Radiology 235:523–529

Kambadakone AR, Prakash P, Hahn PF, Sahani DV (2010) Low-dose CT examinations in Crohn's disease: impact on image quality, diagnostic performance, and radiation dose. AJR 195:78–88

Kamel IR, Goldberg SN, Keogan MT, Rosen MP, Raptopoulos V (2000) Right lower quadrant pain and suspected appendicitis: nonfocused appendiceal CT–review of 100 cases. Radiology 217:159–163

Keyzer C, Tack D, De Maertelaer V, Bohy P, Gevenois PA, Van Gansbeke D (2004) Acute appendicitis: comparison of low-dose and standard-dose unenhanced multi–detector row CT. Radiology 232:164–172

Keyzer C, Cullus P, Tack D, De MV, Bohy P, Gevenois PA (2009) MDCT for suspected acute appendicitis in adults: impact of oral and IV contrast media at standard-dose and simulated low-dose techniques. AJR 193:1272–1281

Krieg AF, Gambino SR, Galen RS (1975) Why are clinical laboratory tests performed? When are they valid? JAMA 233:76–78

Lane MJ, Liu DM, Huynh MD, Jeffrey RB, Mindelzun RE, Katz DS (1999) Suspected acute appendicitis: nonenhanced helical CT in 300 consecutive patients. Radiology 213: 341–346

Leng S, Yu L, McCollough CH (2010) Radiation dose reduction at CT enterography: How low can we go while preserving diagnostic accuracy? AJR 195:76–77

Little MP, Wakeford R, Tawn EJ, Bouffler SD, Berrington de Gonzalez A (2009) Risks associated with low doses and low dose rates of ionizing radiation: why linearity may be (almost) the best we can do. Radiology 251:6–12

Liu W, Esler JS, Kenny BJ, Goh RH, Rainbow AJ, Stevenson GW (2000) Low-dose nonenhanced helical ct of renal colic: assessment of ureteric stone detection and measurement of effective dose equivalent. Radiology 215:51–54

Mulkens TH, Bellinck P, Baeyaert M, Ghysen D, Van Dijck X, Mussen E, Venstermans C, Termote JL (2005) Use of an automatic exposure control mechanism for dose optimization in multi-detector row CT examinations: clinical evaluation. Radiology 237:213–223

Nagel HD (2007) CT parameters that influence radiation dose. In: Tack D, Gevenois PA (eds) Medical radiology: diagnostic imaging. Springer, NY, pp 51–80

Paul JF, Abada HT (2007) Dose in cardiac and vascular MDCT. In: Tack D, Gevenois PA (eds) Medical radiology: diagnostic imaging. Springer, NY, pp 171–184

Platon A, Jlassi H, Rutschmann OT, Becker CD, Verdun FR, Gervaz P, Poletti PA (2009) Evaluation of a low-dose CT protocol with oral contrast for assessment of acute appendicitis. Eur Radiol 19:446–454

Rogers LF (2001) Radiation exposure in CT: why so high? AJR 177:277

Rusinek H, Naidich DP, McGuinness G, Leitman BS, McCauley DI, Krinsky GA, Clayton K, Cohen H (1998) Pulmonary nodule detection: low-dose versus conventional CT. Radiology 209:243–249

Seo H, Lee KH, Kim HJ, Kim K, Kang SB, Kim SY, Kim YH (2009) Diagnosis of acute appendicitis with sliding slab ray-sum interpretation of low-dose unenhanced CT and standard-dose IV contrast-enhanced CT scans. AJR 193:96–105

Shrimpton PC, Hillier MC, Lewis MA, et al (2003). Data from computed tomography (CT) examinations in the UK-2003 review. Chilton: NRPB-67, National Radiological Protection Board

Singh S, Kalra MK, Hsieh J, Licato PE, Do S, Pien HH, Blake MA (2010) Abdominal CT: comparison of adaptive statistical iterative and filtered back projection reconstruction techniques. Radiology 257:373–383

Tack D (2007) Methods and strategies for radiation dose optimization- and reduction-in MDCT with special focus on the image quality. In: Tack D, Gevenois PA (eds) Medical radiology: diagnostic imaging. Springer, NY, pp 99–116

Tack D, Sourtzis S, Delpierre I, De Maertelaer V, Gevenois PA (2003) Low-dose unenhanced multidetector CT of patients with suspected renal colic. AJR 180:305–311

Tack D, Bohy P, Perlot I, De Maertelaer V, Alkeilani O, Sourtzis S, Gevenois PA (2005) Suspected acute colon diverticulitis: imaging with low-dose unenhanced multi–detector row CT. Radiology 237:189–196

Tubiana M, Feinendegen LE, Yang C, Kaminski JM (2009) The linear no-threshold relationship is inconsistent with radiation biologic and experimental data. Radiology 251:13–22

UNSCEAR (2000) Sources and effects of ionizing radiation. NY: United Nations Scientific Committee on the Effects of Atomic Radiation Report to the General Assembly United Nations

Part VI

Concluding Remarks

Summary and Perspectives

Caroline Keyzer and Pierre Alain Gevenois

One should believe that the appendix is so insignificant and that acute appendicitis is so common that almost everything about it is well established and widely known would be as ignorant as the surgeons of the nineteenth century who rejected its central role in acute inflammatory disease of the right lower quadrant of the abdomen. This worm-shaped (*vermiform* appendix) organ is indeed still subject of many questions, controversies, and researches.

The role of the appendix in human is still unknown. It could have an immune role but for many decades nobody reported that appendectomy induces any immune deficiency. Recent studies even showed that removing the appendix might protect against ulcerative colitis. As discussed by van den Broek in "Negative Appendectomy Rate and Implications of Removing a Normal Appendix" however, there is much debate about what to do with a normal appendix found during a laparoscopic intervention. It appears indeed safe to leave it in place in order to avoid additional morbidity and costs. As negative appendectomy rate (NAR) should be as low as possible, imaging is thus ordered in an attempt to reduce it. Whether imaging indeed reduces NAR or not is also a matter of debate as discussed by Coursey and Moreno in "Impact of Imaging on Negative Appendectomy Rate".

The diagnosis of acute appendicitis can be difficult but surgeons are reluctant to any delay in its definitive treatment as acute appendicitis can progress to appendiceal perforation with both morbidity and mortality subsequently increased. Scoring systems based on clinical signs and laboratory findings have been developed in order to increase the clinical diagnostic accuracy. These systems are extensively presented by Humes and Simpson in "Clinical Presentation of Acute Appendicitis: Clinical Signs—Laboratory Findings—Clinical Scores, Alvarado Score and Derivate Scores". As discussed by Menes and Bickell in "Appendicitis Perforation Rates and Time Interval between Symptom Onset and Surgery", while long delay between symptoms onset and treatment has been associated with high perforation rate, studies have however shown that delaying surgery to regular working hours has no impact on the patient's outcome. There is also a debate on whether appendiceal perforation is a different disease process than nonperforated acute appendicitis which questions the importance of time.

Despite the fact that appendectomy is the most commonly performed surgical procedure, there is still no consensus on the best approach to appendectomy as discussed by Mamidanna and Faiz in "Laparoscopy and Laparotomy". There are also controversies about conservative treatment with antibiotic therapy when perforation has been carefully excluded. The treatment of appendiceal perforation is also subject to considerable debate, particularly the role of interval appendectomy as explained by Almoudaris and Faiz in "Treatment of Appendiceal Perforation". Finally, there are also controversies about the management of patients presenting spontaneously resolving appendicitis that can be treated conservatively but with a high rate of recurrence as detailed by Cobben and

C. Keyzer (✉) · P. A. Gevenois
Department of Radiology, Hôpital Erasme,
Université libre de Bruxelles, Route de Lennik,
808, 1070 Brussels, Belgium
e-mail: caroline.keyzer@erasme.ulb.ac.be

C. Keyzer and P. A. Gevenois (eds.), *Imaging of Acute Appendicitis in Adults and Children*,
Medical Radiology. Diagnostic Imaging, DOI: 10.1007/174_2011_247, © Springer-Verlag Berlin Heidelberg 2011

Puijlaert in "Spontaneously Resolving and Chronic Appendicitis". Although relatively uncommon, primary appendiceal neoplasms may present with clinical symptoms that lead to order imaging. The imaging features of these benign and malignant tumors are extensively described by Potretzke and Pickhardt in "Imaging of Primary Appendiceal Neoplasms".

Concerning imaging issues, there is still no consensus for the best imaging approach in patients—children as well as adults—suspected of acute appendicitis. It is now widely accepted that there is no indication anymore for barium enema in acute appendicitis as it was done till the eighties before the age of cross-sectional imaging. Although plain radiography has been shown to be of little diagnostic value in patient suspected of acute appendicitis, it is still frequently performed and traditionally regarded as a useful initial imaging procedure. As discussed by Eisenberg in "Imaging of Acute Appendicitis in Adults: Radiography", it is unclear whether the emergency physicians expect to detect features of acute appendicitis or if they want to reassure the patients who have a clinical low probability of disease. Plain radiographic findings of acute appendicitis are extensively described by Eisenberg in "Imaging of Acute Appendicitis in Adults: Radiography", and by Vinocur and Lee in "Imaging of Acute Appendicitis in Children: Radiography" with special emphasis on the preparation needed in children to minimize their motions and subsequent re-takes and increased radiation dose.

Ultrasonography (US) is nowadays widely used in patients—adults as well as children—with suspected acute appendicitis. US is very efficient, accessible, and nonionizing. This technique has to be done in a correct manner (graded compression and color Doppler) as explained by Jeffrey in "Imaging of Acute Appendicitis in Adults: Ultrasonography" and Holscher in "Imaging of Acute Appendicitis in Children: Ultrasonography", respectively in adults and children. Computed tomography (CT) is also widely used in these patients—adults as well as children—but is still considered as "invasive" because of the radiation and the possibly used contrast agents. Nevertheless, as discussed by ourselves in "Imaging of Acute Appendicitis in Adults: Computed Tomography" and by Spencer, Saettele, and Lowe in "Imaging of Acute Appendicitis in Children: Computed Tomography Including Radiation Issues", respectively in adults and children, the choice of which protocol to use at CT in terms of contrasts is very wide despite little impact on accuracy. On the other hand, radiation issues are discussed and dose optimization for abdomino-pelvic CT in adults and children is provided by Tack and ourselves in "Radiation Dose from MDCT Examinations for Suspected Acute Appendicitis". The choice between US and CT is also still a matter of debate, and several staged imaging strategies are to be evaluated in terms of cost effectiveness as extensively discussed by ourselves in "Ultrasonography Versus Computed Tomography: Evidence-Based Imaging" and by Kamat, Garcia Peña, Blackmore, and Medina in "US versus CT: Evidence-Based Medicine and Cost-Effectiveness in Imaging Acute Appendicitis in Children", respectively in adults and children. An important issue arising this last decade is related to overweight patients who are susceptible to influence the imaging strategy.

MR imaging (MRI) provides multiplanar evaluation of the entire abdomen with excellent anatomic resolution and allows identification of the etiology of acute abdominal pain without any radiation or contrast agent. The acquisition protocols and MR signs of acute appendicitis are extensively described by Schmid-Tannwald and Oto in "Imaging of Acute Appendicitis in Adults: MRI" and by Hörmann in "Imaging of Acute Appendicitis in Children: MRI", respectively in adults and children. The major issue of MRI is still its accessibility, in particular in emergency settings. When accessible, it is the preferred method of imaging pregnant women. However, although MRI does not expose the mother or fetus to ionizing radiation and unenhanced MR images are often diagnostic, the safety of MRI (and especially Gadolinium administration) with respect to the fetus has not been definitely established, as discussed by Schmid-Tannwald and Oto in "Imaging of Acute Appendicitis in Adults: MRI" and by Jaffe in "Imaging of Acute Appendicitis in Adults: Current Practices in Pregnant Women". Current recommendations in pregnant women are discussed by Jaffe and involve initial imaging with US. If the diagnosis remains inconclusive, a thoughtful discussion with the referring clinician is warranted before going on a next imaging modality (i.e. CT or MRI). In conclusion, acute appendicitis is a disease that continues to raise questions and is still susceptible to remain a subject of research for many years.

Index

C. Keyzer and P. A. Gevenois (eds.), *Imaging of Acute Appendicitis in Adults and Children*, Medical Radiology. Diagnostic Imaging, DOI: 10.1007/978-3-642-17872-6, © Springer-Verlag Berlin Heidelberg 2011

GPSR Compliance

The European Union's (EU) General Product Safety Regulation (GPSR) is a set of rules that requires consumer products to be safe and our obligations to ensure this.

If you have any concerns about our products, you can contact us on ProductSafety@springernature.com

In case Publisher is established outside the EU, the EU authorized representative is:

Springer Nature Customer Service Center GmbH
Europaplatz 3
69115 Heidelberg, Germany

Batch number: 10733268

Printed by Printforce, the Netherlands